Drug Treatment Issues in Depression

Editor: Katharine J Palmer

Adis International

Auckland • Buenos Aires • Chester • Hong Kong • Madrid • Milan • Osaka • Paris • Philadelphia • São Paulo • Sydney

Drug Treatment Issues in Depression

Editor: Katharine J Palmer

adis INTERNATIONAL
A Wolters Kluwer Company

Commercial Manager: Gordon Mallarkey
Publication Manager: Lorna Venter-Lewis
Adis International Limited
 ISBN 0-86471-075-5

Earlier versions of some articles in this book were published in Adis International's peer-reviewed medical journals. The editor has collated the articles and worked with the authors to adapt and update the information for this publication.

Printed in Hong Kong.

Foreword

Depression is a common, costly and frequently chronic psychiatric disorder. Although a variety of effective antidepressants are available, the most appropriate approach to the treatment of initial episodes of depression and the prevention of relapse and recurrence are still matters of debate.

The articles in this book explore issues in the management of depression, with a focus on drug therapy. The book begins with an article summarising currently available options and outlining unmet needs. The other articles focus on important specific issues such as prevention of relapse and recurrence, approaches to managing treatment-resistant depression, the suboptimal use and risks/benefits of antidepressants, and the cost-effectiveness and effects on quality of life of these agents.

The articles in this collection are current and forthright. The intention is to stimulate further debate on how best to manage patients with depression.

Katharine J Palmer
Editor, *CNS Drugs*

May 2000

***CNS Drugs** is a highly-regarded international medical journal. The journal promotes rational pharmacotherapy and disease management within the disciplines of clinical psychiatry and neurology by publishing a regular programme of review articles in the subject area.*

Drug Treatment Issues in Depression

Contents

Achievements and Future Possibilities in the Drug Treatment of Depression

Hans-Jürgen Möller[1] and *Hans-Peter Volz*[2]

1 Psychiatric Department, Ludwigs-Maximilians-Universität, Munich, Germany

2 Psychiatric Department, Friedrich-Schiller-Universität, Jena, Germany

Almost 40 years ago, the antidepressive properties of imipramine were first described. The drug belongs to a group of compounds later called the tricyclic antidepressants (TCAs), including substances such as amitriptyline and clomipramine. Only a short time later the monoamine oxidase inhibitors (MAOIs) were discovered, exemplified by phenelzine and pargyline. Both classes of compounds are very effective in the treatment of major depression (TCAs) and atypical depression (MAOIs), but possess considerable disadvantages because of their adverse effect profile. TCAs carry a high incidence of anticholinergic effects and cardiotoxicity, extremely important in (suicidal) overdoses; MAOIs may cause hypertensive crises if sympathomimetic agents, e.g. certain other drugs or tyramine in foodstuffs, are additionally taken. These problems precipitated the search for new, effective antidepressants that were better tolerated and less toxic.

In the following decades, noradrenaline (norepinephrine) reuptake inhibitors (NARIs), selective serotonin (5-hydroxytryptamine; 5-HT) reuptake inhibitors (SSRIs) and reversible and selective inhibitors of monoamine oxidase (MAO) type A (RIMAs) were developed. The advent of mirtazapine added a further mode of action to the pharmacological spectrum: via α_1- auto- and heteroadrenoceptor antagonism, an increase in both noradrenaline and serotonin release is achieved. Further research with the aim of augmenting the mode of action of SSRIs by adding noradrenaline reuptake inhibiting properties led to the development of serotonin and noradrenaline reuptake inhibitors (SNRIs) such as venlafaxine. Nefazodone combines serotonin reuptake inhibition with the blockade of the postsynaptic serotonin 5-HT_2 receptor. The time course of antidepressant research is summarised in table I.

This article provides an overview of these psychopharmacological approaches and remarks on some still unmet medical needs and alternative principles of action of future antidepressants.

1. Selective Serotonin Reuptake Inhibitors (SSRIs)

At present there are 5 marketed SSRIs: fluoxetine, fluvoxamine, paroxetine, sertraline and citalopram. Although the main mechanism of action is similar in all of these compounds, there do exist differences in clinical criteria which seem to be decisive for their application (table II),[1] the most important being their elimination half-life.

This half-life is nearly 330 hours for fluoxetine and its active metabolite, norfluoxetine, whereas for other SSRIs it lies between 15 and 30 hours. The half-life is of particular importance if patients are switched from an SSRI to another antidepressant medication or if severe adverse effects emerge. On the other hand, a long half-life could be advantageous for long term treatment compliance because of the possibility of administering one dose only every second or third day. Further clinically relevant points address nausea and vomiting, with figures on incidence for the individual SSRIs lying between 20 and 37%, also dependent on the dose and the speed of dose increase.

Table I. Development of antidepressive mode of action in the past 40 years

Time	Principle and examples
1957-1979	Tricyclic antidepressants (TCAs): imipramine, clomipramine, amitriptyline
1960-1965	Monoamine oxidase inhibitors (MAOIs): phenelzine, pargyline, tranylcypromine
1970-1980	Newer generation TCAs: lofepramine
1970-1980	Noradrenaline (norepinephrine) reuptake inhibitors (NARIs): maprotiline, levoprotiline
1970-1980	'Atypical antidepressants': mianserin, trazodone
1980-1990	Selective serotonin (5-hydroxytryptamine; 5-HT) reuptake inhibitors (SSRIs): fluoxetine, fluvoxamine, sertraline, paroxetine, citalopram
1980-1995	Reversible and selective inhibitors of monoamine oxidase type A (RIMAs): moclobemide, brofaromine, cimoxatone
1975-2000	Noradrenergic and specific serotonergic antidepressant (NASSA): mirtazapine
1985-2000	Serotonin and noradrenaline reuptake inhibitors (SNRIs): venlafaxine

In comparison with TCAs, all SSRIs possess a favourable adverse effect profile, which is characterised by a lack of anticholinergic and sedating properties. As an example, the adverse effect profile of citalopram is presented in table III.[2] Beside these adverse reactions, no direct cardiotoxicity is described, an advantage especially in (suicidal) overdoses.

SSRIs inhibit the hepatic cytochrome P450 (CYP) 2D6 system, thus causing interactions, e.g. with TCAs, resulting in increased plasma TCA concentrations. As has been shown recently,[3] fluoxetine and paroxetine inhibit CYP2D6 considerably more strongly than fluvoxamine or sertraline.

Apart from basic pharmacological and adverse effect issues, the antidepressive efficacy of these new compounds is, of course, a matter of interest. For all of these drugs, many controlled clinical trials are available. Their superior efficacy over placebo is beyond any doubt.[4-7] Comparative trials versus TCAs and tetracyclic antidepressants have also been published. In this context, the viewpoint of the Danish University Antidepressant Group (DUAG)[8,9] is noteworthy; they showed the TCA clomipramine to be more effective than SSRIs (citalopram, paroxetine).

For an overall impression, the results of a recently published meta-analysis by Anderson and Tomeson[10] should be discussed here in more detail. Since a sufficient number of trials could not be evaluated for sertraline and citalopram, the following considerations are limited

Table II. Pharmacokinetics, dosage in patients with depression and adverse effects of the selective serotonin (5-hydroxytryptamine; 5-HT) reuptake inhibitors[1]

Compound	$t_{1/2\beta}$ (h)	Active metabolite	Active metabolite $t_{1/2\beta}$ (h)	Dosage (mg/day)	Nausea and/or vomiting (%)
Fluoxetine	70	Yes	330	20-40	25
Fluvoxamine	15	No		100-200	37 (15.7)[a]
Paroxetine	12-20	No		10-50	29
Citalopram	33	No		20-60	20
Sertraline	25	Yes	66	50-200	21

a The first value refers to a daily dose of 300mg, the value in parentheses to a daily dose of 150mg.
$t_{1/2\beta}$ = elimination half-life.

to fluvoxamine, fluoxetine and paroxetine. The aim of this comprehensive work was to investigate whether the abovementioned SSRIs differ in their efficacy against TCAs and whether there is a difference in effectiveness in severely depressed patients compared with those who are not. The last issue is addressed by looking separately at in- and outpatient studies and by subdividing studies according to initial severity of depression (for the details regarding the included and excluded studies, see original paper). The results are summarised in table IV.[10]

For the 3 SSRIs included in this table, a significant superior efficacy over placebo was found. In comparison with TCAs, no differences in efficacy were found for fluvoxamine in the main analysis or in the various subgroups. The only difference in efficacy between fluoxetine and TCAs was in the group with a high score on the Hamilton Depression Rating Scale (HAM-D) where TCAs were just significantly more effective. A similar trend emerged in the two trials on inpatients.

Table III. Adverse events reported during comparative controlled clinical trials of citalopram (n = 682) and tricyclic (TCA) and related antidepressants (amitriptyline, clomipramine, imipramine, maprotiline, mianserin, and nortriptyline) [n = 389]. Listed are only those adverse events occurring with an incidence of >5% in any one patient group[2]

Symptoms	Citalopram (%)	TCA	Difference (%)
Significant difference			
Citalopram > TCA			
Nausea	18.8	12.9	+5.9
Ejaculation failure	5.3	0.8	+4.5
TCA > Citalopram			
Dry mouth	28.3	48.6	–20.3
Increased sweating	20.4	29.6	–9.2
Tremor	15.1	26.2	–11.1
Somnolence	13.9	19.8	–5.9
Constipation	13.0	28.8	–15.8
Abnormal accommodation	9.5	18.3	–8.8
Dizziness	9.4	21.6	–12.2
Postural hypotension	8.9	17.2	–8.3
Palpitations	6.9	13.1	–6.2
Taste perversion	3.7	7.5	–3.8
Nonsignificant difference			
Insomnia	17.7	13.4	+4.3
Headache	15.4	15.7	–0.3
Asthenia	12.3	10.5	+1.8
Diarrhoea	6.5	3.9	+2.6
Agitation	6.3	9.3	–3.0
Micturation disorder	5.0	8.0	–3.0
Paraesthesia	5.0	5.4	–0.4
Tachycardia	3.5	5.1	–1.6

For paroxetine, matters were somewhat different. This agent was moderately less effective than TCAs in inpatient studies, including a comparative trial by the DUAG (versus clomipramine; effect size –0.43, $p < 0.01$) and in a comparison against the serotonergic TCAs clomipramine and amitriptyline (effect size –0.37, $p < 0.01$). The effect sizes indicate a clinically important difference. In their conclusion, the authors nevertheless state that, in general, SSRIs are as effective in the treatment of depression as standard TCAs. Considering the number of studies and patients included, efficacy is best established for fluoxetine, fluvoxamine and paroxetine.

The only SSRI that has been tested adequately in inpatients is fluvoxamine, and this is therefore regarded by the authors[10] as the SSRI of choice for this patient group. Paroxetine was found to be less effective than TCAs in inpatient studies and in the trial versus the serotonergic TCAs. Although discussing the possibility of this being a chance finding, the authors do not recommend paroxetine as the antidepressant of choice for inpatients or as an alternative to clomipramine. However, two trials not included in this meta-analysis[11,12] found in a younger adult and elderly depressed inpatient sample no differences between paroxetine and amitriptyline.

Table IV. Relative efficacy of SSRIs against TCAs.[10] Effect sizes (ES) only are given. Since for sertraline and citalopram too few studies (3 and 5, respectively) were published in comparison with fluvoxamine (17), fluoxetine (20) and paroxetine (10), these results are not reported

Results group	All SSRIs	Fluvoxamine	Fluoxetine	Paroxetine
Studies with complete data[a]				
no.	22	6	9	3
ES	–0.05	–0.04	–0.02	0.00
95% CI	(–0.14-0.04)	(–0.26-0.19)	(–0.16-0.11)	(–0.33-0.33)
Placebo-controlled studies[a]				
no.	11	5	3	1
ES	0.02	0.02	0.01	0.03
95% CI	(–0.11-0.15)	(–0.16-0.20)	(–0.23-0.24)	(–0.16-0.23)
All studies[a]				
no.	55	17	20	10
ES	0.00	0.00	0.03	–0.06
95% CI	(–0.08-0.08)	(–0.13-0.12)	(–0.10-0.17)	(–0.23-0.10)
Inpatients[a]				
no.	17	8	2	5
ES	–0.20*	0.07	–0.25	–0.43**
95% CI	(–0.38 - –0.02)	(–0.14-0.28)	(–0.62-0.13)	(–0.72 - –0.13)
Outpatients[a]				
no.	30	7	16	4
ES	0.06	–0.19	0.07	0.10
95% CI	(–0.05-0.16)	(–0.42-0.05)	(–0.07-0.21)	(–0.04-0.24)
High initial HAM-D score[a]				
no.	16	7	4	3
ES	–0.10*	0.00	–0.17*	–0.09
95% CI	(–0.20-0.00)	(–0.22-0.22)	(–0.35-0.00)	(–0.31-0.14)
Low initial HAM-D score[a]				
no.	23	5	10	5
ES	0.00	–0.05	0.17	–0.20
95% CI	(–0.13-0.12)	(–0.23-0.13)	(–0.03-0.37)	(–0.50-0.11)
Serotonergic TCAs[a]				
no.	23	5	10	5
ES	–0.16*	–0.16	0.06	–0.37**
95% CI	(–0.30 - –0.01)	(–0.46-0.13)	(–0.12-0.23)	(–0.64 - –0.09)
Noradrenergic TCAs[a]				
no.	32	12	12	4
ES	0.07*	0.03	0.02	0.10
95% CI	(0.00-0.14)	(–0.11-0.17)	(–0.14-0.18)	(–0.04-0.24)

a Since sertraline and citalopram are not included in this table, the total number is higher than the sum of the trials with fluvoxamine, fluoxetine and paroxetine.

CI = confidence intervals; **HAM-D** = Hamilton Depression Rating Scale; **SSRIs** = selective serotonin (5-hydroxytryptamine; 5-HT) reuptake inhibitors; **TCAs** = tricyclic antidepressants; * $p < 0.05$; ** $p < 0.01$.

The last and perhaps most important conclusion is that '[T]he common clinical practice of using clomipramine or amitriptyline when it is important to maximise efficacy (for example in treatment resistant inpatients) is not rebutted, particularly as many of the studies used relatively modest doses of TCA'.

Two further meta-analyses[13,14] compared the drop-out rate in controlled clinical trials of TCA- versus SSRI-treated patients. In the first paper, including 67 published studies, 4.5% fewer patients in the SSRI groups discontinued because of adverse effects; in the second, including 62 trials, there was a 25% lower drop-out rate. Both results were statistically highly significant. Regarding the drop-out rate resulting from lack of efficacy, Montgomery and Kasper[13] reported no difference between SSRIs and TCAs; Anderson and Tomenson[14] reported only the total drop-out rate, which was 10% less in the SSRI group. No clear differences were reported between the individual SSRIs.

Two clinical trials have been performed regarding the option for paroxetine in treatment-resistant patients. The first[15] included 24 patients and was placebo-controlled, the second[16] included 28 patients and was open-labelled. Therapy resistance was not adequately defined. In both trials, paroxetine (30 mg/day) reduced depressive symptomatology.

For fluoxetine, the only data available are those from controlled trials versus TCAs with patients who experienced tolerability problems with TCAs and who then received fluoxetine in an open fashion.[17] Approximately 60% of these patients responded under fluoxetine. For the remaining SSRIs, no data about the management of therapy-resistant depression have been published so far as we know.

Short term antidepressant efficacy is only one aspect of the choice of pharmacological treatment; the second aspect encompasses the recurrence prevention properties of different compounds. Figure 1[18-21] summarises the results obtained up to now.

The prophylactic activity of SSRIs of up to 1 year in monopolar major depression seems to be validated. However, a prophylactic trial of SSRIs against either lithium or a TCA such as imipramine would be necessary to gather more information about their specific advantages and disadvantages for prophylaxis. At any rate, since the SSRIs possess a preferable adverse effect profile, i.e. are free from sedating properties and do not decrease psychomotor performance or cognitive abilities – especially important for outpatients in their normal social and professional situation – they represent a valuable alternative in recurrence prophylaxis.

2. Reversible Inhibitors of Monoamine Oxidase A (RIMAs)

MAO exists in two functional forms, MAO-A and MAO-B. Classical MAOIs inhibit both isoenzymes nonselectively and irreversibly. MAO-A preferentially deaminates noradrenaline, adrenaline and serotonin, MAO-B preferentially 2-phenylethyl-amine, whereas tyramine and dopamine are substrates of both isoenzymes.

Inhibition of MAO-A is regarded as the decisive factor for the antidepressant effect. Classical MAOIs nonselectively and irreversibly block both functional forms. Therefore, the intake of high amounts of tyramine in food during treatment with these compounds may lead to hypertensive crises (the so-called 'cheese effect', since cheese was often thought to be the main source of exogenous tyramine). This interaction potential, to-

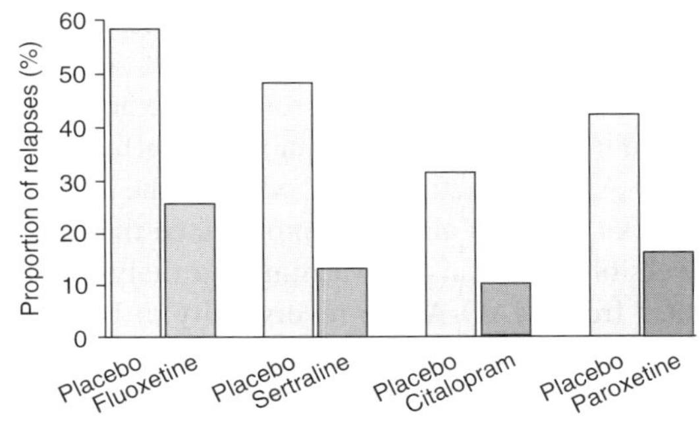

Fig. 1. Overview of prophylactic trials with selective serotonin (5-hydroxytryptamine; 5-HT) uptake inhibitors (SSRIs) [according to Montgomery et al.[18] (fluoxetine); Doogan & Caillard[19] (sertraline); Montgomery & Rasmussen[20] (citalopram); Montgomery & Dunbar[21] (paroxetine)]. All studies were performed for 12 months with the exception of study of citalopram, which lasted only 6 months. This is also the reason for the relatively small placebo-relapse rate in this trial. The mean relapse rates in the SSRI groups amount to 16% and in the placebo groups to 45%.

Table V. Comparison of the inhibitory potencies of reversible versus irreversible monoamine oxidase (MAO) inhibitors on rat brain MAO activity *in vitro* and *ex vivo*[25]

Drug	MAO					
	IC_{50} (μmol/L)			ED_{50} (μmol/kg)		
	A[a]	B[b]	B/A[c]	A[a]	B[b]	B/A[c]
Moclobemide	6	>1000	>170	8	78	10
Brofaromine	0.013	31	2400	5	>1000	>200
Phenelzine	0.015	0.033	2.20	72	91	1.3
Isocarboxazid	0.30	0.018	0.06	17	7	0.4
Tranylcypromine	0.18	0.740	4.10	12	4	0.3

a Serotonin (5-hydroxytryptamine; 5-HT) used to determine specific MAO-A activity.

b Phenylethylamine used to determine specific MAO-B activity.

c Enzyme selectivity is expressed as the ratio of IC_{50} or ED_{50} values for MAO-A and MAO-B.

ED_{50} = oral dose causing 50% inhibition of brain MAO activity 2h after drug administration; **IC_{50}** = concentration that inhibits MAO activity *in vitro* by 50%.

gether with the initial observation that classical MAOIs are therapeutically less effective than TCAs in the treatment of severe depression,[22] has led to a very cautious use of these agents, at least in Europe.[23]

With the discovery of 2 functional forms, which took place only in 1968,[24] the development of new MAOIs for the treatment of depression focused on (a) the selective inhibition of MAO-A, thus allowing MAO-B to remain active and deaminate the potentially hazardous tyramine, and (b) the reversible and competitive property of this inhibition, allowing other substrates (like tyramine) to displace the inhibitor from the binding position. These compounds are called RIMAs. The first drug of this class to be registered was moclobemide, the second intended to be registered was brofaromine. Cimoxatone is registered only in France and is not considered here because of its relatively weak MAO-A inhibitory properties.

As can be gathered from table V,[25] which lists data on the inhibition of irreversible MAOIs as well as RIMAs on rat brain MAO activity *in vitro* and *ex vivo*, moclobemide and brofaromine strongly inhibit MAO-A selectively, whereas the standard MAOIs phenelzine, isocarboxazid and tranylcypromine cause inhibition of both isoenzymes.

After a single oral dose, brofaromine and moclobemide rapidly inhibit MAO-A activity in rat brain and liver, with the maximum effect occurring within 30 minutes.[26] After 16 hours, MAO-A is fully active again, whereas the inhibition with classical MAOIs lasts for more than 3 weeks. It could also be demonstrated that the binding of moclobemide and brofaromine is reversible by means of washing and dialysis techniques. While moclobemide readily dissociates from MAO-A, the reversibility of brofaromine is initially time-dependent, leading to the characterisation of this drug as being selective and reversible, but tightly binding.[27]

Regarding the tyramine-potentiating effects of RIMAs, interaction studies were performed to determine the tyramine dose leading to a systolic blood pressure increase of 30mm Hg. This dose is 450mg of tyramine in untreated volunteers, 65mg for brofaromine and moclobemide, but 8mg for tranylcypromine.[28-30] These data demonstrate that RIMAs have a reduced interaction potential compared with the standard MAOIs, but still pose a certain safety problem, at least in cases of very high tyramine intake.

Regarding clinical efficacy, only the moclobemide data are considered here since the development of brofaromine has been stopped (for reasons outlined by Volz et al.[31]). For a comprehensive review of the brofaromine data, see Volz et al.[32]

Clinical efficacy in the treatment of depression was established in five placebo-controlled trials.[33-37] Four of these showed statistically significant superior efficacy with moclobemide, while the fifth[35] demonstrated no difference. In the latter trial, patients with reactive depression were included and treated either with moclobemide 300 mg/day, clomipramine 150 mg/day or placebo. Clomipramine in this trial was also not superior to placebo. Therefore, the interpretation of this trial remains difficult.

A total of 40 controlled trials of moclobemide versus TCAs and tetracyclic antidepressants have been performed (for a review, see Laux[38]). In nearly all trials, moclobemide was as effective as the comparators. In 2 trials clomipramine was more effective than moclobemide in severely depressed patients. The first[39] included primarily patients with atypical depression, the other investigation[40] was published by the DUAG, who had already demonstrated the weaker action of citalopram and paroxetine *vs* clomipramine (which seems to be the most effective antidepressant). In the latter trial, a fixed-dose design (moclobemide 400 mg/day, clomipramine 150mg/day) was used in inpatients. This rather low moclobemide dosage might be responsible for the unfavourable outcome regarding the moclobemide recipients and raises the issue of the minimum effective dosage of moclobemide in severely depressed inpatients.

Moclobemide was compared with SSRIs in eight trials, three versus fluvoxamine and five versus fluoxetine (for a review see Laux[38]). Moclobemide was either superior (in two trials) or as effective as the SSRI (in six trials).

In the trials comparing moclobemide with classical MAOIs, the results remain somewhat inconclusive (see table VI).[25,41-44] Moclobemide was either more (2 trials), equally (1 trial) or less (1 trial) effective in comparison to tranylcypromine. In these trials, only endogenously depressed patients were included.

In a meta-analysis including data of most controlled clinical trials, Angst and Stabl[45] could demonstrate that moclobemide showed comparable overall antidepressant efficacy in unipolar and bipolar affective disorders, and in patients with major depressive disorder superimposed on dysthymia (double depression). As with classical antidepressants, response rates tended to be lower in psychotic depression. No differences were found for agitated and nonagitated depressed patients. Patients meeting DSM-III-R criteria for major depression with melancholia responded slightly better than nonmelancholics.

Placebo-controlled recurrence-preventing studies have so far not been performed. Open long term trials document good tolerability of moclobemide in long term use (up to 12 months[46]).

Table VI. Summary of comparative, controlled clinical studies of moclobemide (MCL) 100 to 350 mg/day versus tranylcypromine (TCP) 5 to 30 mg/day in patients with major depression (endogenous)[25]

Reference	No. of patients	HAM-D reduction	Overall efficacy	Overall tolerability
Heinze[41]	42	73 (MCL) 76 (TCP)	MCL = TCP	MCL = TCP
Heinze et al.[42]	160	63 (MCL) 58 (MCL)	TCP ≥ MCL	MCL ≥ TCP
Gabelic & Kuhn[43]	40	66 (MCL) 41 (TCP)	MCL > TCP	MCL ≥ TCP
Rossel & Moll[44]	40	59 (MCL) 66 (TCP)	TCP ≥ MCL	MCL = TCP

HAM-D = Hamilton Depression Rating Scale.

As with SSRIs, clear advantages with moclobemide regarding anticholinergic adverse effects and sedating properties become apparent, especially in comparison to TCAs. Table VII summarises the most important aspects.[47] As in the case of SSRIs, the lack of cardiotoxicity is an essential additional advantage of moclobemide over TCAs.

Table VII. Percentage frequency of adverse drug events as determined from premarketing trials comparing moclobemide (1291 patients) with tricyclic antidepressants (TCAs) [1288 patients]. Only events occurring with an incidence of greater than 5% in 1 patient group are listed[47]

Adverse drug event	Moclobemide	TCA
Blurred vision	3.9	6.1*
Constipation	6.4	12.0
Dizziness	7.8	11.8*
Dry mouth	16.6	40.0*
Headache	13.1*	9.7
Insomnia/sleep disturbance	9.8*	8.0
Nausea	8.6	8.1
Sleepiness/somnolence	5.4	11.9*
Sweating	6.5	13.7*
Tachycardia/palpitations	5.2	6.8
Tremor	5.4	13.8*

* $p < 0.05$.

3. Serotonin and Noradrenaline Reuptake Inhibitors (SNRIs)

The only SNRI currently available is venlafaxine. Compared with other antidepressants it has a unique molecular structure. It exists as a racemic mixture of *R*- and *S*-enantiomers, both of which are biologically active.[48,49] The major metabolite, *O*-demethyl-venlafaxine (ODV), has similar antidepressant effects.[50] The serum half-life is 5 hours for venlafaxine and 11 hours for ODV. Protein binding is only 27%, which is much lower than for SSRIs (for example fluoxetine 94%, paroxetine 95%).[51]

Pharmacodynamically, venlafaxine resembles the TCAs since it possesses both serotonin and noradrenaline reuptake inhibiting properties, but lacks their muscarinic-cholinergic, histaminergic and α-adrenergic effects.[52,53] Table VIII gives an overview of drug potency and selectivity for blocking neurotransmitter uptake for venlafaxine, SSRIs and TCAs.[53]

Table VIII. Drug potency and selectivity for blocking neurotransmitter reuptake into rat brain synaptosomes for various antidepressants[53]

Drug	Potency at reuptake blockade (K_i [nmol/L])		
	5-HT	NA	5-HT/NA selectivity
Venlafaxine	39 ± 3	210 ± 20	0.18
Sertraline	3.4 ± 0.4	220 ± 40	0.016
Paroxetine	0.73 ± 0.04	33 ± 2	0.022
Fluoxetine	143 ± 6	14 ± 3	0.10
Imipramine	41 ± 3	14 ± 1	2.9
Amitriptyline	84 ± 1	13.9 ± 1	6.0
Desipramine	180 ± 10	0.6 ± 0.0	300.0

5-HT = serotonin (5-hydroxytryptamine); **K_i** = inhibition constant; **NA** = noradrenaline (norepinephrine).

The clinical efficacy of venlafaxine was established in premarketing double-blind, controlled clinical trials including more than 2000 patients with major depression. In outpatient placebo-controlled studies 323 patients with major depression were included and treated for 6 weeks. Venlafaxine was administered on a 3 times daily basis with dosages of either 75, 150 to 225 or 300 to 375 mg/day. All dosage groups showed statistically superior efficacy of venlafaxine over placebo, the best response being observed if 150 to 225 or 300 to 375mg was given. This result was also confirmed with a twice-daily dosage regimen.

In a comparative outpatient trial versus imipramine (venlafaxine and imipramine 75 to 225 mg/ day, depending on initial improvement), venlafaxine was at least as effective as imipramine. In the end-point analysis superior efficacy for venlafaxine could be established. These results were robust also in inpatient trials. In one of these trials venlafaxine was compared with fluoxetine and showed better efficacy.[54] Inpatient trials in comparison with TCAs have not been published.

The observation that venlafaxine shows a fairly fast onset of effect seems to be of special interest. Already after 4 to 7 days of treatment, a statistically significant treatment effect of 4 points on the Montgomery-Åsberg Depression Rating Scale emerged.[55]

Table IX. Incidence (%) of adverse effects occurring in 10% or more of patients and twice as often with venlafaxine than with placebo[51]

Adverse effect	Venlafaxine (n = 1033)	Placebo (n = 609)
Nausea	37	11
Somnolence	23	9
Dry mouth	22	11
Dizziness	19	7
Constipation	15	7
Nervousness	13	6
Asthenia	12	6
Sweating	12	3
Abnormal ejaculation[a]	12	0
Anorexia	11	2

a 836 men.

Eighty-two patients with rigorously defined treatment-refractory depression were enrolled in an open-label study at two study sites. Study participants received venlafaxine up to a maximum of 450 mg/day and were followed for at least 6 months. Approximately 40% of patients showed a clinically meaningful response to venlafaxine.[51] Of the 222 patients receiving venlafaxine on a long term basis (up to 1 year), only 8% terminated treatment prematurely compared with 6% on placebo. This result can be taken to indicate favourable long term tolerability. The predominant adverse effects were nausea, somnolence, dry mouth, dizziness and constipation, and are summarised in table IX.[51]

A dose-response relationship seems to exist with blood pressure increase: the maximal mean increase for patients treated with 75 mg/day was 1mm Hg, 2mm Hg for 225 mg/day, and 7.5mm Hg for those receiving 375 mg/day.[51] Overall, about 3% of patients receiving venlafaxine experienced blood pressure elevation. This adverse effect mostly occurred in the second month of treatment, but could not be predicted by patient characteristics such as sex, age, renal or hepatic function. Venlafaxine and cimetidine act synergistically in patients with pre-existing hypertension, decreased drug clearance, or liver dysfunction. Since venlafaxine weakly inhibits CYP2D6, it may interact with other drugs metabolised by this enzyme.[51]

4. Mirtazapine

Mirtazapine, which has recently been registered in a number of European countries, is a new antidepressant with yet another mode of action. It acts via two mechanisms: (i) it blocks α_2-adrenergic auto- and heteroreceptors and thus increases noradrenaline and serotonin release; and (ii) it enhances serotonergic neurotransmission via two synergistic points of influence. First, the increased noradrenaline release leads to an increased firing rate of serotonergic raphe cells, mediated via the stimulation of α_1-adrenoceptors on the serotonergic cell body. This increase is facilitated by the simultaneous blockade of α_2-adrenergic heteroreceptors on the serotonergic nerve terminal, preventing a counteraction against enhanced cell firing. Secondly, 5-HT_2 and 5-HT_3 receptors, responsible for some of the adverse events caused by high serotonergic tone, are blocked by mirtazapine, so that only the antidepressive 5-HT_1 receptor effect is left.[56-58]

Although mirtazapine is structurally related to mianserin (6-aza analogue) the two compounds show different interactions with noradrenergic and serotonergic transmission. While mirtazapine potently increases noradrenergic and serotonergic transmission, mianserin does not affect serotonin release and only weakly enhances noradrenergic transmission. This is probably caused by the higher affinity for α_1-adrenoceptors and the pronounced noradrenaline reuptake blockade of mianserin compared with mirtazapine.[59]

Mirtazapine possesses low *in vitro* affinity for muscarinic, cholinergic and dopaminergic receptors, and does not inhibit dopamine reuptake.[60] It has a high affinity for histamine H_1 receptors, which may cause drowsiness and sedation.[61]

The elimination half-life of this compound is 20 to 40 hours, the plasma protein binding 85% and the bioavailability 50%. The main biotransformation routes in humans are demethylation and oxidation, followed by conjugation. One pharmacologically active demethyl metabolite has been identified, demethyl-mirtazapine, which seems to be 3- to 4-fold less active than the parent compound.

The clinical efficacy of mirtazapine has been demonstrated in a series of controlled clinical trials. A total of 249 patients received mirtazapine and 246 placebo. In an unpublished meta-analysis comprising all these patients investigated in different individual trials, a clear-cut superiority of mirtazapine over placebo, which had already been shown for each individual trial, was apparent, starting from week 1 on. The mean HAM-D score (17-item form) at the start of the trials was approximately 24; after a 6-week observation period the score in the active treatment group dropped to about 11, in the placebo group to about 14.5.[56]

732 patients, mostly severely depressed in patients, were included in comparative trials versus amitriptyline and analysed in a meta-analysis with comparable methodology to that of the placebo-controlled data. Most dosages used were near 50 mg/day of mirtazapine and 150 to 200 mg/day of amitriptyline. The end-point analysis revealed a decrease of the HAM-D score of 16.0 and 16.2 for mirtazapine and amitriptyline recipients, respectively.[56] Comparative trials versus clomipramine,[62] doxepin[63] and trazodone[64] confirmed these results.

A meta-analysis of the comparative trials versus amitriptyline in the treatment of severely depressed patients (baseline HAM-D score $\geq$25) was performed. Included were approximately 200 patients in each group. In both groups a reduction of the HAM-D score of nearly 18 was observed, hinting at a good efficacy of the newly developed compound also in this subgroup.[56]

In a further meta-analysis of the HAM-D factor III (anxiety somatisation factor) and the sum score of the HAM-D items 4 to 6 (sleep-items), mirtazapine was clearly superior to placebo and as effective as amitriptyline.[56]

In two trials,[65,66] double-blind treatment with mirtazapine, amitriptyline and placebo was continued for up to 6 months. Mirtazapine (mean daily dose 27mg) in these trials was as effective in continuation treatment as amitriptyline (mean daily dose 168mg) and both compounds were superior to placebo. In these trials, only a moderate number of patients (mirtazapine 43, amitriptyline 48, placebo 27) was included.

Studies evaluating therapy-resistant depressions have not yet been published.

The adverse effect profile of mirtazapine in comparison to placebo is summarised in table X.[56] As can be seen, sedation, drowsiness and fatigue on the one hand, and increased appetite and bodyweight on the other, might be a problem. In comparison with amitriptyline, the anticholinergic and neurological (tremor, vertigo) adverse effects are less pronounced.[56] These results were confirmed in a recently published meta-analysis[67] including 1378 patients receiving mirtazapine, 348 on placebo and 514 receiving amitriptyline. 5% of mirtazapine recipients complained of any adverse clinical experience compared with 76 and 87% in the placebo and amitriptyline groups, respectively. The percentage of patients withdrawn because of adverse events was statistically significantly lower in mirtazapine (4.9%) compared with amitriptyline recipients (9.1%).

The analysis of the data of clinical trials where often-prescribed drugs were coadministered has to date revealed no high interaction potential of mirtazapine.[56]

Table X. Incidence (%) of adverse effects occurring in 10% or more of patients or twice as often with mirtazapine than with placebo[56]

Adverse effect	Mirtazapine (n = 359)	Placebo (n = 328)
Dry mouth	25.3*	15.9
Drowsiness	23.4*	14.2
Excessive sedation	18.7*	5.2
Constipation	18.1	11.9
Fatigue	16.2	11.9
Appetite		
decrease	12.8	12.2
increase	10.6*	2.1
Bodyweight increase	10.3*	1.2
Headache	5.4	10.4**
Hypotension	1.7	0.6

* $p < 0.05$ *vs* placebo; ** $p < 0.05$ *vs* mirtazapine.

5. Nefazodone

Nefazodone, a phenoxyethyl triazoline phenylpiperazine derivate structurally related to trazodone, acts as a selective serotonin inhibitor and as a 5-HT_2 receptor antagonist.[68] In comparison with trazodone, the compound binds considerably less to α_1-receptors. No clinically relevant muscarinic receptor interactions occur.[69]

Oral nefazodone is well absorbed, resulting in peak plasma concentrations approximately 1 hour after intake. Twice-daily administration produces a steady-state within 4 to 5 days. Nefazodone undergoes extensive first-pass metabolism, resulting in a bioavailability of only 15 to 23%. During long term administration, this first-pass metabolism becomes saturated. This results in larger rises of plasma concentration with dosage increases later in treatment. The main metabolites are hydroxy-nefazodone, methyl-chlorophenylpiperazine (mCPP) and desethyl-hydroxy-nefazodone. The last compound accumulates more than the parent compound, resulting in a four times higher plasma concentration than nefazodone.[69]

The dual synaptic effects of nefazodone, reuptake inhibition and 5-HT_2 receptor blockade, may influence both its efficacy and its tolerability. *Ex vivo* studies have shown that nefazodone inhibits serotonin reuptake to the same degree as fluoxetine,[70] but does not appear to cause SSRI-associated adverse effects. In *in vivo* studies the serotonin reuptake inhibition potential was considerably less than with fluoxetine [nefazodone K_i (inhibition constant) 149 nmol/L, fluoxetine 5 nmol/L].[68] Unfortunately, nefazodone has not yet been evaluated in direct comparison with an SSRI.[71]

Nefazodone possesses an IC_{50} (concentration producing 50% inhibition) for the α_1-receptor of 144 nmol/L, compared with 23 nmol/L for trazodone and more than 100 000 nmol/L for fluoxetine.[69] This means that the risk of inducing priapism with nefazodone should be reduced and, in fact, this risk has not been thought to be significant.[72,73]

Nefazodone is an inhibitor of CYP3A4; caution is therefore indicated if nefazodone is coadministered with any drugs known to be metabolised by CYP3A4. In particular, the combination of nefazodone with either terfenadine or astemizole is contraindicated. Nefazodone is an extremely weak inhibitor of CYP2D6; therefore, it is not likely to decrease the clearance of drugs metabolised by this isoenzyme.[74]

At a dosage of 300 to 600 mg/day, nefazodone is as effective as imipramine and superior to placebo for the treatment of severe depression and depression with comorbid anxiety disorders, and prevents recurrence of depression.[75-80] Recurrence of depression was analysed in approximately 700 depressed patients in comparison with imipramine. Nefazodone was as efficacious in preventing relapse as imipramine. Both compounds were statistically significantly superior to placebo at the end of the 1-year observation period.

Table XI. Incidence (%) of adverse effects occurring in 10% or more of patients and more than twice as often with nefazodone than with placebo[81]

Adverse effect	Nefazodone	Placebo
Headache	36	33
Dry mouth	25	13
Nausea	22	12
Dizziness	17	5
Somnolence	15	14
Constipation	14	8
Insomnia	11	9
Asthenia	11	5
Lightheadedness	10	3
Blurred vision	9	3
Confusion	7	2
Abnormal vision	7	1
Postural hypotension	4	1
Decreased concentration	3	1
Ataxia	2	0

Tolerability of nefazodone is regarded as good. The most common adverse events (reported at ≥5% and significantly different from placebo) are asthenia, dry mouth, nausea, constipation, somnolence, dizziness, lightheadedness, confusion, blurred vision and abnormal vision (table XI[81]).

It is tempting to speculate that the absence of SSRI-like adverse effects may be the result of 5-HT_2 antagonism, which may neutralise some of the more activating effects of unopposed reuptake inhibition.[71] In animal studies, it was shown that 5-HT_2 antagonism inhibited the manifestation of serotonergic overactivity.[75] The absence of typical SSRI adverse effects may also be linked to the fact that *in vivo* serotonin reuptake inhibition of nefazodone is considerably less than that of fluoxetine, for example.

The absence of activating effects may be linked to the observation that, unlike any other antidepressant, nefazodone does not suppress, and in some studies increases, rapid eye movement (REM) sleep.[72,73] It also increases stages 3 and 4 sleep.[65] Therefore, treatment of depression-related insomnia and night-time awakenings should be especially effective with this compound.[69]

Nefazodone possesses an interaction potential with alprazolam, triazolam, haloperidol, antihypertensives and MAOIs; no interactions were observed for alcohol and lorazepam.[74]

6. Conclusion: Open Questions

Our overview provides the impression that the newly developed antidepressants seem to possess certain advantages in comparison to TCAs, especially as far as adverse effect profiles and reduced toxicity are concerned. Regarding efficacy, the discussion still does not focus on the issue of which new antidepressant may be superior to TCAs, but on the question of whether the new generation is as effective as TCAs. This implies that two major medical needs for treating depressed patients have not yet been met: (i) superior efficacy in comparison with TCAs; and (ii) faster onset of action.

The demand for a reliably effective agent for treating resistant depression also remains to be realised. As far as these issues are concerned, a major advantage of the most recently developed compounds, venlafaxine and mirtazapine, has not yet become apparent. Perhaps certain patient subgroups respond better to these compounds because they possess a broader spectrum of influence on neurotransmission in comparison with the SSRIs, but this seems to be the only additional benefit to which we can look forward.

Since no major efficacy advantages are obvious, the adverse effect profile gains special interest. Undoubtedly, the new compounds starting with the SSRIs show advantages in comparison with TCAs: no sedation (except mirtazapine), no anticholinergic activity, and no cardiotoxic effects. However, certain adverse effect problems still exist, e.g. nausea and vomiting with the SSRIs, insomnia and headache with moclobemide, nausea, somnolence and dry mouth with venlafaxine, and drowsiness, increased appetite, dry mouth and weight increase with mirtazapine. The least to be demanded of future antidepressants – if superior efficacy cannot be attained – is exemption from these potentially disabling adverse effects.

To us, it seems questionable whether a so-called 'ideal' antidepressant can be developed on the basis of the principles of action established up to now. New pharmacological mechanisms should be further investigated to overcome the efficacy disadvantages shared by all existing antidepressants. In this context, some thought might be given to the modulation of neuropeptides. These molecules play a key role in the regulation of CNS functions, and although specific neuropeptides which have antidepressive properties have not yet been identified, preliminary evidence suggests that their existence is likely. Further systematic research is warranted, which is, however, complicated by the low blood-brain barrier permeability and chemical lability of these compounds.

A new point of attack of future antidepressants might be the direct influence on second messenger systems, e.g. via cyclic adenosine monophosphate (cAMP) or the phosphatidylinositol system. The first step in this direction was rolipram, the development of which was stopped some years ago. Interestingly, lithium acts on this system, and part of its efficacy is determined by this influence.

A very different antidepressant treatment approach, which might fulfil some of the stated features of an 'ideal' antidepressant, is *S*-adenosyl-L-methionine (SAMe; ademetionine), a naturally occurring substance produced in mammals from L-methionine and adenosine triphosphate. In a recently published meta-analysis,[83] a clear-cut superiority of this molecule in comparison with placebo and even promises of better efficacy and faster onset of action compared with traditional antidepressants have emerged. Interestingly, almost no adverse effects have been observed. SAMe increased the conversion of phosphatidyl-ethanolamine to phosphatidyl-choline, improving the fluidity of cell membranes and possibly facilitating neurotransmission by increasing the density of available receptors or heightening the efficiency of receptor-effector coupling[84]. After a further clarification of the mode of action, a new antidepressant approach might become possible with this agent.

These are only some very preliminary considerations, indicating that the investigation of new possibilities in the future development of antidepressants is necessary to overcome adverse effect problems and – perhaps even more important – efficacy problems, where no major progress has been achieved since the discovery of imipramine in the late 1950s.

Acknowledgements

We gratefully thank Dr Kreitschmann-Andermahr for her excellent assistance in preparing the English version of this paper.

References

1. Kasper S, Möller HJ. Antidepressive Psychopharmakatherapie: selektive Serotonin-Wiederaufnahmehemmer (SSRI) als neues Wirkprinzip. Deutsches Arzteblatt 1995; 92: A428-34
2. Baldwin D, Johnson FN. Tolerability and safety of citalopram. Rev Contemp Pharmacother 1995; 6: 315-25
3. Harvey AT, Preskorn SH. Interactions of serotonin reuptake inhibitors with tricyclic antidepressants. Arch Gen Psychiatry 1995; 52: 783-4
4. Bech P. A meta-analysis of the antidepressant properties of serotonin reuptake inhibitors. Int Rev Psychol 1990; 2: 207-11
5. Grimsley SR, Jann MW. Paroxetine, sertraline, and fluvoxamine: new selective serotonin reuptake inhibitors. Clin Pharm 1992; 11: 930-56
6. Kasper S, Fuger J, Möller HJ. Comparative efficacy of antidepressants. Drugs 1992; 43 Suppl. 2: 11-23
7. Davis JM, Wang Z, Janicak PG. A quantitative analysis of clinical drug trials for the treatment of affective disorders. Psychopharmacol Bull 1993; 29: 175-81
8. Danish University Antidepressant Group. Citalopram: clinical effective profile in comparison with clomipramine. A controlled multicenter study. Psychopharmacol 1986; 90: 131-8
9. Danish University Antidepressant Group. Paroxetine: a selective serotonin reuptake inhibitor showing better tolerance, but weaker antidepressant effect than clomipramine in a controlled multicentre study. J Affect Disord 1990; 18: 289-99
10. Anderson IM, Tomenson BM. The efficacy of selective serotonin re-uptake inhibitors in depression: a meta-analysis of studies against tricyclic antidepressants. J Psychopharmacol 1994; 8: 238-49
11. Stuppaeck CH, Geretsegger C, Whitworth AB, et al. A multicenter double-blind trial of paroxetine versus amitriptyline in depressed inpatients. J Clin Psychopharmacol 1994; 14: 241-6
12. Geretsegger C, Stuppaeck CH, Mair M, et al. Multicenter double blind study of paroxetine and amitriptyline in elderly depressed inpatients. Psychopharmacology 1995; 119: 277-81
13. Montgomery SA, Kasper S. Comparsion of compliance between serotonergic reuptake inhibitors and tricyclic antidepressants: a meta-analysis. Int Clin Psychopharmacol 1995; 9 Suppl. 4: 33-40
14. Anderson IM, Tomenson BM. Treatment discontinuation with selective serotonin reuptake inhibition compared with tricyclic antidepressants: a meta-analysis. BMJ 1995; 310: 1433-8
15. Tyrer P, Marsden CA, Casey P, et al. Clinical efficacy of paroxetine in resistant depression. J Psychopharmacol 1987; 1: 251-7
16. Gagiano CA, Müller PGM, Fourie J, et al. The therapeutic efficacy of paroxetine: (a) an open study in patients with major depression not responding to antidepressants; (b) a double-blind comparision with amitriptyline in depressed outpatients. Acta Psychiatr Scand 1989; 80 Suppl. 350: 130-1
17. Beasley CM, Syler ME, Cunningham GE, et al. Fluoxetine in tricyclic refractory major depressive disorder. J Affect Disord 1990; 20: 193-200
18. Montgomery SA, Dufour H, Brion S, et al. The prophylactic efficacy of fluoxetine in unipolar depression. Br J Psychiatry 1988; Suppl. 3: 69-76
19. Doogan DP, Caillard V. Sertraline in the prevention of depression. Br J Psychiatry 1992; 160: 217-22
20. Montgomery SA, Rasmussen JG. Citalopram 20mg, citalopram 40mg and placebo in the prevention of relapse of major depression. Int Clin Psychopharmacol 1992; 6 Suppl. 5: 71-3
21. Montgomery SA, Dunbar G. Paroxetine is better than placebo in relapse prevention and the prophylaxis of recurrent depression. Int Clin Psychopharmacol 1993; 8: 189-95
22. Raskin A, Schulterbrandt JG, Reatig N, et al. Depression subtypes and response to phenelzine, diazepam and placebo. Arch Gen Psychiatry 1974; 30: 66-75
23. Paykel ES, White JL. A European study of views on the use of monoamine oxidase inhibitors. Br J Psychiatry 1989; 155 Suppl. 6: 9-17
24. Johnston JP. Some observations upon a new monoamine oxidase inhibitor in brain tissue. Biochem Pharmacol 1968; 17: 1285-97
25. Laux G, Volz HP, Möller HJ. Newer and older monoamine oxidase inhibitors: a comparative profile. CNS Drugs 1995; 3: 145-58
26. Waldmeier PC. On the reversibility of reversible MAO inhibitors. Naunyn Schmiedebergs Arch Pharmacol 1985; 169: 305-10
27. Anderson C, Waldmeier PC, Tipton KF. The inhibition of monoamine oxidase by brofaromine. Biochem Pharmacol 1991; 41: 1871-7
28. Bieck PR, Antonin KH. Oral tyramine pressor test and the safety of monoamine oxidase inhibitor drugs: comparison of brofaromine and tranylcypromine in healthy subjects. J Clin Psychopharmacol 1988; 8: 237-45
29. Bieck PR, Antonin KH. Tyramine potentiation during treatment with MAO inhibitors: brofaromine and moclobemide vs. irreversible inhibitors. J Neural Transm 1989; 28 Suppl.: 21-31
30. Gleiter CH, Mühlbauer B, Schulz RM, et al. Monoamine oxidase inhibition by the MAO-A inhibitors brofaromine and clorgyline in healthy volunteers. J Neural Transm Gen Sect 1994; 95: 241-5
31. Volz HP, Gleiter CH, Struck M, et al. Brofaromine: insight into the nature of drug development. CNS Drugs 1995; 3: 1-8

32. Volz HP, Gleiter CH, Waldmeier PC, et al. Brofaromine – a review of its pharmacological properties and therapeutic use. J Neural Transm Park Dis Dement Sect 1996; 103: 217-45
33. Versiani M, Oggero U, Alterwain P, et al. Moclobemide in the treatment of major depressive episodes – a double-blind comparative multicenter trial vs. imipramine and placebo. Br J Psychiatry 1989; 155: 72-9
34. Bakish D, Bradwejn N, Nair N, et al. A comparison of moclobemide, amitriptyline and placebo in depression: a Canadian multicentre study. Psychopharmacol 1992; 106: 98-101
35. Larsen JK, Holm P, Hoyer E, et al. Moclobemide and clomipramine in reactive depression: a placebo-controlled randomized clinical trial. Acta Psychiatr Scand 1989; 79: 530-6
36. Casacchia M, Carolei A, Barba C, et al. A placebo-controlled study of the antidepressant activity of moclobemide, a new MAO-A inhibitor. Pharmacopsychiatry 1994 17: 122-5
37. Botte L, Evrard JC, Gilles C, et al. Controlled comparison of RO 11-1163 (moclobemide) and placebo in the treatment of depression. Acta Psychiatr Belg 1992; 92: 355-69
38. Laux G. Kontrollierte Vergleichsstudien mit Moclobemid in der Depressionsbehandlung. Psychopharmakotherapie 1994; 1: 9-18
39. Larsen JK, Gjerris A, Holm P, et al. Moclobemide in depression: a randomized trial against isocarboxazide and clomipramine emphazising atypical depression. Acta Psychiatr Scand 1991; 84: 564-70
40. Danish University Antidepressant Group. Moclobemide: a reversible MAO-A inhibitor showing weaker antidepressant effect than clomipramine in a controlled multicentre study. J Affect Disord 1993; 28: 105-16
41. Heinze C. Moclobemide versus tranylcypromine in the treatment of depression: a double-blind comparative study [abstract]. Psychopharmacol 1988; Suppl 96.: 11.41.10
42. Heinze G, Rossel L, Gabelic I, et al. Double-blind comparison of moclobemide and tranylcypromine in depression. Pharmacopsychiatry 1993; 26: 240-5
43. Gabelic I, Kuhn B. Moclobemide (Ro 11-1163) versus tranylcypromine in the treatment of endogenous depression [abstract]. Acta Psychiatr Scand 1990; 82 Suppl. 360: 63
44. Rossel L, Moll E. Moclobemide versus tranylcypromine in the treatment of depression. Acta Psychiatr Scand 1990; 82 Suppl. 360: 61-2
45. Angst J, Stabl M. Efficacy of moclobemide in different patient groups: a meta-analysis of studies. Psychopharmacol 1992; 106: S109-13
46. Moll E, Neumann N, Schmidt-Burgk W, et al. Safety and efficacy during long-term treatment with moclobemide. Clin Neuropharmacol 1994; 17 Suppl. 1: S74-87
47. Chen D, Ruck R. Safety of moclobemide in clincal use. Clin Neuropharmacol 1993; 16 Suppl. 2: S63-8
48. Wang CP, Howell SR, Scatina J, et al. The disposition of venlafaxine enantiomers in dogs, rats, and humans receiving venlafaxine. Chirality 1992; 4: 84-90
49. Muth ES, Haskins JT, Moyer HA, et al. Antidepressant biochemical profile of the novel bicyclic compound WY-45,030, an ethyl cyclohexanol derivative. Biochem Pharmacol 1986; 35: 4493-7
50. Muth EA, Moyer JA, Haskins JT, et al. Biochemical, neurophysiological, and behavioral effects of Wy-45.233 and other identified metabolites of the antidepressant venlafaxine. Drug Develop Res 1991; 23: 191-9
51. Feighner JP. The role of venlafaxine in rational antidepressant therapy. J Clin Psychiatry 1994; 55 Suppl. A: 62-8
52. Howell SR, Husbands GE, Scatina JA, et al. Metabolic disposition of ^{14}C-venlafaxine in mouse, rat, dog, rhesus monkey and man. Xenobiotica 1993; 23: 349-59
53. Bolden-Watson C, Richelson E. Blockade by newly-developed antidepressants of biogenic amine uptake into rat brain synaptosomes. Life Sci 1993; 52: 1023-9
54. Bouchard JM, Peze E, Daurignac I. The Venlafaxine French Inpatient Study Group: a double-blind comparison of venlafaxine and fluoxetine in patients hospitalized for major depression and melancholia. Int Clin Psychopharmacol. In press
55. Preskorn SH. Antidepressant drug selection: criteria and options. J Clin Psychiatry 1994; 55: Suppl. A: 6-22
56. Sitsen JMA, Zivkov M. Mirtazapine: clinical profile. CNS Drugs 1995; 4 Suppl. 1: 39-48
57. Clement HH, Gemsa D, Weseman W. The effect of noradrenergic drugs on serotonin metabolism in the nucleus raphe dorsalis of the rat, studied by *in vitro* voltometry. Eur J Pharmacol 1992; 217: 43-8
58. de Boer T, Nefkens F, Van Helvoirt A. The α_2 antagonist ORG 3770 enhances serotonin transmission *in vivo*. Eur J Pharmacology 1994; 253: R5-6
59. de Boer T, Ruigt GSF, Berendsen HHG. The α_2-selective adrenoceptor antagonist Org 3770 (mirtazapine, Remeron®) enhances noradrenergic and serotonergic transmission. Hum Psychopharmacol 1995; 10: S107-18
60. de Boer T, Ruigt SF. The selective α_2-adrenoreceptor antagonist mirtazapine (Org 3770) enhances noradrenergic and 5-HT_{1A}–mediated serotonergic neurotransmission. CNS Drugs 1995; 4 Suppl.1: 29-38
61. de Boer T, Maura G, Raiteri M, et al. Neurochemical and autonomic pharmacological profiles of the 6-aza-analogue of mianserin: Org 3770 and its enantiomers. Neuropharmacology 1988; 27: 399-408
62. Richou H, Ruimy P, Charbaut J, et al. A multicentre, double-blind, clomipramine-controlled efficacy and safety study of Org 3770. Hum Psychopharm 1995 Jul-Aug; 10: 263-71
63. Marttila M, Jaaskelainen J, Jarvi R, et al. A double-blind study comparing the efficacy and tolerability of mirtazapine and doxepin in patients with major depression. Eur Neuropsychopharmacol 1995 Dec; 5: 441-6
64. van Moffaert M, de Wilde J, Verreecken A, et al. Mirtazapine is more effective than trazodone: a controlled study in hospitalized patients with major depression. Int Clin Psychopharmacol 1995; 10: 3-9
65. Bremner JD. A double-blind comparison of Org 3770, amitriptyline, and placebo in major depression. J Clin Psychiatry 1995 Nov; 56: 519-25
66. Smith WT, Glaudin V, Panagides J, et al. Mirtazapine vs amitriptyline vs placebo in the treatment of major depressive disorder. Psychopharmacol Bull 1990; 26: 191-6

67. Montgomery SA. Safety of mirtazapine: a review. Int Clin Psychopharmacol 1995; 10 Suppl. 4: 37-45
68. Taylor DP, Carter RB, Eison AS, et al. Pharmacology and neurochemistry of nefazodone, a novel antidepressant. J Clin Psychiatry 1995; 54 Suppl. 6: 3-11
69. Dubobsky SL, Thomas M. Serotonergic mechanisms and current and future psychiatric practice. J Clin Psychiatry 1995; 56 Suppl. 2: 38-48
70. Eison AS, Eison MS, Torrente JR, et al. Nefazodone: preclinical pharmacology of a new antidepressant. Psychopharmacol Bull 1990; 26: 311-5
71. Sussman N. The potential benefits of serotonin receptor–specific agents. J Clin Psychiatry; 55 Suppl.: 45-51
72. Sharpley AL, Walsh AE, Cowan PJ. Nefazodone – a novel antidepressant – may increase REM sleep. Biol Psychiatry 1992; 31: 1070-3
73. Armitage R, Roffwarg H, Cain J, et al. The effect of nefazodone on sleep EEG in major depression. Neuropsychopharmacol 1994; 10: 123-7
74. Nefazodone: the latest FDA approved antidepressant [editorial]. Int Drug Ther Newslett 1995; 30: 17-20
75. Gammans R, Schwiderski U, O'Brien K, et al. Nefazodone efficacy in severe depression [abstract]. Clin Neuropharmacol 1992; 15 Suppl. 1 Pt B: 332B
76. Feighner JP, Pambakian R, Fowler RC, et al. A comparison of nefazodone, imipramine and placebo in patients with moderate to severe depression. Psychopharmacol Bull 1989; 25: 219-21
77. Dassylva B, Fontaine R, Gammans D, et al. Efficacy of nefazodone in patients suffering from major depressive disorder and panic disorder [abstract]. Biol Psychiatry 1992; 31: 169A
78. Rickels K, Schweitzer E, Clary C, et al. Nefazodone and imipramine in major depression: a placebo-controlled trial. Br J Psychiatry 1994; 164: 802-5
79. Fontaine R, Ontiveros A, Elle R, et al. A double-blind comparison of nefazodone, imipramine, and placebo in major depression. J Clin Psychiatry 1994; 55: 234-41
80. Anton SF, Robinson DS, Roberts DL, et al. Long-term treatment of depression with nefazodone. Psychopharmacol Bull 1994, 30: 165-9
81. Serzone®. Product information. Bristol-Myers Squibb, Princeton, New Jersey, USA, 1995
82. Peroutka SJ, Sleight AJ, McCarthy BG, et al. The clinical utility of pharmacological agents that act at serotonin receptors. J Neuropsychiatry 1989; 1: 253-62
83. Bressa GM. S-adenosyl-l-methionine (SAMe) as antidepressant: a meta-analysis of clinical studies. Acta Neurol Scand 1994; Suppl. 154: 7-14
84. Cimino M, Vantini G, Algeri S, et al. Age-related modification of dopaminergic and beta-adrenergic receptor system: restoration to normal activity by modifying membrane fluidity with S-adenosylmethionine. Life Sci 1984; 34: 2029-39

Correspondence: Prof. Dr *H.J. Möller*, Psychiatric Department, Ludwigs-Maximilians-Universität München, Nussbaumstrasse 7, D-80336 Munich, Germany.

Suboptimal Use of Antidepressants in the Treatment of Depression

John Donoghue[1] and *David M. Taylor*[2]

1 PCS Health, Liverpool, England

2 South London & Maudsley NHS Trust, Denmark Hill, London, England

Effective treatments for depression have been available for over 40 years. However, reports of the suboptimal use of antidepressant agents have been a feature of the literature on depression for the past quarter century.[1] Depression is a major healthcare problem with a high incidence and prevalence,[2] a recurrent and chronic natural history,[3] high burdens of morbidity, poor quality of life and impaired functioning,[4,5] a suicide rate of 12 to 25%[2] and disproportionately high costs in both health and social care sectors.[6,7] Despite the enormous public health impact and well established treatability of depression,[8] consensus on treatment is still lacking.[1] The health gains which might be expected to accrue from the widespread availability of treatments with well recognised efficacy do not appear to have been realised in practice.[8]

This review describes the attempts that have been made to develop a consensus on how to achieve effective treatment with antidepressants, and the reports of and the outcomes associated with suboptimal antidepressant use.

1. Consensus and Treatment Guidelines

As the number of available antidepressants has grown so has the range of pharmacological activities, adverse effects and, perhaps to a lesser extent, therapeutic benefits. This, along with increasing demand for treatment to be 'evidence-based', has led to the production of treatment guidelines or protocols which are intended to promote optimal management of depression. Some of the more important guidelines for drug treatment in depression are summarised in table I.

Among these guidelines, all published in the last 10 years, there is broad agreement in most areas. For example, a majority of organisations did not clearly specify a first-line drug, but recommended careful selection based on patient characteristics. The UK Department of Health[14] was alone in clearly recommending that selective serotonin (5-hydroxytryptamine; 5-HT) reuptake inhibitors (SSRIs) should be considered second-line agents. More recently in Texas, USA,[17] SSRIs were preferred as first-line drugs with tricyclic antidepressants (TCAs) relegated essentially to third-line agents.

The evidence base for these recommendations is somewhat contradictory. Initially, SSRIs were largely accepted as being as effective as TCAs and related drugs,[18,19] but were not considered to be better tolerated, at least in terms of withdrawals from clinical trials.[18] Other analyses have strongly suggested that SSRIs are better tolerated than the older tricyclic

Table I. Summary of guidelines for the drug treatment of depression

Year	Organisation	Drugs recommended	Dose recommendations	Duration of treatment	Comments	Reference
1989	World Health Organization	None: advice to practitioners to become familiar with 2 or 3 compounds	None: advice to increase dose or change drug if no response after 3wk	6mo after recovery, then slow discontinuation	'Long term' therapy suggested for prophylaxis of recurrent episodes. Antidepressants or lithium recommended	9
1992	Royal College of Psychiatrists and Royal College of General Practitioners (UK)	None: 'newer compounds' suggested for patients at risk of suicide or when adverse effects are likely to be problematic	TCAs 125-150 mg/day. Vague statement about the effectiveness of 75 mg/day doses of TCAs	4-6mo after 'initial treatment phase' at treatment doses	'Long term prophylaxis' suggested for patients with recurrent episodes. Other, nondrug treatments are also recommended and discussed	10
1993	British Association for Psychopharmacology (UK)	None: indirect suggestions that 'newer antidepressants' should be used, especially where there is suicide risk or where poor tolerability is likely to affect compliance	'Full therapeutic doses'	4mo following apparent response, at 'full antidepressant dose'	Patients with 2 or more episodes in 5y should receive full treatment doses for 3y or more	11
1993	The Scottish Office, National Health Service (Scotland)	TCAs and SSRIs first choice (long discussion of which might be preferred), MAOIs second-line	TCAs – 150 mg/day	'About 6 months'. Doses not stated	Recommendations not clearly stated	12
1993	Agency for Healthcare Policy Research (For US Department of Health)	None: medication chosen individually according to various factors. All available medications scrutinised in great detail	Individual drug doses given. Most TCAs 75-300 mg/day. Plasma concentration monitoring recommended for some drugs	Full acute dose for 4-9mo. Augmentation strategies suggested when full response not achieved	Nondrug measures widely discussed. Maintenance treatment recommended for recurrent episodes	13
1993	Department of Health (UK)	SSRIs second-line. TCAs and related drugs tacitly recommended as first-line agents	Indirectly suggests that lower doses of TCAs may be effective, e.g. amitriptyline 75 mg/day	Not stated	Few clear recommendations given. Data examined exhaustively	14
1995	National Health Service (UK)	TCAs and related drugs or SSRIs according to patient characteristics. Moclobemide second-line	TCAs 'not less than 125 mg/day'	At least 4-6mo after initial response	Decisions on long term prophylaxis made jointly by patient and doctor	15
1996	American Psychiatric Association (US)	Wide range of drugs listed (TCAs and related drugs, SSRIs, MAOIs, lithium, etc.) but none specifically recommended. Clear treatment guidelines given for specific types of depression and for various comorbidities	TCAs generally above 100 mg/day; up to 300 mg/day	At least 4-5mo after full remission of symptoms (at full therapeutic dose)	Nondrug measures also covered by guidelines. Long term prophylaxis (perhaps indefinitely) recommended for recurrent episodes	16
1999	Texas Medication Algorithm Project (US)	First-line: SSRIs Second-line: amfebutamone (bupropion), nefazodone, venlafaxine Third-line: TCAs Fourth-line: MAOIs	TCAs generally 150-300 mg/day. Plasma concentration monitoring recommended for some drugs	Continue at full therapeutic doses for 6-9mo	Maintenance treatment for ≥1y suggested for patients with 2 or 3 prior episodes	17

MAOIs = monoamine oxidase inhibitors; **SSRIs** = selective serotonin (5-hydroxytryptamine; 5-HT) reuptake inhibitors; **TCAs** = tricyclic antidepressants.

compounds.[20,21] Clinically, experience firmly supports the relatively superior tolerability of SSRIs and other newer antidepressants, but doubts remain over the ability of some new antidepressants to match the well known efficacy of older TCAs.

Antidepressant dose recommendations are, of course, of vital importance in depression because of the perceived hazard of using subtherapeutic doses, particularly of TCAs and related drugs (therapeutic doses of other drugs are better defined and readily achieved). It is generally accepted that doses of the TCAs amitriptyline or imipramine should equal or exceed 125 mg/day before any true antidepressant effect is seen.[10,22] Lower doses of these drugs are held to be subtherapeutic. One placebo-controlled study in primary care patients with depression found that the median effective dose of amitriptyline was 125 mg/day with a mean effective dose of 119 mg/day.[23] Another well conducted study found that a daily dose of dothiepin (dosulepin) 75mg was no better than placebo in treating depression in general practice patients.[24] However, at least one other trial has shown low doses to be effective,[25] albeit in patients with mild depression and anxiety. More recently a large meta-analysis strongly indicated that the 'therapeutic dose' of antidepressants is 100 mg/day or more of imipramine or its equivalent.[26] In the US, although the wider use of plasma concentration monitoring renders somewhat redundant the argument surrounding effective doses of TCAs, still, as in other countries, debate continues.

This uncertainty is reflected in doses recommended in official guidelines. Four organisations clearly recommended TCA doses of 125 mg/day or greater.[10,12,15,17] Paykel and Priest,[10] on behalf of two major organisations, noted that doses of TCAs of 125 to 150 mg/day 'are effective' but were less certain about lower doses: 'there is no evidence that doses of 75mg daily or lower are effective, although individual patients may respond to and remain well on such doses and relapse on withdrawal'. In addition, the British Association for Psychopharmacology[11] recommended 'full therapeutic doses' but did not indicate what these might be, and the US Department of Health and Human Services[13] recommended plasma concentration monitoring, but also indicated that therapeutic doses of many TCAs begin at 75 mg/day. Overall, however, there is general, if not total, agreement between organisations that doses of TCAs of 125 mg/day or more are required for clear therapeutic benefit. Moreover, there seems to be more water-tight consensus on the therapeutic doses of newer drugs, with the possible exception of sertraline, for which a range of minimum effective doses (50 to 100 mg/day) is sometimes cited.[16,17]

The recommended duration of treatment with antidepressants ranges from 16 weeks to 9 months after the patient responds to treatment. All organisations providing dose recommendations suggested that treatment over this period should consist of full treatment doses. It is well accepted that relapse is common if pharmacotherapy is withdrawn within 4 months of remission[10,27] and this knowledge clearly forms the basis for the guidelines presented here.

Recommendations on longer term prophylaxis in recurrent depression are less consistent. Most organisations recommend maintenance treatment but the duration of this treatment is poorly defined. This at least partly reflects the paucity of data in this area, although there is some agreement that treatment should be lifelong in patients experiencing 2 to 3 episodes within 5 years.[11,17] The longest study[28] showed that the use of antidepressants (mainly older TCAs) with or without concurrent lithium significantly reduced recurrence of depression over 2 to 5 years. In another study, where the majority of patients were taking an SSRI,[29] continuation of treatment for 2 years significantly reduced recurrence. In this study, the report authored by the Depression Guideline Panel of the Agency for Healthcare Policy and Research[13] was used to guide therapy.

Any straightforward, unequivocal summary of the published guidelines and research data regarding the drug treatment of depression is likely to be subject to censure and debate. Nevertheless, these data and clinical experience strongly suggest that depressed patients should be treated with effective doses of antidepressants (at least 125 mg/day of TCAs) and that this treatment should be continued for at least 4 months after remission. For patients with recurrent depression, maintenance therapy with the full, effective dose of the antidepressant should be instituted. The duration of maintenance therapy is not clearly defined by published research and should be determined on an individual basis.

2. Reports of Suboptimal Use of Antidepressants

Reports of suboptimal use of antidepressants in both primary care and specialist settings have appeared with some regularity in the literature for the past 25 years, covering virtually all aspects of antidepressant use. They include reports of initiation of treatment being inappropriately delayed, treatment being discontinued prematurely and the widespread prescribing of antidepressants in doses which are not considered to be effective for the treatment of major depression.

In 1973 reports of suboptimal antidepressant use in the UK and the US were published.[30,31] In the UK, five primary care medical practices entered patients newly diagnosed with depression (n = 73) into a study which investigated the course of antidepressant treatment. Of patients entering the study, 20% received doses considered to be subtherapeutic. However, what was striking was the rapidity with which patients withdrew from treatment: 41% had stopped their medication within 2 weeks and by 4 weeks this increased to 68% of patients, with the general practitioner (GP) rarely aware that their patient had stopped treatment.[30] In the US, Kotin et al.[31] reported that only 16% of depressed patients admitted to hospital for treatment of depression had received at least 150 mg/day of imipramine or its equivalent before admission. Over half had received no treatment at all.

One year later, the UK study was extended to include chronically depressed general practice attenders and depressed patients (n = 361) referred to psychiatric outpatient clinics. It was found that new patients were more likely to be prescribed a TCA, and only 25% of patients who received a TCA received a dose above 75 mg/day. Only 21 of 73 GPs taking part in the study said they would use a TCA at 100 mg/day or above, the main reason given was the presence of intolerable adverse effects at these doses.[32]

In 1981 Johnson[33] reported the results of a study of antidepressant treatment of 119 patients with depression seen in general practice. Only 25% of all patients received a dose of a TCA above 75 mg/day, with 32% receiving 75 mg/day and 55% receiving less than 75 mg/day. Moreover, 20% of the patients received a TCA at a dose below 30 mg/day. In the patients who remained depressed, the proportion receiving treatment with an antidepressant decreased over time, and in patients who continued with treatment, the dose was not increased despite the lack of response to the subtherapeutic antidepressant dose.

The following year, a large (n = 1000), prospective naturalistic multicentre (in five US cities) study of the psychobiology of depression, developed by the National Institute for Mental Health (NIMH) in the US, found that 66% of patients with major depression had received no antidepressant treatment before entry into the study. Of those who had received treatment, only 3% had received an adequate dose for 4 weeks. Clinical, diagnostic and socio-demographic factors were found not to have had a significant influence on these patterns of treatment.[34] Similar findings were made 1 year later, when data from a large study by Jick et al.[35] became available. In a population of nearly 7000 patients prescribed an antidepressant, 77% of those prescribed a TCA were prescribed less than 100 mg/day, 21% 100 to 150mg/day and 2% 150 mg/day or higher.

Another small study in primary care patients with depression in the UK[36] supported Johnson's findings of 1981.[33] Patients who were compliant with low dose antidepressant treatment were likely to continue to receive the same treatment via a repeat prescription without seeing the doctor, and without an adequate review of their response to treatment. As many as 44% of all prescriptions for psychotropic medicines were prescribed in this manner.[36]

Further reports of similar findings of suboptimal antidepressant use are found in more small studies in the late 1980s.[37,38] Keller et al.[38] reported further on the outcomes of the NIMH study.[34] Depressed patients who entered the study were assessed for the intensity of the treatment they received. Of 250 participants who entered as inpatients, 31% received no antidepressant, a low dose or an inadequate trial (e.g. of too short a duration) of therapy. Of 88 patients who entered the study for outpatient care, 53% had received no antidepressant, a low dose or an inadequate trial of therapy.[38] These patterns could not be related to differences in patient characteristics, and the authors were unable to explain satisfactorily why these patients had received such a low intensity of treatment. Moreover, they found that such low intensity treatment persisted even in those patients who were the most severely ill, and who remained in treatment for the full 8 weeks of the study.[38]

Table II. Antidepressant doses found in population-based studies

Drug	Mean dose (mg/day)			
	Rosholm et al.[44]	Munizza et al.[45]	Bingefors et al.[46]	Donoghue et al.[47]
Amitriptyline	67	50	61	59
Clomipramine	64	56	70	59
Imipramine	67	60		
Dothiepin		78		77

The growing awareness and disquiet about the inadequate use of antidepressants led to the publication in 1989 of an influential review of antidepressant prescribing in the primary care setting.[39] On the basis of several small studies, Thompson and Thompson[39] stated that ‘the majority of general practitioners prescribe antidepressants in subtherapeutic doses’.

By the early 1990s, little had changed. McCombs et al.[40] published the results of a random retrospective database analysis of antidepressant use in the California Medicaid Program. Data for nearly 7000 new patient episodes were identified, but of these 45% were excluded because a minimum daily antidepressant dose expected to effectively treat depression was not achieved. Only 3.5% of the remainder of new patient episodes displayed antidepressent use patterns clearly consistent with successful treatment of major depression and 12.6% of the remainder showed clear indications of treatment failure. In the remaining 84% of new patient episodes, patients received subtherapeutic doses of antidepressants, were noncompliant with treatment, discontinued treatment prematurely or had other medicines co-prescribed which were indicative of treatment of problems other than major depression. The authors concluded that at best, only 20 to 25% of patients with major depressive disorder achieved a minimum therapeutic dose (defined as at least the equivalent of 75 mg/day of imipramine) for a minimum period of 6 months.[40]

In 1992 Katon et al.[41] reported findings from a study in which nearly 800 patients who were high users of primary care services were screened for depression, anxiety and depressive somatisation. Only 11% of patients requiring an antidepressant had received an adequate dose and duration of therapy. An intervention in which study physicians received advice on appropriate treatment from a psychiatrist increased the proportion of patients treated with an antidepressant, but did not significantly improve the adequacy of treatment.[41]

The following year, findings of a survey of pharmacy records of 1030 patients in a large Health Maintenance Organisation who were treated by primary care physicians and of 769 patients who were treated by psychiatrists were reported.[42] Patients treated by psychiatrists were significantly more likely to receive an effective dose of an antidepressant and to continue treatment for more than 30 days. Primary care physicians were more likely to use older TCAs than psychiatrists. Overall, less than 50% of patients received a dose of antidepressant considered to be adequate. Middle-aged patients were most likely to receive an adequate dose of antidepressant.[42]

In the same year (1993), the first of several large patient record database studies was published by Rosholm et al.[43] This study examined a population of about 460 000 in Denmark (table II). The analysis included 14 725 prescriptions of antidepressants issued to 3360 patients (1.6% of the population). Of those patients prescribed an antidepressant, 75% received a TCA. In primary care, both the average doses and the most commonly prescribed doses of antidepressants were below those doses known to be effective in the treatment of depression (table II).[43]

The growing awareness of this problem prompted a number of surveys to investigate the rationale (if any) behind these findings. In a survey of GPs in Scotland,[48] 231 of 318 survey questionnaires were completed. When ranked in order of prescribing preference, six of the top seven antidepressants were TCAs. Less than 25% of respondents expressed a willingness to increase antidepressant doses up to the maximum specified in the British National Formulary. Moreover, 26% admitted that they were not able to make an informed choice when prescribing an antidepressant and 14% prescribed the same drug for every patient with no attempt to select an antidepressant to meet individual patient needs. The authors concluded that primary care physicians were expected to diagnose and treat patients with depression yet had not received adequate training for this body of work.[48]

Another survey published the following year compared the responses of 123 GPs and 97 psychiatrists in South Wales.[49] The response rates were 60 and 67%, respectively. There were important differences between GPs and psychiatrists: 52% of GPs and 17% of psychiatrists would prescribe a lower than recommended dose of antidepressant, and 40% of GPs and 7% of psychiatrists would continue treatment for less than 4 months.

Taken together, these studies suggest that an important element in suboptimal use of antidepressants may be a lack of understanding on the part of primary care physicians of the importance of administration of adequate doses of and continuation of treatment with antidepressants, and that there may be gaps in the physicians' training which need to be addressed.

Further evidence of the pandemic of suboptimal use of antidepressants came from New Zealand in a study involving a review of case notes of patients referred to a community psychiatric unit and who had been prescribed an antidepressant prior to the referral.[50] 163 patients were included, of whom 55 met DSM-III[51] criteria for major depression. Overall, 87% of patients who were prescribed an antidepressant received a TCA; 44% of those who received a TCA were prescribed a dose below 50 mg/day and 34% a dose of 50 to 100 mg/day.[50]

In the same year the first of the large database studies of antidepressant use in the UK was published.[52] Data for prescription of antidepressants in a population in excess of 1 million were obtained from the individual Health Authorities. More than 70 000 such prescriptions were issued over a period of 3 months by approximately 500 primary care physicians. The TCAs amitriptyline, clomipramine and dothiepin accounted for 61% of all prescriptions of antidepressants; less than 14% of prescriptions of these TCAs reached a dose considered to be effective by the UK Consensus Guidelines.[10] Prescriptions for the atypical TCA lofepramine and the SSRIs reached an effective dose in 61 and 98% of cases, respectively. This was the first study to make a direct comparison between TCAs and SSRIs in this way, although it was not possible in this study to relate the prescriptions to a diagnosis of depression.[52]

Also in 1994, in the US, data on medication use in a sample of 634 depressed patients from the Medical Outcomes Study were gathered using structured interviews.[53] Only 23% of patients interviewed had recently been prescribed an antidepressant; 30% had been prescribed a benzodiazepine. The dose was 'inappropriately low' in 39% of those patients who had recently been prescribed an antidepressant.[53]

In 1995, Rosholm and colleagues[44] presented findings from a study in which a random sample of antidepressant users from 12 primary care practices in Denmark was selected. Several parameters were investigated, including the indication for prescription of the antidepressant, the dose and duration of treatment with the antidepressant and the severity of depressive illness. Of the 98 patients randomised, 72 had been prescribed the antidepressant for the treatment of depression. Treatment tended to be long term, but doses were generally low, and moderate to severe major depression persisted in many patients.

Interest in the phenomenon of prescription of low doses of antidepressants continued to grow. Also in 1995, the results of a census study in the Piedmont region of Italy (population of approximately 4.3 million people) were published.[45] Data on 3396 patients attending 66 of a total of 75 psychiatric outpatient clinics were obtained. Of these, 678 patients were prescribed an antidepressant. Average doses were low and similar to doses identified in other large studies. However, newer antidepressants were prescribed within effective dose ranges (table II). This study also found that female patients received lower doses of antidepressants than males.

Studies of antidepressant use have concentrated mainly on the issue of adequacy of dose. However, a different study from Italy investigated the duration of treatment with antidepressants.[54] Antidepressant use in a randomly selected sample of 8743 National Health Service patients in Rome was investigated over a period of 30 months. Of these patients, 473 (5.4%) received at least one prescription for an antidepressant, with more than half (54%) having a duration of treatment of 1 month or less. The mean duration of treatment was 38 days with amitriptyline and 37 days with fluoxetine.[54]

In 1996, three large studies of antidepressant use in the UK were published. Two of these studies[47,55] used a large national primary care medical record database with access to over 750 000 patient records. The third[56] used a record-linkage database of a population of about 400 000 in Scotland.

The first of these studies[55] brought together the findings of what were, in effect, three separate but related investigations. One of these investigations examined a National Health Service database of prescriptions of antidepressants given to patients from a population of about 1 million; individual prescriptions of antidepressants could not be linked to a diagnosis of depression. Part of this investigation had been reported previously.[52] The great majority of the prescriptions for TCAs were at subtherapeutic doses. These findings were compared with those from a national primary care medical record database of about 750 000 patient records from which a diagnosis of depression could be identified. Again, older TCAs were prescribed at low doses. SSRIs were almost always prescribed at effective doses. Finally, medical records in primary care were reviewed to determine whether or not the above findings held true for individual patients and if there was any evidence that TCAs were prescribed at low doses because patients were having doses titrated to effective levels. A similar pattern of low dose prescription of TCAs was observed in this final investigation, and there was no evidence that dose titration could provide an explanation for the widespread use of low doses of TCAs.[55]

Using the same data source, the second study (table II)[47] investigated whether these antidepressant prescribing patterns were changing over time by comparing data from 1993 with that from 1995 The analysis of over 100 000 prescriptions for antidepressants revealed little, if any, change over time in either the doses prescribed or the percentage of TCA-treated patients receiving effective doses (fig. 1).[47] In 1993, average daily doses for the older TCAs amitriptyline, clomipramine and dothiepin were, respectively, 55, 64 and 76mg, compared with 59, 59 and 77mg in 1995.[47]

The third major UK study[56] was published in 1996 and linked patient records between primary and secondary care in a large population in Scotland. It investigated both the use and safety of antidepressants and found that over a 14-month period, 85 315 prescriptions had been issued to 20 195 patients, the majority of whom (14 988) received a prescription for a TCA. At least 72% of those prescribed a TCA received only a subtherapeutic dose. Antidepressants were prescribed for only a short period of time: 38% of patients received 30 days or less and 68% received less than 90 days of treatment.[56]

1996 also saw the publication of the findings on antidepressant use in general practice from a large (n = 25 916 consecutive primary care attenders) World Health Organization epidemiological study in

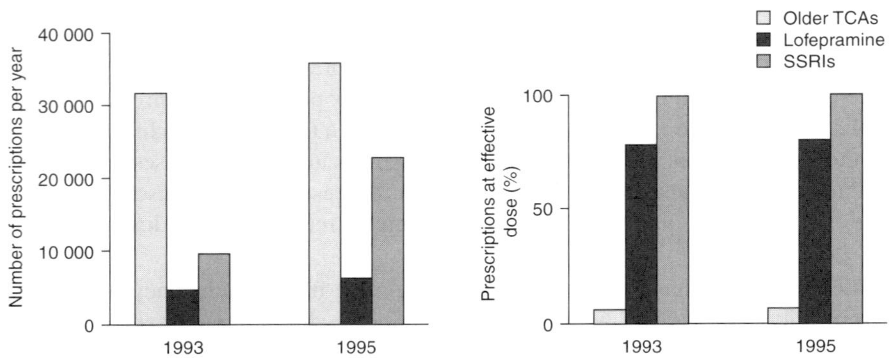

Fig. 1. Antidepressant prescribing patterns in the UK in 1993 and 1995.[47]
SSRIs = selective serotonin (5-hydroxytryptamine; 5-HT) reuptake inhibitors; **TCAs** = tricyclic antidepressants.

15 countries.[2] Consecutive primary care attenders were subjected to a mental health evaluation. 10.4% of these attenders were found to be experiencing a depressive episode, although only approximately 25% of these 10.4% had been given a diagnosis of depression by their primary care physician. Overall, only 13% of patients who met International Classification of Diseases (ICD)-10[57] criteria for a depressive episode had been prescribed an antidepressant. Factors influencing the prescription of an antidepressant were the presence of psychological symptoms (this increased the likelihood of prescription of an antidepressant by 4.7-fold), the presence of physical illness (this decreased the likelihood of prescription of an antidepressant by 2-fold) and age (younger patients were less likely to be prescribed an antidepressant than older patients).[2]

Similar findings have come from smaller studies in France, Sweden, the Netherlands and Finland. A study by Rouillon et al.[58] in France found that only 26% of patients who were treated with a TCA in primary care were prescribed an effective dose compared with 100% of those who were treated with an SSRI. In Sweden, Bingefors et al.[46] found that the average dose of amitriptyline was 47.6 mg/day at initiation of therapy and increased to 61 mg/day if treatment continued; the average doses of clomipramine were 49.6 and 69.6 mg/day at these 2 time-points, respectively (table II). A retrospective longitudinal study of antidepressant use in 2554 patients in the Netherlands found that the mean dose of amitriptyline (the only TCA investigated) was 50mg/day, and that the majority of patients received less than 4 months of therapy.[59] In Finland, a small study found that 71% of prescriptions for TCAs were for doses below 75mg/day.[60]

The possibility that appropriate use of low doses of TCAs in elderly patients could account for the phenomenon of widespread low dose prescribing of these drugs was investigated in a large database study in the UK.[61] In a population of approximately 750 000 primary care patients, the choice and adequacy of dose was compared in patients under or over the age of 65 years. Over 58 000 prescriptions for antidepressants in patients with a diagnosis of depression were included in the analysis. The older patients were more likely than the younger ones to be prescribed a TCA, and were more likely to be prescribed an adequate dose (defined for a TCA as ≥75 mg/day in older patients and ≥125 mg/day in younger patients, as per the UK consensus guidelines[10]). However, 65% of elderly patients failed to receive an effective dose. Therefore, the appropriate use of lower doses in elderly patients could not be considered to account for extensive low dose prescribing of TCAs.[61]

The most recent study to address this problem employed a different method. A logistic regression analysis of longitudinal antidepressant use in patients initiating treatment for a new episode of depression was performed. This analysis compared outcomes in patients who were initiating treatment with TCAs with those who were initiating treatment with an SSRI.[62] Over 10 000 patients started treatment with a TCA but only 6% of them completed 4 months of continuous therapy at an adequate dose. Over 6000 patients initiated treatment with an SSRI and 33% of them completed 4 months of continuous therapy at an adequate dose. After controlling for potential confounding factors through the logistic regression analysis, patients who initiated therapy with an SSRI were much more likely (odds ratio = 7.473) than patients who initiated therapy with a TCA to have a prescribed average daily dose and duration of treatment which were consistent with recommended treatment guidelines. Doses were titrated upward to higher than the initial dose in only 9% of patients who were prescribed a TCA.[62]

Attention has also focused on the prescription of SSRIs. In a 5-year naturalistic study of SSRI use patterns in a population of about 800 000 primary care patients, there were over 93 000 prescriptions for SSRIs associated with a total of 27 210 treatment episodes.[63] Although patients invariably received effective doses and the average number of days of therapy prescribed ranged from 116 days in patients who received sertraline to 125 days in patients who received fluoxetine, the length of continuous treatment was inadequate for the majority of patients; only 31% of patients entered a fourth month of continuous therapy.[63]

More evidence comes from the pan-European survey of depression in the community (second phase), the Depression Research in European Society II (DEPRES II) Study.[64] In this study, 1884 depressed patients who had consulted a healthcare professional about their symptoms in the previous 6 months completed a detailed interview. Only 30% of patients with depression had received treatment with an antidepressant and 17% had received treatment with a benzodiazepine alone. Overall, 63% of 146 patients treated with a TCA received a dose of only 75 mg/day or below. This figure rose to over 80% in patients from Belgium or Germany.

3. Outcomes

Despite an increasing awareness of the prevalence of suboptimal use of antidepressants, there appear to have been relatively few studies which have investigated the outcomes of these patterns of drug use. Most of the studies which have taken place followed patients after admission to or discharge from a hospital setting and few were of naturalistic design in a primary care setting.

As early as 1981, Johnson[33] reported that in primary care in the UK, doses of antidepressants were not increased to effective levels even in patients who failed to respond to low dose treatment. In 1986, Keller and co-workers[65] reported on the course of illness in 101 patients whose illness had recurred following recovery from an index episode of depression. They found a high risk of recurrence and that a longer duration of an episode before effective treatment was implemented predicted significantly greater risk of developing chronic depressive illness, as did a longer duration of a previous episode of depression.[65]

In 1988, several studies and reviews of outcomes of treatment of depression were published. Kiloh et al.[66] reported the findings of a long term study in which patients had been followed for 15 years after an index hospital admission for depression. This study provided an important insight into outcomes. The authors concluded that 'the prognosis of depressive illness in general may be more serious than is generally realised'. Only 20% of patients remained continuously well, 63% recovered from the index episode but experienced further episodes and 17% were continuously incapacitated or committed suicide. However, no conclusions were reached about adequacy of treatment in any of these groups.[66]

In the same year, Goethe et al.[67] noted that despite difficulties in comparing different methods, studies consistently demonstrated higher rates of response in patients receiving 'adequate' treatment. These authors compared the outcomes of two doses of imipramine in a retrospective case study of patients meeting DSM-III[51] criteria for nonbipolar major affective disorder. The intensity of treatment was broadly defined as being 'probably inadequate' (36% of patients), 'possibly adequate' (19% of patients) and 'probably adequate' (45% of patients). Only 29% of patients in the 'probably inadequate' group had a good outcome, similar to response rates achieved with placebo in clinical trials, and 58% of these patients had a poor outcome. These figures were reversed in the 'probably adequate' treatment group, with a good outcome in 54% and a poor outcome in 25% of patients. The authors concluded that their findings were consistent with the results of other studies, they had identified important differences in outcome between adequately and inadequately treated patients, and they supported the observations that many patients with major depression failed to receive effective therapy with an antidepressant.[67]

In a review of chronic depression, Scott (1988)[68] described adequacy and appropriateness of treatment as key factors predicting the development of chronic depression, citing several studies which demonstrated that patients who had developed chronic depression had received suboptimal or no treatment. Scott drew on evidence suggesting a correlation between the time between the onset of depressive illness and the introduction of adequate treatment, and the likelihood that the depression will respond to treatment. The review also indicated that inadequate treatment or absence of treatment in the early stages of the illness may be associated with the development of chronic depression. Scott indicated that inadequate treatment is a preventable cause of poor outcomes.[68]

The results of an intervention study on the Swedish island of Gotland were also published in 1989.[69] The intervention involved an intensive educational programme about depression and its treatment and was aimed at primary care practitioners. It resulted in significant changes in prescribing of psychotropic medicines with associated improvements in outcome measures in patients with depression. The frequency of prescribing of defined daily doses of antidepressants increased, while that of benzodiazepines and antipsychotic agents fell. The frequency and duration of sickness absence certificates issued in primary care for depression decreased, as did the number of days spent in hospital by patients with depression and the number of suicides (this was the reverse of a national trend). Although data were not presented specifically on dose and duration of treatment, this study provided encouraging evidence that 'increasing the competence and stringency in treating and preventing depressive disorders' could have a direct impact on improving outcomes in primary care settings.[69]

By 1989, the issue of the use of low doses of antidepressants to treat depression was receiving increasing attention. One group suggested that low dose treatment may be perpetuated if such treatment achieved a partial response: the patient may come to accept this somewhat improved functioning as a new norm and so not expect or seek further improvement.[70]

Thompson and Thompson[39] provided a wide-ranging review of the suboptimal use of antidepressants in primary care. They hypothesised that depressed patients treated in primary care were different from patients seen in clinical trials, and were more likely to respond to lower doses of antidepressant. They were unable to find studies to support this hypothesis, and presented data suggesting that in primary care, as in clinical trials, full doses of antidepressants were required to produce a therapeutic effect.

In 1990, Frank et al.[71] reported the 3-year outcomes of maintenance therapy in 128 patients with recurrent depression. Patients who had had an acute episode of major depression which responded to imipramine received continuation therapy on full dose imipramine (patients received imipramine in flexible doses, with a mean dose of greater than 200 mg/day). Survival on this dose was compared with an earlier study by Prien et al.[72] in which imipramine responders were maintained on a lower dose of imipramine

(75 to 150mg daily). Frank et al.[71] concluded that treatment with full dose imipramine 'provided protection against recurrence of illness over a longer period of time than in any previous study of maintenance therapy of recurrent depression'. This *post hoc* comparison can be criticised because the earlier study[72] was multicentre, and the patients in the study by Frank et al.[71] received at least 7 months of interpersonal psychotherapy. However, Thase[73] showed that the difference in survival rates between the two studies[71,72] was probably due to the difference between the maintenance doses of imipramine.

In 1991, Scott and Eccleston[74] applied multiple linear regression analysis to investigate factors influencing the development of chronic depression (n = 100). They found that the most important factor predicting the duration of depressive illness was the time between the onset of symptoms and the introduction of treatment – a similar finding to that of Keller et al.[65]

The study by McCombs et al.,[40] which found that only 3.5% of patients in a large sample had antidepressant use patterns consistent with effective treatment, and that at least 12.6% of cases were definite treatment failures, also found that treatment failure resulted in an increased cost of $US1000 (1990 value) per patient in the year following the episode. The authors concluded that 'While the data and methodology used to classify patients are imprecise, the magnitude of the population receiving subtherapeutic doses or abbreviated courses of antidepressants cannot be ignored'.[40]

There was a weak trend toward poorer outcomes in patients who received low doses (≤100 mg/day) of a TCA compared with higher doses of a TCA (≥100 mg/day) or clinical management without an antidepressant in another study.[75] In a series of 130 consecutive patients with new episodes of depression, outcomes were assessed 4 months after initiation of treatment with an antidepressant. This finding was similar to that in a placebo-controlled trial in patients in primary care,[24] in which placebo tended to be superior to dothiepin 75 mg/day, although the difference between placebo and dothiepin 75 mg/day was not significant. Brugha and colleagues[75] pointed out that their study should not be taken as evidence that antidepressants lacked efficacy, but that 'in clinical practice, their advantages may fail to be realised, at least in the longer term'. These authors suggested that their findings were a consequence of the failure to prescribe adequate doses of antidepressant.

In the same year, a meta-analysis of 10 studies[76] of the effect of antidepressant treatment on the ability of depressed patients to work found that the percentage of 827 patients who returned to work reached a maximum after 4 to 6 months of treatment. Work outcomes were correlated with duration of treatment and were not related to improvements in symptom response, suggesting that premature discontinuation of treatment might prolong functional impairment.[76]

The 4-arm study (n = 239) by Shea et al.[77] looked at short and medium term outcomes at 6, 12 and 18 months in patients with depression. In two of the arms patients were treated with psychotherapy alone, in one arm (n = 57) with impramine plus clinical management and in the final arm (n = 62) with placebo plus clinical management. After a 4-month period of treatment with an antidepressant the patients had a high rate of relapse (50%) suggesting that even a 4-month period of treatment was insufficient to both achieve and maintain recovery.[77]

A study of long term outcomes in 72 patients with recurrent depression found that the period of highest risk for re-emergence of depressive symptoms was in the months immediately following recovery, and that continuation of antidepressant treatment significantly reduced this risk.[28] The monthly rate of depressive episodes was 4% in patients who continued treatment after recovery and 9% in those who did not, emphasising the importance of continuing with treatment after recovery. Regression analysis found that the risk of recurrence 2 and 3 years after recovery from a depressive episode was influenced only by the number of previous episodes of depression with a higher risk in patients with more previous episodes.[28] A number of other variables had been included in the analysis: gender, age, education, marital status, age of onset of illness, family history of major affective disorders, in- or outpatient status during the index episode, duration of the index episode, score on the Hamilton Depression Rating Scale at the height of the index episode, Research Diagnostic Criteria subtype of the index episode, pressure or absence of an underlying chronic and intermittent minor depressive disorder or cyclothymic personality, and the response on dexamethasone suppression test at entry.

In 1993, Frank et al.[78] prospectively compared full dose (150 to 300 mg/day) with half dose (75 to 150 mg/day) imipramine in a double-blind study of maintenance treatment of 20 patients with recurrent depression.[78] After resolution of an acute episode, patients were randomised to continue with full or half dose maintenance treatment with imipramine for 3 years. Survival analysis suggested a superior effect with full dose treatment, with a mean survival time (depression-free period) of 135 weeks compared with 75 weeks for half dose therapy.[78]

A 1994 study investigated antidepressant use in Swedish people who had committed suicide.[79] The study involved a total of 3400 cases of suicide (85% of the total suicides) in Sweden in the years 1990 to 1991. Only 16% of these people had detectable concentrations of an antidepressant in their blood post-mortem, although about 50% were depressed (based on findings from earlier studies). This study concluded that treatment failure was a more important factor in suicide than the toxicity of an overdose of antidepressants and suboptimal treatment is a possible reason why the availability of antidepressants had failed to reduce suicide rates.[79]

The question of why the availability of effective treatments for depression had failed to produce the desired health gain was raised by Brugha.[8] This author notes that long term outcomes in depression were dismal even when the disease is treated by specialist services. Although they recognised patients as being depressed, psychiatrists tended to under-use effective treatments even in well-resourced centres. The question was put as to whether enough was yet known about how much under-treatment existed, and why it occurred. The author states "only when we know 'why' and 'how much' [under-treatment of depression exists] will it be possible to devise and reliably assess strategies to reduce under-treatment".[8]

However, other workers were less convinced of a universal need for adequate doses of antidepressant. In a small study of 88 depressed primary care patients starting treatment with an antidepressant, patients who received low intensity treatment had a significantly lower likelihood of an initial clinical response compared with patients who received a higher intensity treatment.[80] However, this difference was not sustained over time: by 4 months after initiation of treatment there were no differences between the low and high intensity treatment groups. A replication sample of 157 patients yielded similar results. The authors suggested that efforts to improve the intensity of treatment for depression should concentrate on patients whose initial response to treatment was poor. However, the study had several limitations including low statistical power, selection bias and the lack of long term follow-up data.[80]

A study that was less methodologically impaired compared standardised antidepressant therapy with treatment 'as usual' in primary care.[81] Primary care patients meeting DSM-III-R[82] criteria for major depression were randomised to receive nortriptyline (n = 91), interpersonal psychotherapy (n = 93) or treatment as usual (n = 92). Treatment outcomes were determined at 8 months. Patients who received nortriptyline or interpersonal therapy responded faster and better than those who received treatment as usual. Among treatment completers, approximately 70% of patients who received nortriptyline or interpersonal therapy were considered to have recovered at 8 months, compared with only 20% of those who received treatment as usual.[81]

A later report by the same group addressed the issue of whether achieving better outcomes with antidepressants or interpersonal therapy was cost effective. No cost offsets were found: improving outcomes consumed more healthcare resources resulting in an overall increase in health-related costs.[83]

In the UK, a study of outcomes in over 200 primary care patients taking long term antidepressants[84] (mean duration of treatment 3.4 years) found that only one-third of patients were prescribed a daily dose of antidepressant equivalent to 125mg of amitriptyline. Over 75% of patients had 'case-level depression' with 62% exhibiting moderate to severe symptoms. The rate of consultation of these patients with their primary care physician was twice as high as that of age- and gender-matched comparators. The author stated that 'the burden of depression on the general practitioner would reduce if patients were successfully treated and became symptom-free' and 'continued use of subtherapeutic doses (of antidepressants) is ineffective and cannot be justified'.[84]

Outcomes from the DEPRES II Study[64] included findings relating to the impairment of activities in depressed patients and patient reports of the results of antidepressant treatment. Depressed patients (n = 1884) who had consulted a healthcare professional about their symptoms in the previous 6 months had been unable to undertake normal activities for a mean period of 30 days, and those in employment had a mean of 20 days lost to depression during the previous 6 months. Significantly more of the patients reported that the antidepressant made them feel like their 'normal self' when they received an SSRI (n = 147 received this treatment) than when they received a TCA (n = 146).

4. Newer Antidepressants

Newer antidepressants such as venlafaxine, mirtazapine, nefazodone, reboxetine, amfebutamone (bupropion) milnacipran have not been included in this review. This is not a reflection on how these drugs are used in practice, but rather reflects the paucity of data in the literature concerning these drugs. Moreover, we are not aware of any data on the use of hypericum (extract of St John's Wort), which is widely used in Germany.

5. Comment

It appears that for many years there has been an awareness that the use of antidepressants to treat depression has not achieved the outcomes that controlled trials would lead one to expect. Both experimental and observational studies have suggested a link between adequacy of antidepressant treatment and outcomes, and many guidelines have been issued in attempts to improve the stringency of treatment and, hence, outcomes. However, the overwhelming tenor of the literature is that the treatment of depression is incongruous with the magnitude of the burden of this serious disorder. In particular, the literature indicates that antidepressants are used in ways that have not been show to confer any benefit, and which, indeed, may put patients at increased risk.

Reports of the suboptimal use of antidepressants have come mainly from primary care or outpatient treatment settings.[2,30,32,33,36,38-49,52-63] Fewer reports of antidepressant prescribing prior to admission to hospital or entry into formal studies are available.[31,34,38,43,50]

It is noteworthy that the suboptimal use of antidepressants is not confined within national boundaries or systems of healthcare: similar findings have been made within individual countries including Denmark,[43,44] Finland,[60] France,[58] Italy,[45,54] The Netherlands,[59] New Zealand,[50] Sweden,[46] the UK,[30,32,33,36,39,48,49,52,55,61-63] the US[31,34,38,40-42,53] and in international studies.[2,64] This suggests that inadequate use of antidepressants is independent of the system of healthcare in which treatment is delivered, international differences in physician training and therapeutic approaches and varying health beliefs and expectations.

Descriptions of the suboptimal use of antidepressants have included inappropriate delays in the initiation of treatment,[2,31,34,38] the use of inadequate antidepressant doses[30-36,38-43,46-50,52,54-62] and premature discontinuation of treatment.[30,33,38,40-42,62,63] The size of studies has ranged from small (less than 1000 prescriptions or patients)[30-34,36,38,39,41] to large (between 1000 and 10 000 prescriptions or patients)[35,40,42,45,54,59] to very large (greater than 10 000 prescriptions or patients).[2,43,47,52,55,56,61-63]

The conclusion seems inescapable: antidepressant use is suboptimal on an enormous scale irrespective of national boundaries. Wherever studies have been conducted, whether small or large scale, whether investigating initiation of treatment, doses prescribed or duration of treatment, the findings are similar. For patients to receive adequate antidepressant therapy – an effective dose for an adequate period of time – is clearly exceptional. This appears to be reflected in poor outcomes.[8,67,68,71,77,79,84]

However, despite the overwhelming weight of evidence, the findings that antidepressants are used suboptimally have been questioned.[22,39,85-87] The studies that have investigated antidepressant use have been mainly descriptive and observational and conducted in nonrandomised populations, and it is impossible to infer direct causal relationships between treatment patterns and outcomes from these studies.[88,89] Clinical trials have been criticised for not being representative of primary care populations. In addition, methodological shortcomings limit the generalisability of their findings.[90] There is thus little direct evidence that these patterns of antidepressant use result in poor outcomes.

However, in the face of the data that are available from clinical trials, the weight of clinical experience and opinion, the universal use of antidepressants in ways that have not been shown to be effective and the evidence of poor outcomes in depression, to insist that poor outcomes are not a result of suboptimal use of antidepressants seems untenable. Although it is not impossible that some patients may indeed have an acceptable response to low antidepressant doses, it seems highly unlikely that this would be the case for the vast majority of patients. We are not aware of any evidence that the suboptimal use of antidepressants confers any benefit. However, it imposes risks from adverse effects and toxicity[91-93] and all the consequences of inadequate treatment including failure to respond,[9-12,14-16] increased risk of relapse[10,11] and the development or perpetuation of recurrent or chronic depressive illness.[65,67,71,77,78,84] Suboptimal antidepressant use may also increase the risk of suicide.[69,79]

As stated earlier, Brugha[8] stated in 1995 that "only when we know 'why' and 'how much' will it be possible to devise and reliably assess strategies to reduce undertreatment". The 'how much' seems now to be well established. The weight of the evidence, confirmed by very large epidemiological studies, is that the vast majority of patients fail to receive effective doses of TCAs.[43,47,55,56,61,62] Even fewer patients receive an effective dose for an adequate period of time.[40,56,62] In terms of the numbers of patients receiving adequate doses there are clear differences between treatment with TCAs and that with SSRIs; virtually all SSRI-treated patients receive an adequate dose.[45-47,52,55,59,61,62] The only study to employ regression analysis to control for the effects of observable influences on treatment patterns found that patients initiating treatment with an SSRI were at least 7 times more likely to complete 4 months of continuous treatment at an effective antidepressant dose than patients who initiated treatment with a TCA.[62] When only older TCAs (amitriptyline, imipramine, dothiepin) were considered, patients initiating treatment with an SSRI were 17 times more likely to complete an episode of treatment.[62] However, this does not mean that there is any room for complacency in the prescribing of SSRIs: although SSRI-treated patients are much more likely to receive an effective dose, less than one-third complete 4 months of continuous therapy.[63] We are not able to make any comments regarding treatment with newer antidepressants because sufficient data are not yet available.

The question that remains unanswered is 'why?'. In the absence of evidence that outcomes for suboptimal antidepressant use are good, possible explanations include: patients cannot tolerate effective doses of TCAs for a long enough period of time,[39] physicians are not adequately aware of the principles of therapeutics in this area,[48] physician training is lacking, or that the health beliefs and expectations of patients may prevent them from receiving and continuing with effective treatment.[94] The remarkable consistency between studies of antidepressant treatment patterns suggests that most patients cannot tolerate treatment doses of TCAs for long enough for treatment to be effective and recovery sustained. Because depression is a relapsing and remitting illness, such outcomes may be hidden in the medium term. Yet long term outcomes are poor in patients with depression.[67,68] Although clinical trials clearly demonstrate the efficacy of antidepressants,[18,19] the availability of these drugs for over 40 years has had little, if any, impact on the prevalence of depressive illness.[8]

An important barrier to improving antidepressant use seems to be the continued use of TCAs in primary care. Although they have been available for 40 years and clinicians are familiar with them,[14] they do not appear to be used effectively. Although it might be said that education is the key to improving the use of these drugs, and indeed 1 study found that an educational programme could improve outcomes,[69] there is little evidence that the necessary educational programmes are being developed. Indeed, the scale of the initiative required suggests that such programmes are not likely to be developed. In the UK, educational initiatives which were part of the national Defeat Depression Campaign appear to have had little impact on the use of TCAs.[47]

An important factor underlying the continuing widespread use of TCAs is cost. These medicines are much lower in cost than newer antidepressants, and claims have been made that increasing the use of these drugs would increase healthcare costs.[14,18,95,96] But there is little evidence to support such assertions. Although it is difficult to apply the findings of cost-effectiveness studies across different systems of healthcare, studies to date have found that the use of SSRIs results in cost offsets, and that the use of SSRIs instead of TCAs is at worst cost neutral, and at best cost effective.[97-108] To perpetuate the use of TCAs because their acquisition cost is lower than that of newer antidepressants, particularly in developed countries, is untenable.

6. Recommendations

It seems almost patronising to make recommendations that appear to us to be so self-evident.

Clear guidance needs to be issued to physicians regarding the crucial importance of recognising depression and, once the disease is recognised, initiating effective treatment without delay.

Clear guidance also needs to be issued regarding the crucial importance of administering an effective antidepressant dose for an adequate period of time to depressed patients. The evidence suggests that this is not likely to be achieved if TCAs are prescribed. Although clinical trials are unable to find differences in efficacy between TCAs and SSRIs, pharmacoepidemiological studies clearly show the clinical advantage of SSRIs in practice.

Clear guidance needs to be issued regarding the importance of identifying patients with recurrent depression and maintaining these patients on long term treatment.

Population-based studies investigating the relationship between antidepressant treatment and outcomes should be a key priority in government research programmes.

References

1. Donoghue JM. Sub-optimal use of tricyclic antidepressants in primary care [editorial]. Acta Psychiatr Scand 1998; 98: 429-31
2. Weiller E, Lecrubier Y, Boyer P. Antidepressant use in general practice. Therapie 1996; 51: 429-30
3. Klerman GL, Weissman MM. The course, morbidity, and costs of depression. Arch Gen Psychiatry 1992; 49: 831-4
4. Wells KB, Stewart A, Hays RD, et al. The functioning and well-being of depressed patients: results from the medical outcomes study. JAMA 1989; 262: 914-9
5. Hays RD, Wells KB, Sherbourne CD, et al. Functioning and well-being outcomes of patients with depression compared with chronic general medical illnesses. Arch Gen Psychiatry 1995; 52: 11-9
6. Simon GE, VonKorff M, Barlow W. Health care costs of primary care patients with recognised depression. Arch Gen Psychiatry 1995; 52: 850-6

7. Kind P, Sorensen J. The costs of depression. Int Clin Psychopharmacology 1993; 7: 191-5
8. Brugha TS. Depression undertreatment: lost cohorts, lost opportunities? Psycholog Med 1995; 25: 3-6
9. Pharmacotherapy of depressive disorders: a consensus statement. WHO Mental Health Collaborating Centres. J Affect Disord 1989; 17 (2): 197-8
10. Paykel ES, Priest RG. Recognition and management of depression in general practice: consensus statement. BMJ 1992; 305: 1198-202
11. Montgomery SA, Bebbington P, Cowen P, et al. Guidelines for treating depressive illness with antidepressants. J Psychopharmacol 1993; 7: 19-23
12. Clinical Resource and Audit Group. Depressive illness: a critical review of current practice and the way ahead. Consensus statement. Edinburgh: The Scottish Office, National Health Service in Scotland, 1993
13. Depression Guideline Panel, Agency for Health Care Policy Research Treatment of Major Depression. Clinical practice guideline. No. 5, Vol. 2. Rockville (MD): US Department of Health and Human Services, 1993 (AHCPR Publication No. 93-0550, 1993. 20)
14. The treatment of depression in primary care: which treatments are effective in the management of depression in primary care? Eff Health Care 1993; 5: 1-12
15. Selecting an antidepressant. MeReC Bulletin 1995; 6 (I): 1-4
16. Karasu TB, Docherty JP, Gelenberg A, et al. Practice guideline for major depressive disorder in adults. In: Practice guidelines. Washington, DC: American Psychiatric Association, 1996: 83-127
17. Crismon ML, Trivedi M, Pigott TA, et al. The Texas medication algorithm project: report of the Texas consensus conference panel on medication treatment of major depressive disorder. J Clin Psychiatry 1999; 60: 142-56
18. Song F, Freemantle N, Sheldon TA, et al. Selective serotonin reuptake inhibitors: meta-analysis of efficacy and acceptability. BMJ 1993; 306: 683-7
19. Anderson IM, Tomenson BM. The efficacy of selective serotonin re-uptake inhibitors in depression: a meta-analysis of studies against tricyclic antidepressants. J Psychopharmacol 1994; 8: 238-49
20. Montgomery SA, Henry J, McDonald G, et al. Selective serotonin reuptake inhibitors: meta-analysis of discontinuation rates. Int Clin Psychopharmacol 1994; 9: 47-53
21. Hotopf M, Hardy R, Lewis G. Discontinuation rates of SSRIs and tricyclic antidepressants: a meta-analysis and investigation of heterogeneity. Br J Psychiatry 1997; 170: 120-7
22. Kendrick T. Prescribing antidepressants in general practice: watchful waiting for minor depression, full dose treatment for major depression. BMJ 1996; 313: 829-30
23. Paykel ES, Hollyman JA, Freeling P, et al. Predictors of therapeutic benefit from amitriptyline in mild depression: a general practice placebo-controlled trial. J Affect Disord 1988; 14: 83-95
24. Thompson C, Thompson CM. The prescribing of antidepressants in general practice: II. A placebo-controlled trial of low-dose dothiepin. Hum Psychopharmacol 1989; 4: 191-204
25. Tyrer P, Murphy S, Kingdon D, et al. The Nottingham study of neurotic disorder: comparison of drug and psychological treatments. Lancet 1988; I: 235-40
26. Bollini P, Pampallona S, Tibaldi G, et al. Effectiveness of antidepressants: meta-analysis of dose-effect relationships in randomised clinical trials. Br J Psychiatry 1999; 174: 297-303
27. Thase ME, Sullivan LR. Relapse and recurrence of depression: a practical approach for prevention. CNS Drugs 1995; 4: 261-77
28. Maj M, Vietro F, Pirozzi R, et al. Pattern of recurrence of illness after recovery of an episode of major depression: a prospective study. Am J Psychiatry 1992; 149: 795-800
29. Melfi CA, Chawla AJ, Croghan TW, et al. The effects of adherence to antidepressant treatment guidelines on relapse and recurrence of depression. Arch Gen Psychiatry 1998; 55: 1128-32
30. Johnson DAW. Treatment of depression in general practice. BMJ 1973; 1: 18-20
31. Kotin J, Post RM, Goodwin FK. Drug treatment of depressed patients referred for hospitalisation. Am J Psychiatry 1973; 130: 1139-41
32. Johnson DAW. A study of the use of antidepressant medication in general practice. Br J Psychiatry 1974; 125: 186-92
33. Johnson DAW. Depression: treatment compliance in general practice. Acta Psychiatr Scand 1981; 63 Suppl. 290: 447-53
34. Keller MB, Klerman GL, Lavori PW, et al. Treatment received by depressed patients. J Am Med Assoc 1982; 248: 1848-55
35. Jick H, Dinan BJ, Hunter JW, et al. Tricyclic antidepressants and convulsions. J Clin Psychopharmacol 1983; 3: 182-5
36. Jones L, Simpson D, Brown AC, et al. Prescribing psychotropic drugs in general practice: three year study. BMJ 1984; 289: 1045-8
37. Pollock BG, Perel JM. Tricyclic antidepressants: contemporary issues for therapeutic practice. Can J Psychiatry 1989; 34: 609-17
38. Keller MB, Lavori PW, Klerman GL, et al. Low levels and lack of predictors of somatotherapy and psychotherapy received by depressed patients. Arch Gen Psychiatry 1986; 43: 458-66
39. Thompson C, Thompson CM. The prescription of antidepressants in general practice: I. A critical review. Hum Psychopharmacol 1989; 4: 91-102
40. McCombs JS, Nichol MB, Stimmel GL, et al. The cost of antidepressant drug therapy failure: a study of antidepressant use patterns in a medicaid population. J Clin Psychiatry 1990; 51 Suppl. 6: 60-9
41. Katon W, VonKorff M, Lin E, et al. Adequacy and duration of antidepressant treatment in primary care. Med Care 1992; 30: 67-76
42. Simon GE, VonKorff M, Wagner EH, et al. Patterns of antidepressant use in community practice. Gen Hosp Psychiatry 1993; 15: 399-408
43. Rosholm J-U, Hallas J, Gram LF. Outpatient utilisation of antidepressants: a prescription database analysis. J Affect Disord 1993; 27: 21-8
44. Rosholm JU, Gram LF, Damsbo N, et al. Antidepressant treatment in general practice – an interview study. Scand J Prim Care 1995; 13: 281-6
45. Munizza C, Tibaldi G, Bollini P, et al. Prescription pattern of antidepressants in out-patient psychiatric practice. Psychologic Med 1995; 25: 771-8
46. Bingefors K, Isacson D, von Knorring L. Antidepressant dose patterns in Swedish clinical practice. Int Clin Psychopharmacol 1997; 12 (5): 283-90

47. Donoghue JM, Tylee A, Wildgust HJ. Cross sectional database analysis of antidepressant prescribing in general practice in the United Kingdom, 1993-5. BMJ 1996; 313: 861-2
48. Matthews K, Eagles JM, Matthews CA. The use of antidepressant drugs in general practice: a questionnaire survey. Euro J Clin Pharmacol 1993; 45: 205-10
49. Kerr MP. Antidepressant prescribing: a comparison between general practitioners and psychistrists. Br J Gen Pract 1994; 44: 275-6
50. Thomson RJ. Antidepressant prescribing among referrals to a community mental health unit in New Zealand. Psychiatr Bull 1994; 18: 461-2
51. American Psychiatric Association. Diagnostic and statistical manual of mental disorders. 3rd ed. Washington, DC: American Psychiatric Association, 1980
52. Donoghue JM. The prescribing of antidepressants in general practice: the use of PACT data (brief report). Postgrad Med J 1994; 70 Suppl. 2: S23-S24
53. Wells KB, Katon W, Rogers B, et al. Use of minor tranquillisers and antidepressant medications by depressed outpatients: results from the Medical Outcomes Study. Am J Psychiatry 1994; 151: 694-700
54. Arpino C, Da Cas R, Donini G, et al. The use and misuse of antidepressant drugs in a random sample of the population of Rome, Italy. Acta Psychiatr Scand 1995; 92: 7-9
55. Donoghue JM, Tylee A. The treatment of depression: prescribing patterns of antidepressants in primary care in the United Kingdom. Br J Psychiatry 1996; 168: 164-8
56. MacDonald TM, McMahon AD, Reid IC, et al. Antidepressant drug use in primary care: a record linkage study in Tayside, Scotland. BMJ 1996; 313: 860-1
57. World Health Organization. International classification of diseases. 10th ed. Geneva: World Health Organization, 1992
58. Rouillon F, Blachier C, Dreyfus JP, et al. Etude pharmaco-epidemiologique de la consommation des antidepresseurs en population generale L'encephale Sp 1996; 1: 39-48
59. Gregor KJ, Hylan TR, van Dijk PCM, et al. Outpatient antidepressant utilisation in a Dutch sick fund. Am J Manage Care 1998; 4: 1150-60
60. Isometsa E, Seppala I, Henriksson M, et al. Inadequate dosaging in general practice of tricyclic vs. other antidepressants for depression. Acta Psychiatr Scand 1998; 98: 451-4
61. Donoghue J, Katona C, Tylee A. The treatment of depression: antidepressant prescribing for elderly patients in primary care. J Pharm 1998; 260: 500-2
62. Dunn RL, Donoghue JM, Ozminkowski RJ, et al. Longitudinal patterns of antidepressant prescribing in primary care in the UK: comparison with treatment guidelines. J Psychopharmacol 1999; 13 (2): 136-43
63. Donoghue JM. Selective serotonin re-uptake inhibitor use in primary care: a five year naturalistic study. Clin Drug Invest 1998 Dec; 16 (6): 453-62
64. Tylee A, Gastpar M, Lepine J-P, et al. DEPRES II (Depression Research in European Society II): a patient survey of the symptoms, disability, and current management of depression in the community. DEPRES Steering Committee. Int Clin Psychopharmacol 1999; 14 (3): 139-51
65. Keller MB, Klerman GL, Lavori PW, et al. The persistent risk of chronicity in recurrent episodes of non-bipolar major depressive disorder: a prospective follow-up. Am J Psychiatry 1986; 143: 24-8
66. Kiloh LG, Andrews G, Neilson M. The long-term outcome of depressive illness. Br J Psychiatry 1988; 153: 752-7
67. Goethe JW, Szarek BL, Cook WL. A comparison of adequately vs. Inadequately treated depressed patients. J Nerv Ment Dis 1988; 176: 465-70
68. Scott J. Chronic depression. Br J Psychiatry 1988; 153: 287-97
69. Rutz W, Walinder J, Eberhard G, et al. An educational programme on depressive disorders for general practitioners in Gotland: Background and evaluation. Acta Psychiatr Scand 1989; 79: 19-26
70. Bacani-Oropilla T, Lippman SB. Chronic depression: issues in long-term management. Postgrad Med 1989; 85: 171-5
71. Frank E, Kupfer DJ, Perel JM, et al. Three year outcomes for maintenance therapies in recurrent depression. Arch Gen Psychiatry 1990; 47: 1093-9
72. Prien RF, Kupfer DJ, Mansky PA, et al. Drug therapy in the prevention of recurrences in unipolar and bipolar affective disorders. Report of the NIMH collaborative study group comparing lithium carbonate, imipramone, and a lithium carbonate-imipramine combination. Arch Gen Psychiatry 1984; 41: 1096-104
73. Thase ME. Relapse and recurrence in umipolar major depression: short-term and long-term approaches. J Clin Psychiatry 1990; 51 Suppl.: 51-7
74. Scott J, Eccleston D. Prediction, treatment and prognosis of chronic primary major depression. Int Clin Psychopharmacol 1991; 6 Suppl. 1: 41-9
75. Brugha TS, Bebbington PE, MacCarthy B, et al. Antidepressants may not assist recovery in practice: a naturalistic prospective survey. Acta Psychiatr Scand 1992; 86: 5-11
76. Mintz J, Mintz LI, Arruda MJ, et al. Treatments of depression and the functional capacity to work. Arch Gen Psychiatry 1992; 49 (10): 761-8
77. Shea MT, Elkin I, Imber SD, et al. Course of depressive symptoms over follow-up. Arch Gen Psychiatry 1992; 49: 782-7
78. Frank E, Kupfer DJ, Perel JM, et al. Comparison of full-dose versus half-dose pharmacotherapy in the maintenance treatment of recurrent depression. J Affect Disord 1993; 27: 139-45
79. Isacsson G, Holmgren P, Wassermen D, et al. Use of antidepressants among people committing suicide in Sweden. Br Med J 1994; 308: 506-9
80. Simon GE, Lin EHB, Katon W, et al. Outcomes of 'inadequate' antidepressant treatment. J Gen Intern Med 1995; 10: 663-70
81. Schulberg HC, Block MR, Madonia MJ, et al. Treating major depression in primary care practice. Eight month clinical outcomes. Arch Gen Psychiatry 1996; 53: 913-9
82. American Psychiatric Association. Diagnostic and statistical manual of mental disorders. 3rd rev. ed. Washington, DC: American Psychiatric Association, 1987

83. Lave JR, Frank RG, Schulberg HC, et al. Cost-effectiveness of treatments for major depression in primary care practice. Arch Gen Psychiatry 1998; 55: 645-51
84. Ali IM. Long-term treatment with antidepressants in primary care. Psychiatr Bull 1998; 22: 15-9
85. Fish D. What is an effective dose [letter]? BMJ 1997; 314: 826
86. Moore MV. More on what is an effective dose [letter]. BMJ 1997; 314: 826
87. Tan RS. Low dose tricyclic antidepressants are effective in treating major depression [letter]. BMJ 1997; 314: 827
88. Dodd GK, Berti C. A critical appraisal of a naturalistic study to support cost effective prescribing patterns of selective serotonin reuptake inhibitors in primary care. J Serotonin Res 1997; 3: 169-72
89. Donoghue JM. Response to: a critical appraisal of a naturalistic study to support cost effective prescribing patterns of selective serotonin reuptake inhibitors in primary care. J Serotonin Res 1997; 4: 233-7
90. Hotopf M, Lewis G, Normand C. Putting trials on trial – the costs and consequences of small trials in depression: a systematic review of methodology. J Epidemiol Community Health 1997; 51: 354-8
91. Freeman HL, O'Hanlon JF. Acute and subacute effects of antidepressants on performance. J Drug Dev Clin Pract 1995; 7: 7-20
92. Ray WA. Psychotropic drugs and injuries among the elderly: a review. J Clin Psychopharmacol 1992; 12: 386-96
93. Henry JA, Alexander CA, Sener EK. Relative mortality from overdose of antidepressants. BMJ 1995; 310: 221-4
94. Demyttenaere K. Compliance during treatment with antidepressants. J Affect Disord 1997; 43: 27-39
95. Freemantle N, House A, Mason J, et al. Economics of treatment of depression [letter]. Br J Psychiatry 1995; 166: 397
96. Hotopf M, Lewis G, Normand C. Are SSRIs a cost effective alternative to tricyclics? Br J Psychiatry 1996; 168: 404-9
97. Jonsson B, Bebbington PE. What price depression? The cost of depression and the cost-effectiveness of pharmacological treatment. Br J Psychiatry 1994; 164: 665-73
98. Le Pen C, Levy E, Ravily J, et al. The cost of treatment dropout in depression. A cost-benefit analysis of fluoxetine vs tricyclics. J Affect Disord 1994; 31: 1-18
99. Sclar DA, Robison LM, Skaer TL, et al. Antidepressant pharmacotherapy: economic outcomes in a health maintenance organisation. Clin Ther 1994; 16: 715-30
100. Stewart A. Antidepressant pharmacotherapy: cost comparison of SSRIs and TCAs. BMJ Economics 1994; 7: 67-79
101. Lapierre Y, Bentkover J, Schainbaum S, et al. Direct cost of depression: analysis of treatment costs of paroxetine versus imipramine in Canada. Can J Psychiatry 1995; 40: 370-7
102. Simon G, Wagner E, VonKorff M. Cost-effectiveness comparisons using 'real world' randomised trials: the case of new antidepressant drugs. J Clin Epidemiol 1995; 48: 363-73
103. Skaer TL, Sclar DA, Robison LM, et al. Economic evaluation of amitriptyline, desipramine, nortriptyline and sertraline in the management of patients with depression. Curr Ther Res 1995; 56: 556-67
104. Forder J, Kavanagh S, Fenyo A. A comparison of the cost-effectiveness of sertraline versus tricyclic antidepressants in primary care. J Affect Disord 1996; 38: 97-111
105. Simon GE, VonKorff M, Heiligenstein JH, et al. Initial antidepressant choice in primary care. J Am Med Assoc 1996; 275: 1897-902
106. Thompson D, Buesching D, Gregor KJ, et al. Patterns of antidepressant use and their relation to costs of care. Am J Manage Care 1996; 2: 1239-46
107. Donoghue JM. Costs of treating depression: policy should be evidence-based [commentary]. In: Maj M, Sartorius N, editors. Depressive disorders. Vol. 1. Chichester: John Wiley & Sons Ltd, 1999: 459-61 (Evidence and Experience in Psychiatry Series, World Psychiatric Association)
108. Rosenbaum JF, Hylan TR. Costs of depressive disorders: a review. In: Maj M, Sartorius N, editors. Depressive disorders. Vol. 1. Chichester: John Wiley & Sons Ltd, 1999: 401-49 (Evidence and Experience in Psychiatry Series, World Psychiatric Association)

Correspondence: *John Donoghue*, Pharmaceutical Consultant, PCS Health, 4 Wrenfield Grove, Liverpool L17 9QD, England.
E-mail: john@donoghue.u-net.com

Relapse and Recurrence of Depression
An Updated Practical Approach for Prevention

Michael E. Thase

Western Psychiatric Institute and Clinic, Department of Psychiatry, University of Pittsburgh School of Medicine, Pittsburgh, Pennsylvania, USA

The major affective disorders are increasingly recognised as recurrent and potentially chronic conditions. Each new episode of major depressive disorder is punctuated by renewed risks of chronicity, suicide and psychosocial impairment. As a result, treatment strategies with a long term, prophylactic focus are recommended for many patients. This article will review issues pertaining to the use of long term, preventative treatment strategies for depressive states.

1. Natural History of Depression

Epidemiological evidence suggests that the age at onset of a first episode of mood disorder is becoming progressively younger.[1] Moreover, the incidence of affective disorder appears to be increasing among younger cohorts.[1,2] Thus, the already considerable public health impact of the affective disorders will most certainly increase in the future.

The point prevalence of chronic and recurrent cases of major affective disorder exceeds that for acute, first-episode disorders.[3,4] In the 1970s, Angst et al.[5] and Zis and Goodwin[6] documented the likelihood of relapse and recurrence in the major affective disorders. These findings were prospectively confirmed in a series of studies conducted under the auspices of the National Institute of Mental Health Collaborative Study on the Psychobiology of Depression (as summarised by Keller and Hanks[7]). At the least, 50% of those who have experienced one episode of major depression will experience another at some later point. Thus, assuming a lifetime risk of major depression of 5%,[8] an individual who has recovered from an initial episode of depression has at least a 10-fold greater risk of having another episode when compared with a person of similar age and sex who has never been clinically depressed. For recurrent (unipolar) major depression and bipolar depression, where recurrence rates of at least 70 to 90% are expected, the increase in risk of recurrence is 14- to 18-fold when compared with that in the general population.[5,7,9-11] Chronic minor depressive disorders (i.e. dysthymia) are similarly associated with a marked increase in the risk of subsequent major depressive episodes.[7]

Despite vigorous public education efforts, many depressed individuals are still likely to be either untreated or incorrectly diagnosed and/or inadequately treated.[12,13] This state of affairs, while undoubtedly reinforced by societal attitudes and stigma, underscores the generally favourable short term prognosis of the mood disorders.[5-11,14] For example, most episodes of acute major depression will last no longer than 1 year, and between 80 and 90% will have remitted within 2 years, without specific treatment.[7,15]

However, even episodes of depression of such limited duration convey many adverse economic, interpersonal and medical consequences.[7,14,16-19] For example, family dysfunction is quite common and may persist after the episode has remitted.[17] Impairment of leisure time and vocational functioning may similarly persist long after resolution of a depressive episode.[18,19] Furthermore, substance abuse, including that of alcohol (ethanol) and hypnosedatives, may develop during an untreated depressive episode,[20,21] and depressed patients are, on average, heavier tobacco users than nondepressed individuals.[22] Thus, for those whose depression remains untreated and who do not remit spontaneously, an ingrained pattern of chronic depression conveys even more negative prognostic implications.[7,21]

While most initial episodes of depression occur at times of stress, only a minority of persons encountering such difficulties develop persistent depressive syndromes. This highlights the role of underlying psychobiological vulnerability factors in the aetiology of depression.[14,23] Such risk factors include:[14,16,21,23]

- a family history of affective disorder or alcoholism
- a long established pattern of maladaptive cognitions or interpersonal difficulties
- chronic medical problems
- a history of early trauma or abuse.

Interestingly, the relationship between stress and episodes of recurrent depression appears to be less pronounced in highly recurrent cases, in which new episodes may appear to occur 'out-of-the-blue'. Further, individuals who have dysthymic disorder prior to the onset of a major depressive episode typically have a significantly greater number of vulnerability factors than acutely depressed patients whose depression is not preceded by other mood disorders.[14,21]

In other major depressive episodes, the onset of the syndrome develops insidiously, i.e. over a matter of weeks or even months.[7,24] Prodromal symptoms such as anxiety, irritability, decreased hedonic capacity and poor concentration may be identified that herald the onset of a depressive episode.[24] In more protracted depressive syndromes, it is often difficult to distinguish between those psychosocial and interpersonal factors that precede the affective illness and those factors that are consequences of it.[16]

2. Phases of Treatment of Unipolar Depressive Disorder

A clear conceptualisation of the course of depressive illness and its treatment provides a framework for a coherent, long term treatment plan. Such an approach has been proposed by Frank et al.[25] using the '5 Rs': response, remission, relapse, recovery and recurrence (see fig. 1). The relationship between these outcomes and 3 interlocking phases of treatment – acute, continuation and maintenance – are described in sections 2.1 to 2.3.

2.1 Acute Treatment

The acute phase of treatment begins with the selection of a strategy. The treatment modality first chosen for a depressive episode is generally predetermined by the patient's choice of mental health providers. For example, depressed persons treated by family practitioners are likely to receive pharmacotherapy and practical advice, whereas the clients of psychologists, social workers and other therapists are almost certain to receive counselling or psychotherapy.[26] At present, most psychiatrists prefer to use a combination of both modalities.[26,27] Identifying better means of matching patients with potentially effective treatments would be preferred.

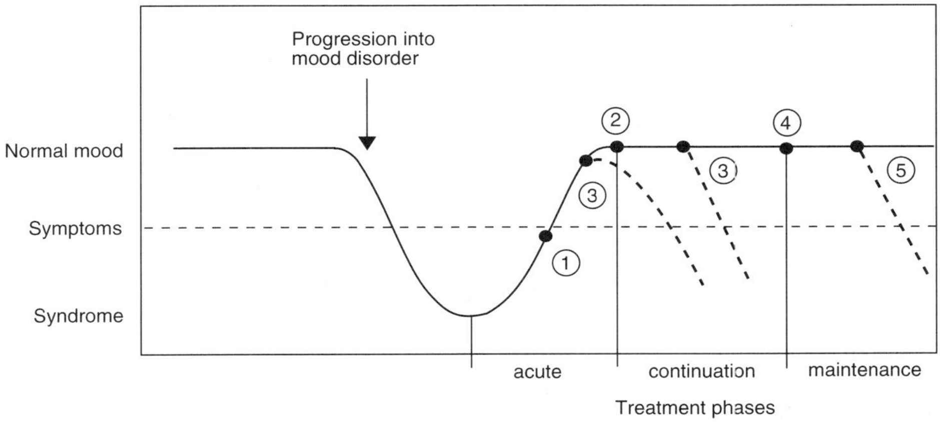

Fig. 1. A diagram of five possible outcomes (1. response; 2. remission; 3. relapse; 4. recovery; and 5. recurrence) across the three phases of treatment of depression (acute, continuation and maintenance).

The term 'treatment response' is used to categorise the initial therapeutic goal for depressed patients. Response may encompass both spontaneous remissions of symptoms and placebo responses, in addition to specific responses to active treatments. A response generally corresponds to at least a 40 to 60% reduction of symptoms.[28] This is often achieved within 3 to 6 weeks after the initiation of antidepressant pharmacotherapy. In controlled studies of mild to moderately depressed outpatients, specified, time-limited psychotherapies [such as Beck's model of cognitive behavioural therapy (CBT)[29] and Klerman and colleagues interpersonal psychotherapy (IPT)[30]] appear to achieve results comparable with those of tricyclic antidepressants when given over 12 to 16 weeks.[31,32]

With either type of treatment, however, failure to achieve a treatment response after a trial of appropriate duration (e.g. 6 to 8 weeks for pharmacotherapy and 12 to 16 weeks for psychotherapy) should result in a switch to an alternative first-line treatment. Thus, sequential courses of acute phase therapy should be provided until patients achieve a clear response.[33]

2.2 Continuation Therapy

The acute phase of therapy ends and continuation therapy begins when a patient has achieved a significant response to treatment. During continuation therapy, medication dosage typically remains constant and visits to the clinician become less frequent. The goals of continuation therapy are: (i) prevention of relapse; and (ii) conversion of a response into a remission.[14]

Remission is defined by a substantial reduction of symptoms and a return to a level of functioning equal to the patient's premorbid state.[14,25] A patient who achieves a stable remission for at least 4 to 6 months may be said to have recovered from the index depressive episode.[25] It is of note that the risk of relapse in patients not receiving continuation therapy is as high in first episode cases as it is in recurrent depression.[34,35]

Relapse is defined as an increase of depressive symptoms back to a syndromal level at any point between the initial treatment response and the end of continuation therapy.[14,25] Reviews of empirical studies of pharmacological treatments indicate that the risk of relapse is particularly high if an antidepressant is discontinued within the first 4 months of achieving response, with relapse rates typically ranging from 40 to 60%.[14,34,35] By contrast, relapse rates of only 10 to 20% are observed during continuation pharmacotherapy.[14,34,35] In our experience at the University of Pittsburgh,[14] a relapse rate of only 5% was observed over a 4-month period of continued pharmacotherapy with a maximum dose of antidepressant in combination with IPT.[14]

Continuation pharmacotherapy is often compromised by noncompliance. In many cases, this is attributable to drug-induced adverse effects. The newer antidepressants, such as the selective serotonin (5-hydroxytryptamine; 5-HT) reuptake inhibitors (SSRIs), have been well received as treatments for outpatients, largely because of their more favourable adverse effect profiles compared with older agents. Controlled studies of the use of SSRIs for up to 2 years of therapy have yielded promising findings.[35] For example, Doogan and Caillard[36] reported the results of a multicentre study in which patients were randomly assigned to either placebo or active medication after first responding to 8 weeks of sertraline. They found a highly significant advantage of continuation therapy with sertraline over placebo, with no discernable difference in adverse effects between the 2 treatment groups. These findings parallel those of studies on continuation treatment with fluoxetine,[37] citalopram[38] and paroxetine.[39]

Only a few systematic studies involving patients with chronic, treatment-resistant and/or atypical disorders have been performed. Small studies of continuation pharmacotherapy with imipramine,[40] phenelzine[41] and tranylcypromine[42] in patients with such disorders indicate a similar prophylactic effect with continuation pharmacotherapy to that seen in more mild conditions. However, Stewart et al.[43] failed to confirm the preventive efficacy of imipramine in relation to phenelzine in a larger placebo-controlled study of atypical depression.

Besides premature discontinuation of pharmacotherapy and noncompliance, other risk factors for relapse include:[14,23,44-46]

- severity of the index depressive episode
- presence of persistent residual (subsyndromal) depressive symptoms
- severe personality pathology
- older age
- high levels of dysfunctional attitudes
- poor social support
- ongoing or renewed psychosocial stressors.

Patients who do not achieve stable remissions during continuation treatment represent a particularly high risk group.[14] The presence of residual symptoms conveys increased risk of relapse despite continuation therapy, suggesting the need for more vigorous pharmacotherapy and/or the adjunctive use of psychotherapy.[47]

Depressive relapse has also been documented following termination of short term psychotherapy.[48-51] In a study conducted by our group at the University of Pittsburgh,[49] patients treated with CBT had a 31% relapse rate overall during the first year of follow-up. However, only 10% of the 'responders' relapsed if they had a remission of 8 weeks duration before discontinuing treatment. By contrast, the relapse rate of the incompletely remitted patients was 52%. Moreover, relapsers were found to be more severely ill at baseline, had higher levels of dysfunctional attitudes and were less likely to be married.[49]

The outcomes of patients followed-up after termination of cognitive therapy provide some support for the notion that cognitive therapy has a prophylactic value comparable to continuation pharmacotherapy.[50] However, across numerous studies of psychotherapy, only a fraction of patients who entered the trial both responded to treatment *and* remained well over 12 to 18 months of follow-up.[49-51] Hence, many patients may need longer courses of psychotherapy. To this end, models of 'continuation psychotherapy' are being developed to lessen the risk of relapse in high-risk cases following termination of a short term psychotherapy treatment protocol.[52]

Conventionally, continuation therapy ends when the patient meets criteria for recovery (i.e. after 4 to 6 months of sustained euthymia).[14,25] A recovery is presumed to represent a qualitatively distinct state when compared with remission. For example, it is hypothesised that the psychobiological correlates of the acute depressive state become quiescent during recovery.[14] A recurrent or renewed period of depressive symptoms following recovery is thus conceptualised as the onset of a distinctly new episode of affective illness. However, because 10 to 15% of apparently recovered patients have recurrences within the first 8 weeks of discontinuing antidepressant medication,[53] it appears that time alone may not provide an adequate definition of recovery.

Anticholinergic withdrawal symptoms, provoked by too rapid a reduction in the dosage of selected heterocyclic agents, such as amitriptyline, maprotiline, imipramine or clomipramine, sometimes make it difficult to distinguish between withdrawal symptoms and a precipitous symptomatic recurrence.[54] Hence, it is generally not prudent to taper a heterocyclic antidepressant at a rate faster than 25% of the total dose each week. The emergence of antidepressant withdrawal symptoms will generally respond in rapid fashion to a resumption of the antidepressant at a dosage that was previously effective.[14] Similar tapering strategies are needed for several of the SSRIs and venlafaxine.[55] Slow tapering is usually not necessary for fluoxetine because of the long elimination half-life of the metabolite, norfluoxetine.[55]

2.3 Maintenance Therapy

Maintenance pharmacotherapy should be considered after continuation therapy for all patients at a high risk of recurrence. The characteristics of such patients include a history of recurrent episodes of depression.[56,57] This is especially true for patients who have experienced episodes of depression within 2 or 3 years prior to the onset of the index episode.[49,53] Other risk factors for recurrent depression include both early and late onset of depression (i.e. before age 25 or after age 60 years), chronicity, gender (i.e. rates may be higher in women), severity of the index episode, a seasonal pattern of mood disturbance, and a family history of affective disorder.[56]

The need for maintenance therapy is illustrated by the findings of studies of patients with highly recurrent unipolar depression. In 1 study, an 85% recurrence rate was observed within 3 years after the withdrawal of imipramine.[58] Conversely, 80% of patients receiving maintenance pharmacotherapy remained well. Most other studies have also documented a superior outcome for patients receiving active maintenance therapy, although the magnitude of the drug-placebo differences is generally smaller.[56,57] As discussed in section 3.2, the higher recurrence rate observed in earlier studies may have been attributable to the use of lower dosages of maintenance pharmacotherapy.

3. Considerations in Maintenance Therapy

Prescribing a course of maintenance antidepressant therapy involves a careful assessment of the risks of recurrent illness, the expected benefits of continued treatment and the potential costs of such treatment (in terms of both drug acquisition costs and the costs of adverse effects).[56,57] Optimal results of maintenance treatment are achieved when the clinician and patient have established a strong, collaborative alliance. One of the best ways to achieve this is to reach a shared conclusion that the benefits of maintenance treatment outweigh the costs.[59]

Questions such as 'Do I need to take antidepressants forever?' and 'How long should pharmacotherapy be maintained?' often surface when clinicians and patients consider a maintenance treatment plan. The analogy of controlling hypertension with ongoing medication provides one vehicle by which to discuss long term treatment. Moreover, this model offers the opportunity to discuss potential reductions of vulnerability through psychosocial and behavioural interventions (i.e. using the hypertension analogy, bodyweight loss, salt restriction, exercise and smoking cessation are widely recognised methods of reducing vulnerability).

As with the pharmacological treatment of hypertension, reassessment of the cost : benefit ratio of maintenance therapy for depression should be performed collaboratively on a periodic basis, such as annually or biannually. During these collaborative discussions, it is helpful to explore and address certain common, but maladaptive, attitudes that may be associated with noncompliance during maintenance pharmacotherapy (e.g. 'I don't want to get hooked on this stuff', 'I feel dependent on this drug', or 'For once, I'd like to be normal and not have to rely on these pills to stay well').[59] In such discussions, it may be useful to include a spouse, parent or significant other. In our experience, the well-meaning, but misguided, pressure from family members often provides the impetus for patients' requests to discontinue medication.

3.1 Drug Choice

Maintenance pharmacotherapy is typically provided using the same antidepressant agent(s) as that used during acute and continuation therapy.[56,57] Patients are initially seen monthly and, after a period of sustained recovery, the frequency of visits is often reduced to every other month or even less frequently.

3.1.1 Tricyclic Antidepressants and Lithium

The agents that have been most extensive studied as maintenance treatments are the tricyclic antidepressants and lithium. In earlier reviews,[56,57,60] both modalities have been shown to convey about a 2- or 3-fold protective effect over 18 to 36 months when compared with placebo.

A meta-analysis of earlier studies indicated that lithium is effective in preventing depressive relapses and recurrences.[61] Schou[62] reached a similar conclusion in a qualitative review of older studies of maintenance phase treatment. European studies tend to provide the strongest support for the efficacy of long term lithium prophylaxis of unipolar depression.[63,64]

However, in one well conducted, multicentre American study,[65] unipolar patients, who were first stabilised on both imipramine and subsequently randomly assigned to lithium maintenance treatment, had a significantly poorer outcome than patients randomised to treatment with imipramine, either with or without concomitant lithium therapy. Moreover, lithium was only marginally more effective than placebo in this study.[65] Similarly, in a more recent trial conducted in the UK,[66] the combination of lithium and amitriptyline was found to be no more effective than amitriptyline alone.

Therefore, evidence for the routine use of lithium as maintenance therapy does not appear as compelling as that for tricyclic antidepressants. On the other hand, for many patients with bipolar depression, lithium is still warranted as the 'foundation' maintenance therapy.[11,57] Moreover, lithium maintenance therapy of unipolar depression also would appear to be useful for patients who have responded to lithium, have previously benefitted from lithium prophylaxis, and/or not responded to antidepressant monotherapy.[62]

On the basis of available published literature, it could be argued that tricyclic antidepressants are the treatment of choice for the prophylaxis of recurrent unipolar depression.[14,57] However, this is specifically because tricyclics: (i) have been in use longer than other agents such as the SSRIs; and (ii) were used with greater frequency than monoamine oxidase (MAO) inhibitors (MAOIs) in the 1960s and 1970s.

3.1.2 Selective Serotonin Reuptake Inhibitors

There are still only a handful of trials of the use of SSRIs as maintenance therapy. Zimeldine, which was withdrawn from the market because of the induction of Guillain-Barré syndrome, showed significant prophylactic efficacy (relative to placebo) in an 18-month study.[67] Montgomery et al.[37] found a 26% 1-year recurrence rate (23 of 88 patients) for fluoxetine, compared with a 57% recurrence rate (54 of 94) for placebo. The efficacy of fluvoxamine,[68] sertraline,[68,69] and paroxetine[70] has been studied in protocols lasting 1 to 2 years.

3.1.3 Monoamine Oxidase Inhibitors

Three published studies have examined the efficacy of nonselective MAOIs when used as maintenance therapy.[43,71,72] As noted earlier, phenelzine but not imipramine was an effective preventive treatment in a study of atypical depression.[43] In a placebo-controlled study, phenelzine, but not nortriptyline, prevented recurrent episodes of late-life depression.[71] Phenelzine (45 or 60 mg/day) was also found to be more effective than placebo in preventing recurrence in a young patient sample characterised by anxious and atypical depressive features.[72] Although phenelzine was well tolerated in one study,[71] a high dropout rate largely offset the efficacy of the drug in the other.[72] Because of evidence confirming the value of MAOIs as short term strategies for atypical,[73] anergic[74] and imipramine-resistant recurrent depression,[75,76] these agents should not be considered obsolete. Nevertheless, dietary restrictions and multiple adverse effects limit the older, nonselective MAOIs to third- or fourth-line use.

Reversible and selective MAOIs have been under development for some time. One such agent, the MAO-A selective drug moclobemide, is available in most of the Western world (aside from the US). In a controlled 4-month study of continuation therapy,[77] moclobemide was found to be as effective and as well tolerated as fluoxetine. In an open-label, maintenance phase study, moclobemide was found to be associated with a modest relapse rate (25%) over 1 year, as well as a favourable long term adverse effect profile.[78] Although concerns about the efficacy of moclobemide linger, the reversible inhibitors of MAO-A (RIMAs) may ultimately prove to be significantly better for long term treatment than their nonselective predecessors.

3.2 Dosage

Many clinicians reduce the dosage of antidepressants during long term treatment, often to a 'maintenance dose' of about one-half of that used during acute therapy.[56,57] The results of earlier studies document that the maintenance dose strategy is more effective than placebo (see, for example, Prien[57]). However, several lines of evidence suggest that this practice may be less effective than the full dose prophylactic strategy for preventing recurrent affective disorders.[56]

For example, in a retrospective examination of patients treated in a university-affiliated mood disorders clinic, patients with recurrences were found to have been maintained on significantly lower dosages of antidepressants than those who remained well.[79] A retrospective examination of our own group's experiences in conducting long term treatment trials over the past 15 years yielded a similar conclusion.[56] We found that the recurrence rate of patients maintained on lower dosages of imipramine (mean dosage = 137 mg/day) was significantly higher than the rate observed in a later study using higher maintenance dosages (mean dosage = 216 mg/day). In a controlled study that compared low (75 mg/day) and ultra-low (37.4 mg/day) dosages of maprotiline as maintenance therapy, significantly more recurrences occurred in the ultra-low dosage group.[80]

Prospective confirmation of the greater efficacy of full dose maintenance tricyclic treatment is provided by data from a double-blind study conducted by our group.[81] Patients with highly recurrent unipolar depression (i.e. 4 or more lifetime episodes) were randomly assigned to either full-dose (approximately 200 mg/day, n = 10) or half-dose (approximately 100 mg/day, n = 10) imipramine maintenance pharmacotherapy. The recurrence rate over 36 months in the full-dose group was only 30%, compared with 70% in the half-dose group. Franchini and colleagues[70] conducted a similar study of 68 patients who had responded to paroxetine 40 mg/day. The recurrence rate of patients switched to a 20 mg/day maintenance therapy dosage was significantly higher than the recurrence rate of the patients maintained on the full dosage (i.e. 52 *vs* 24%). Thus, both retrospective and prospective comparisons of heterocyclic antidepressants indicate that the full-dose maintenance treatment strategy is significantly more effective than lower dosage strategies.

3.3 Adverse Effects

The long term toll of persistent, dose-dependent adverse effects probably underlie clinicians' predilection for use of lower dosage maintenance strategies mentioned in section 3.2.[9,14]

While long term pharmacotherapy with heterocyclic agents is tolerated by a majority of patients, ongoing problems with bodyweight gain, dental caries (caused by chronic xerostomia), sedation, constipation and sexual dysfunction all may complicate maintenance treatment. Patients undergoing long term therapy with nonselective MAOIs may experience comparable problems with bodyweight gain, oedema, insomnia and sexual dysfunction.[14,57,82] One study suggests that dropout due to intolerable adverse effects may actually be higher during long term MAOI treatment than typically observed during maintenance therapy with tricyclic antidepressants.[72] Bodyweight gain, acne, diarrhoea, polyuria, tremor and hypothyroidism are well documented complications of long term lithium therapy,[9,57] along with the spectre of chronic renal interstitial fibrosis.[83] In practice, such adverse experiences often lead to noncompliance, dosage reduction and/or premature discontinuation of medication.[9,57] Therefore, there is a clear need for continued development of alternative treatments for maintenance therapy.

Clinical experience suggests that the SSRIs are generally well tolerated during long term therapy.[36,55,68-70] Perhaps the most common persistent problem with these agents is sexual dysfunction, which may require dosage reduction or trials of various adjunctive medications.

The so-called 'second generation' heterocyclics (i.e. trazodone, maprotiline and amoxapine) and the newer monocyclic antidepressants [i.e. nefazodone, amfebutamone (bupropion), mirtazapine and venlafaxine] are effective treatments for many depressed outpatients. However, while several studies document efficacy in prevention of relapse and/or recurrence, maprotiline[80,84] and amoxapine[85] may not offer substantial advantages over the tricyclics with respect to the incidence of adverse effects. Some data also support the potential utility of trazodone[86] and amfebutamone[87] as long term preventative treatments, although such studies are not definitive. Amfebutamone, mirtazapine and venlafaxine share the SSRIs' relative safety in overdose.

3.4 Duration of Treatment

There is no single correct answer to the important question of 'How long should pharmacotherapy be maintained?' While continuation therapy is indicated for virtually all patients for a relatively narrow time frame, maintenance treatment may extend indefinitely.[9,14,57] The best answer to the question would be 'for as long as the benefits outweigh the risks'. There are few empirical data, however, to support a maintenance treatment plan beyond the first 24 or 36 months of pharmacotherapy.[9,10,56,57]

On one hand, many thousands of patients have taken tricyclic and MAOI antidepressants and/or lithium as maintenance for 10, 15 or even 20 years without marked adverse effects, and nothing has emerged to date to suggest anything as worrisome as the risk of tardive dyskinesia that is associated with long term antipsychotic therapy. On the other hand, the meta-analysis conducted by Belsher and Costello[23] suggests that the annual risk of subsequent depressive episodes becomes rather small after 2 years of sustained recovery. Thus, the risk-benefit equation may slowly shift over time.

A small, but informative, study completed by our Pittsburgh group[88] examined the outcome of 20 patients with unipolar depression who had experienced 3 depression-free years during maintenance treatment with imipramine. These patients subsequently were randomly assigned to either 2 more years of full dose imipramine treatment or double-blind placebo substitution. The 2-year recurrence rate among 9 placebo-treated patients was 67%, compared with only 9% in 11 patients receiving ongoing imipramine treatment ($p < 0.006$).

Although the highly recurrent nature of depression in this sample may bias the placebo group's recurrence rate upward, the clinical implication is clear: even after 3 years of sustained recovery there remains a significant risk of recurrent depression following withdrawal of pharmacotherapy. Findings such as this could suggest that the 'price' of antidepressant prophylaxis is sustained vulnerability off medication.[89]

3.5 Role of Psychotherapy in Maintenance Therapy

While a modest body of empirical evidence exists to support the popular strategy of combining psychotherapeutic and pharmacological approaches during acute treatment of affective disorders,[90] strong empirical justification for the routine combination of these forms of therapy as maintenance treatment strategies is lacking. Similarly, the efficacy of psychotherapy alone as a maintenance treatment has not been definitely established.

Only three studies have addressed the efficacy of IPT as continuation[91] or maintenance treatments.[58,92] In a study of continuation therapy,[91] 150 depressed women who responded to acute phase pharmacotherapy with amitriptyline were subsequently randomised to one of four treatment strategies: (i) individual IPT; (ii) placebo pharmacotherapy; (iii) maintenance amitriptyline; or (iv) a combination of psychotherapy and pharmacotherapy. No additional prophylaxis was conferred by combined psychotherapy and pharmacotherapy when compared with amitriptyline only. Moreover, the relapse risk of those withdrawn from pharmacotherapy and treated only with psychotherapy was not significantly different to that of the group treated with only placebo.[91] There was, however, evidence of improved interpersonal functioning in the women who were treated with psychotherapy and who remained well.[93]

In the second study, Frank and associates[58] found that a systematised form of maintenance IPT (IPT-M), provided on a monthly basis following an initial course of weekly sessions (in combination with pharmacotherapy), was significantly more effective than placebo in preventing recurrence. However, IPT-M was significantly less effective than maintenance imipramine pharmacotherapy.[58] Further, patients randomly assigned to receive the combination of IPT-M and imipramine did not show significantly superior prophylaxis when compared with those receiving pharmacotherapy alone (see fig. 2).[58]

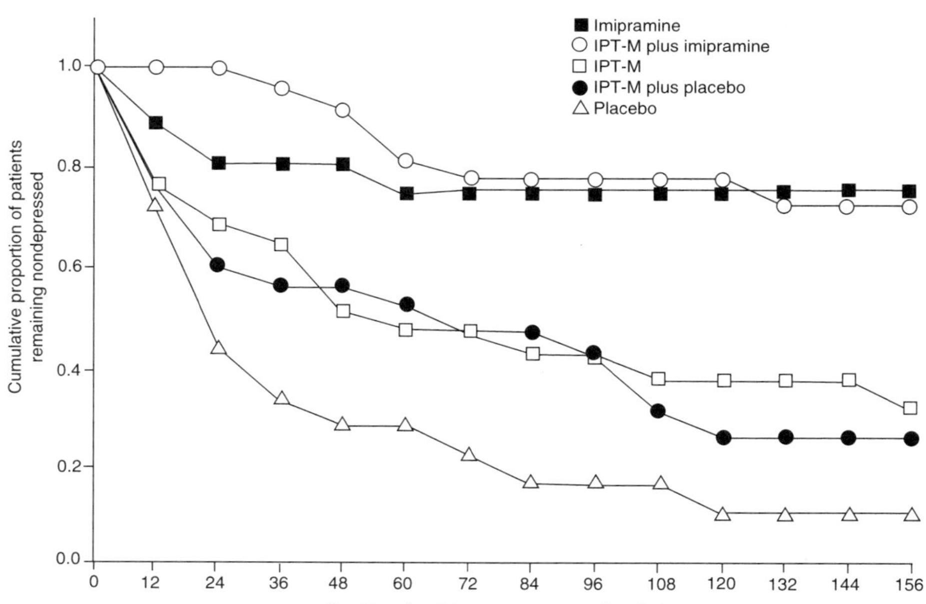

Fig. 2. 3-year survival rates of patients with recurrent major depression.
IPT-M = maintenance interpersonal psychotherapy (adapted from Frank et al.,[58] with permission).

In the third study, Reynolds et al.[92] found that the combination of nortriptyline and monthly IPT had an additive benefit (relative to the monotherapies) in preventing recurrent depression among an older sample. Both monotherapies were superior to the placebo control group and nortriptyline alone and IPT-M alone did not differ significantly.

The prophylactic success of IPT-M was found to be linked to the quality of the therapeutic relationship.[94,95] Specifically, those patients who participated in high quality therapy (i.e. defined by above average scores on a measure that assessed the quality of therapy) were at significantly lower risk of relapse than patients whose therapy scores were below the mean on this measure. In fact, recurrence rates for those patients undergoing high quality therapy did not differ from those who received pharmacotherapy until the third year of the study. In contrast, the fate of the patients in the low quality therapy group was virtually identical to that of patients treated with placebo alone. In a subsequent report, Spanrer et al.[95] found that higher quality IPT actually partially offset the increased recurrence risk associated with EEG sleep disturbance. Thus, IPT-M was either a potent prophylactic therapy or was ineffective, depending on the fidelity of the therapy.

It remains to be seen if more frequent psychotherapeutic contact enhances the efficacy of IPT-M. A study by Frank and colleagues is currently underway at the University of Pittsburgh to determine if continued weekly or twice-monthly psychotherapeutic contact is superior to monthly sessions of therapy.

Several recent studies have investigated CBT as a longer term treatment. As noted in section 2.2, the results of most naturalistic follow-up studies suggest that patients treated with CBT have lower relapse rates over the first 6 to 24 months of follow-up than patients withdrawn from short term treatment with tricyclic antidepressants.[50,96-98] Recent studies by Fava et al.[99] and Paykel et al.[100] further indicated that a relatively brief course of CBT after acute-phase pharmacotherapy may reduce the subsequent risk of recurrent depression.

4. Relapse and Recurrence in Specific Situations

4.1 Recurrent Depressive Episodes During Maintenance Therapy

Naturalistic and controlled studies suggest that between 20 and 70% of patients with recurrent unipolar depression will ultimately experience recurrences despite maintenance antidepressant pharmacotherapy.[9,57,101] Our group's experience suggests that noncompliance and other factors leading to inadequate blood drug concentrations are the leading reasons for recurrent episodes.[14,102] If feasible, obtaining a blood drug concentration is a prudent first step in the evaluation of a 'breakthrough' depressive episode. Increasing the dosage may also be a useful option, particularly with the newer agents for which valid blood concentration determinations are not yet available. For example, the value of a dosage increase has been shown in patients who relapse despite ongoing fluoxetine pharmacotherapy.[103]

Routinely adopting a dosage increase strategy, however, does not address the possibility that noncompliance triggered the recurrence. In this case, a dosage increase may lead to increased toxicity if the patient also tries to remedy the problem by improving his or her compliance without informing the attending physician. An unexplained reduction in blood drug concentrations usually points to a compliance problem, which warrants prompt psychoeducational and psychotherapeutic interventions.[33,59] It is imperative to ask patients directly about their medication compliance.

Identifying other potential psychosocial correlates of the clinical worsening, such as relationship difficulties or other stresses, may also provide cues for additional changes in the treatment plan. As with schizophrenia, high levels of criticism and/or expressed emotion in the households of patients receiving maintenance medication may hasten recurrences.[46,104,105] Therapy for individuals, couples or families may be added to pharmacotherapy. Medication noncompliance related to life stresses is another potential indication for concurrent psychotherapy during long term drug treatment.[14,106]

It is also important not to overlook the potential role of concomitant medication in depressive relapse. Changes in blood concentrations may reflect drug interactions and/or alterations in hepatic metabolism. This is particularly relevant for patients taking an antidepressant medication that has a therapeutic 'window' of efficacy, such as nortriptyline. Smokers, for example, may metabolise tricyclic antidepressants more rapidly than nonsmokers due to nicotine-induced hepatic enzyme induction. This will cause a marked increase in blood drug concentrations following cessation of smoking. Other important interactions include increases of tricyclic drug concentrations in patients concomitantly treated with fluoxetine, phenothiazines or cimetidine.

Recurrence of depressive episodes has been linked to the concept of neurophysiological tolerance to the therapeutic effects of antidepressants.[107] However, evaluation of the role of tolerance in the loss of therapeutic effects is difficult, as it is not possible to know with absolute certainty that a patient had specifically responded to pharmacotherapy in the first place. For example, a presumed 'true' medication response may have actually been due to spontaneous remission, seasonal variation, placebo response and/or a coincidental change in life circumstances. As placebo response rates may reach up to 40% in some groups of depressed patients, a significant proportion of relapses or recurrences attributed to drug 'failure' may be due to other causes.

Besides increasing dosage, many clinicians manage breakthrough episodes by augmenting the antidepressant medication with lithium or switching to another antidepressant. Unfortunately, no empirical data exist to guide such decisions. In our clinical experience, it is generally useful to defer making major changes in the treatment plan for at least 1 to 2 weeks in order to differentiate a more transient reduction in drug efficacy from a genuine recurrent episode.[14] In any case, patients who experience breakthrough episodes despite compliance with pharmacotherapy require close follow-up, specifically because such renewed depressive symptomatology is often associated with demoralisation and/or emergence of suicidal ideation. Moreover, in the case of tricyclic or MAOI treatment, prescribing a large supply of maintenance medication provides patients with a particularly lethal method of suicide.

4.2 Psychotic Depression

Most psychotically depressed patients who respond to pharmacotherapy require concurrent treatment with both an antidepressant and an antipsychotic.[108] However, few empirical data exist to guide strategies for continuation and maintenance treatment of psychotic depression. Although some patients relapse upon withdrawal of an antipsychotic from a combined treatment strategy,[109] most clinicians still prefer to try to discontinue the antipsychotic agent as soon as is feasible. This is mainly done to reduce the risk of tardive dyskinesia. The availability of novel antipsychotics with apparently lower risks for the induction of tardive dyskinesia, including clozapine, risperidone and olanzapine, provide a welcome alternative for long term treatment of patients who require maintenance antipsychotics.

Until more definitive data are available, the strategy outlined in figure 3 can be considered for continuation and maintenance treatment of psychotic depression. This has been extrapolated from long term treatment strategies of severe nonpsychotic depression. As noted above, the novel antipsychotics clearly deserve consideration,[110] particularly when previously unaffected patients begin to manifest signs of tardive dyskinesia.

4.3 Relapse and Recurrence Following Electroconvulsive Therapy

The risk of relapse is particularly high following successful treatment with electroconvulsive therapy (ECT).[111,112] In fact, a successful course of ECT may provide little

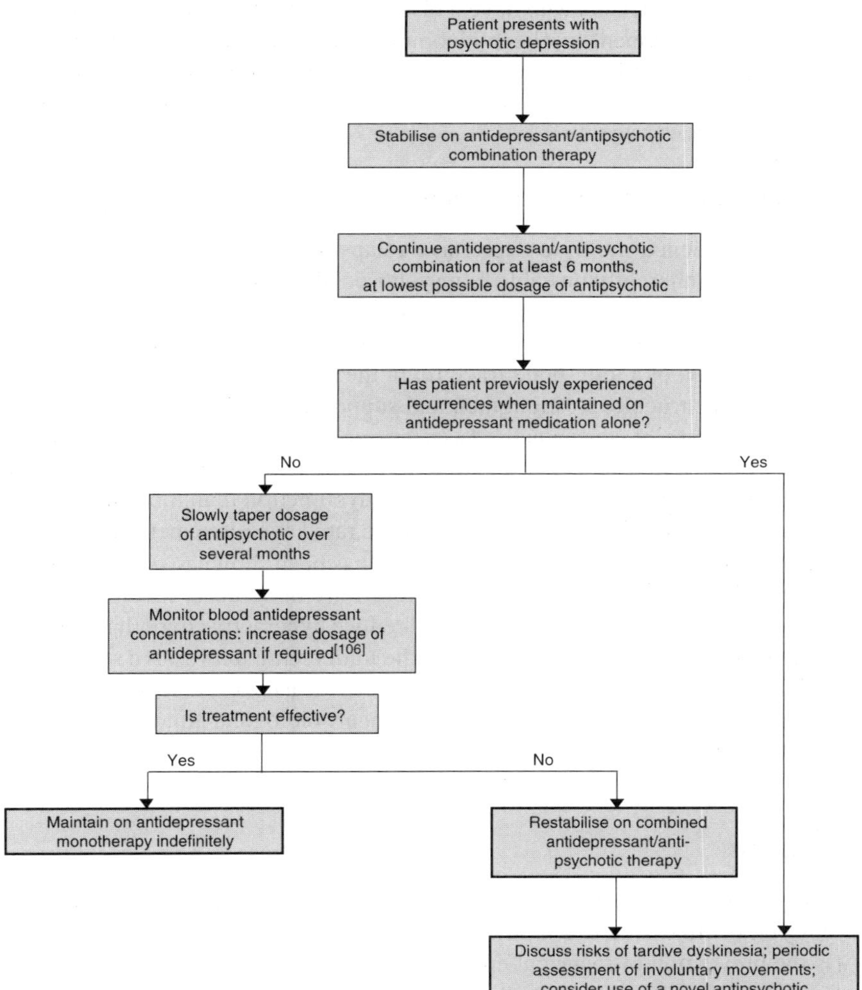

Fig. 3. Treatment strategy for the prevention of relapse and recurrence in patients with psychotic depression.

protection against subsequent episodes of depression.[9,10] These risks of relapse are heightened by the criteria used for selection of ECT, which skew the population of treated patients to include an over-representation of highly vulnerable patients, including those who are psychotically depressed, elderly and have treatment-resistant disorders.[113]

Most patients should receive continuation and maintenance pharmacotherapy following ECT. However, recent evidence tempers enthusiasm for this strategy. Sackheim et al.[114] found that patients with tricyclic-resistant depression who had responded to ECT had a high risk of relapse when they resumed taking previously administered agents for continuation treatment. Therefore, patients who are resistant to one or more classes of antidepressants before receiving ECT should probably be placed on a novel form of antidepressant for prophylaxis.

Antidepressant/lithium combinations have been used for prophylaxis by some clinicians following ECT, while others prefer using a MAOI or an alternative novel antidepressant, with or without lithium.[115] In patients who have a history of multiple relapses, a sustained course of 'maintenance' ECT treatment has been recommended on a weekly or biweekly basis.[116] Ironically, as their use as first-line therapy diminishes, tricyclic antidepressants may ultimately be established as the best choice for post-ECT treatment for patients who have failed to respond to the SSRIs or other newer agents.

5. Psychobiology of Depressive Vulnerability

Patients who experience multiple depressive relapses or recurrences may be viewed as functioning within an inherently unstable biopsychosocial milieu. Although the hypertension analogy was used to illustrate some aspects of recurrent affective illness in section 3, perhaps the issues pertaining to sustained depressive vulnerability may be better understood in the context of the non-union of a long-bone fracture. In the same way that a cast or brace is worn to provide an external structure to strengthen and support a bone that will not heal, so might long term pharmacotherapy be conceptualised as necessary to stabilise persistently dysregulated neurobiological systems. Indeed, evidence suggests that patients with recurrent depression are more likely to manifest objective signs of biological dysfunction than those in a first episode, including hypercortisolaemia[117] and increased phasic rapid eye movement (REM) sleep.[118]

In this regard, effective antidepressant treatment has been shown to correct inefficiencies in noradrenergic neurotransmission, reverse alterations in cerebral metabolism, suppress aberrant electroencephalographic sleep indices and reduce hyperactive hypothalamic-pituitary-adrenocortical axis function.[119] Research into the underlying depressive state, such as the examination of neurobiological disturbances, may provide a means to identify those patients who require long term pharmacotherapy. Persistent neurobiological abnormalities, in spite of ongoing maintenance antidepressant therapy may thus reveal the highest level of illness vulnerability.[14,119]

6. Conclusions

The majority of patients with depression will experience recurrent episodes of illness. As each new episode of illness carries a new risk of chronicity, the best plan to minimise such morbidity is the prevention of recurrent episodes.

As such, all patients who respond to antidepressant medications warrant at least 6 months of continuation pharmacotherapy. Moreover, patients who respond to antidepressants should *not* be tapered from continuation therapy unless their remission has been complete and sustained. An indefinite course of maintenance pharmacotherapy provides a substantial and ongoing prophylactic advantage for patients at high risk of recurrent depressive episodes. It is likely that similar guidelines apply to patients who have responded to treatment with acute phase psychotherapy in lieu of medication.

A rapidly growing database suggests that SSRIs are effective long term preventative treatments, with tricyclic antidepressants, MAOIs, lithium and other antidepressant agents providing useful options for patients who do not respond to SSRIs.

Maintenance models of psychotherapy may also be considered for patients unwilling or unable to take long term pharmacotherapy, although the research support for such efforts is less substantial.

Acknowledgements

This research was supported by grants MH-41884 and MH-30915 from the National Institute of Mental Health. We wish to thank Ms Lisa Stupar and Ms Leslie Vasey for their assistance in the preparation of this manuscript.

References

1. Klerman GL. The current age of youthful melancholia: evidence for increase in depression among adolescents and young adults. Br J Psychiatry 1988; 152: 4-14
2. Klerman GL, Weissman MM. Increasing rates of depression. JAMA 1989; 261: 2229-35
3. Weissman MM, Leaf PJ, Tischler GL, et al. Affective disorders in five United States communities. Psychol Med 1983; 18: 141-53
4. Weissman MM, Leaf PJ, Bruce ML, et al. The epidemiology of dysthymia in five communities: rates, risks, comorbidity, and treatment. Am J Psychiatry 1988; 145: 815-9
5. Angst J, Baastrup P, Grof P, et al. The course of monopolar depression and bipolar psychoses. Psychiatr Neurol Neurochir 1973; 76: 489-500
6. Zis AP, Goodwin FK. Major affective disorder as a recurrent illness: a critical review. Arch Gen Psychiatry 1979; 36: 835-9
7. Keller MB, Hanks DL. The natural history and heterogeneity of depressive disorders: implications for rational antidepressant therapy. J Clin Psychiatry 1994; 55 (9 Suppl.): 25-31
8. Robins LN, Helzer JE, Weissman MM, et al. Lifetime prevalence of specific psychiatric disorders in 3 sites. Arch Gen Psychiatry 1984; 41: 949-58
9. Consensus Development Panel. Mood disorders: pharmacologic prevention of recurrences [NIMH/NIH Consensus Development Conference Statement]. Am J Psychiatry 1985; 142: 469-76
10. Consensus statement: WHO mental health collaborating centers. J Affect Disord 1989; 17: 197-8
11. Goodwin FK, Jamison KR. Manic-depressive illness. New York: Oxford University Press, 1990
12. Keller MB, Klerman GL, Lavori PW, et al. Treatment received by depressed patients. JAMA 1982; 248: 1848-55
13. Keller MB, Lavori PW, Klerman GL, et al. Low levels and lack of predictors of somatotherapy and psychotherapy received by depressed patients. Arch Gen Psychiatry 1986; 43: 458-66
14. Thase ME. Relapse and recurrence in unipolar major depression: short-term and long-term approaches. J Clin Psychiatry 1990; 51 (6 Suppl.): 51-7
15. Sargeant JK, Bruce ML, Florio LP, et al. Factors associated with 1-year outcome of major depression in the community. Arch Gen Psychiatry 1990; 47: 519-26
16. Barnett PA, Gotlib IA. Psychosocial functioning and depression: distinguishing among antecedents, concomitants, and consequences. Psychol Bull 1988; 104: 97-126
17. Keitner GI, Miller IW. Family functioning and major depression: an overview. Am J Psychiatry 1990; 147: 1128-37
18. Bauwens F, Tracy A, Pardoen D, et al. Social adjustment of remitted bipolar and unipolar outpatients: a comparison with age- and sex-matched controls. Br J Psychiatry 1991; 159: 239-44
19. Perugi G, Maremmani I, McNair D, et al. Differential changes in areas of social adjustment from depressive episodes through recovery. J Affect Disord 1988; 15: 39-43
20. Buydens-Branchey L, Branchey MG, Noumair D. Age of alcoholism onset. I: Relationship to psychopathology. Arch Gen Psychiatry 1989; 46: 225-30
21. Akiskal HS. Factors associated with incomplete recovery in primary depressive illness. J Clin Psychiatry 1982; 43: 266-71
22. Bresalau N, Kilbey MM, Andreski P. Nicotine dependence, major depression, and anxiety in young adults. Arch Gen Psychiatry 1991; 48: 1069-74
23. Belsher G, Costello CG. Relapse after recovery from unipolar depression: a critical review. Psychol Bull 1988; 104: 84-96
24. Fava GA, Kellner R. Prodromal symptoms in affective disorders. Am J Psychiatry 1991; 148: 823-30

25. Frank E, Prien RF, Jarrett RB, et al. Conceptualization and rationale for consensus definitions of terms in major depressive disorder: remission, recovery, relapse, and recurrence. Arch Gen Psychiatry 1991; 48: 851-5
26. Orleans CT, George LK, Houpt J, et al. How primary care physicians treat psychiatric disorders: a national survey of family practitioners. Am J Psychiatry 1985; 142: 52-7
27. Karasu TB. Psychotherapy and pharmacotherapy: toward an integrative model. Am J Psychiatry 1982; 139: 1102-13
28. Prien RF, Carpenter LL, Kupfer DJ. The definition and operational criteria for treatment outcome of major depressive disorder: a review of the current research literature. Arch Gen Psychiatry 1991; 48: 796-800
29. Beck AT, Rush AJ, Shaw BG, et al. Cognitive therapy of depression. New York: Guilford Press, 1979
30. Klerman GL, Weissman MM, Rounsaville BJ, et al., editors. Interpersonal psychotherapy of depression. New York: Basic Books, 1984
31. Dobson KS. A meta-analysis of the efficacy of cognitive therapy for depression. J Consult Clin Psychol 1989; 57: 414-9
32. Robinson LA, Berman JS, Neimer RA. Psychotherapy for treatment of depression: a review of the controlled outcome research. Psychol Bull 1990; 108: 30-49
33. Simons AD, Thase ME. Mood disorders. In: Thase ME, Hersen M, Edelstein BA, editors. Handbook of outpatient treatment in adults. New York: Plenum Press, 1990: 91-138
34. Prien RF, Kupfer DJ. Continuation drug therapy for major depressive episodes: how long should it be maintained? Am J Psychiatry 1986; 143: 18-23
35. Montgomery SA, Doogan DP, Burnside R. The influence of different relapse criteria on the assessment of long-term efficacy of sertraline. Int Clin Psychopharmacol 1991 Dec 6; Suppl. 2: 37-46
36. Doogan DP, Caillard V. Sertraline in the prevention of depression. Br J Psychiatry 1992; 160: 217-22
37. Montgomery SA, Dufour H, Brion S, et al. The prophylactic efficacy of fluoxetine in unipolar depression. Br J Psychiatry 1988; 153 Suppl.: 69-76
38. Montgomery SA, Rasmussen JGC, Tanghoj P. A 24-week study of 20 mg citalopram, 40 mg citalopram, and placebo in the prevention of relapse of major depression. Int Clin Psychopharmacol 1993; 8: 181-8
39. Montgomery SA, Dunbar G. Paroxetine is better than placebo in relapse prevention and the prophylaxis of recurrent depression. Int Clin Psychopharmacol 1993; 8: 189-95
40. Kocsis JH, Sutton BM, Frances J. Long-term follow-up of chronic depression treated with imipramine. J Clin Psychiatry 1991; 52: 56-9
41. Harrison W, Rabkin J, Stewart JW, et al. Phenelzine for chronic depression: a study of continuation treatment. J Clin Psychiatry 1986; 47: 346-9
42. Thase ME, Trivedi MH, Rush AJ. MAOI's in the contemporary treatment of depression. Neuropsychopharmacology 1995; 12: 185-219
43. Stewart JW, Tricamo E, McGrath PJ, et al. Prophylactic efficacy of phenelzine and imipramine in chronic atypical depression: likelihood of recurrence of discontinuation after 6 months' remission. Am J Psychiatry 1997; 154: 31-6
44. Faravelli C, Ambonetti A, Pallanti S, et al. Depressive relapses and incomplete recovery from index episode. Am J Psychiatry 1986; 143: 888-91
45. Hammen C, Ellicott A, Gitlin M, et al. Sociotropy-autonomy and vulnerability to specific life events in patients with unipolar depression and bipolar disorders. J Abnorm Psychol 1989; 98: 154-60
46. Hooley JM, Teasdale JD. Predictors of relapse in unipolar depressives: expressed emotion, marital distress, and perceived criticism. J Abnorm Psychol 1989; 98: 229-35
47. Fava GA, Grandi S, Zielezny M, et al. Cognitive behavioral treatment of residual symptoms in primary major depressive disorder. Am J Psychiatry 1994; 151: 1295-9
48. Weissman MM, Klerman GL, Prusoff BA, et al. Depressed outpatients: one year after treatment with drugs and/or interpersonal psychotherapy. Arch Gen Psychiatry 1981; 38: 51-5
49. Thase ME, Simons AD, McGeary J, et al. Relapse following cognitive behavior therapy of depression: potential implications for longer-term forms of treatment? Am J Psychiatry 1992; 149: 1046-52
50. Evans MD, Hollon SD, DeRubeis RJ, et al. Differential relapse following cognitive therapy and pharmacotherapy for depression. Arch Gen Psychiatry 1992; 49: 802-8
51. Shea MT, Elkin I, Imber SD, et al. Course of depressive symptoms over follow-up: findings from The National Institute of Mental Health Treatment of Depression Collaborative Research Program. Arch Gen Psychiatry 1992; 49: 782-7
52. Jarrett RB, Kraft D. Prophylactic cognitive therapy for major depressive disorder. In Session: Psychotherapy in Practice 1997; 3: 65-79
53. Frank E, Kupfer DJ, Perel JM. Early recurrence in unipolar depression. Arch Gen Psychiatry 1989; 46: 397-400
54. Dilsaver SC, Greden JF. Antidepressant withdrawal phenomena. Biol Psychiatry 1984; 19: 237-56
55. Coupland NJ, Bell CJ, Potokar JP. Serotonin reuptake inhibitor withdrawal. J Clin Psychopharmacol 1996; 16: 356-62
56. Thase ME. Long-term treatments of recurrent depressive disorders. J Clin Psychiatry 1992; 53 Suppl.: 33-44
57. Prien RF. Long-term treatment of affective disorders. In: Meltzer HY, editor. Psychopharmacology: the third generation of progress. New York: Raven Press, 1987: 1051-8
58. Frank E, Kupfer DJ, Perel JM, et al. Three-year outcomes for maintenance therapies in recurrent depression. Arch Gen Psychiatry 1990; 47: 1093-9
59. Wright JH, Thase ME. Cognitive and biological therapies: a synthesis. Psychiatric Ann 1992; 22: 451-8
60. Prien RF, Kocsis JH. Long-term treatment of mood disorders. In: Bloom FE, Kupfer DJ, editors. Psychopharmacology: the fourth generation of progress. New York: Raven Press, 1995: 1067-79
61. Davis JM. Overview: maintenance therapy in psychiatry. II: Affective disorders. Am J Psychiatry 1976; 133: 1-3
62. Schou M. Lithium as a prophylactic agent in unipolar affective illness. Arch Gen Psychiatry 1979; 36: 849-51

63. Coppen A, Ghose K, Rao R, et al. Mianserin and lithium in the prophylaxis of depression. Br J Psychiatry 1978; 133: 206-10
64. Glen AIM, Johnson AL, Shepherd M. Continuation therapy with lithium and amitriptyline in unipolar depressive illness: a randomized double-blind, controlled trial. Psychol Med 1984; 14: 37-50
65. Prien RF, Kupfer DJ, Manskey PA, et al. Drug therapy in the prevention of recurrences in unipolar and bipolar affective disorders. Arch Gen Psychiatry 1984; 41: 1096-104
66. Johnstone WC, Owens DGC, Lambert MT, et al. Combination tricyclic antidepressant and lithium maintenance medication in unipolar and bipolar depressed patients. J Affect Disord 1990; 20: 225-33
67. Bjork K. The efficacy of zimelidine in preventing depressive episodes in recurrent major depressive disorders – a double-blind placebo-controlled study. Acta Psychiatr Scand 1983; 308: 182-9
68. Franchini L, Gasperini M, Perez J, et al.. A double-blind study of long-term treatment with sertraline or fluvoxamine for prevention of highly recurrent unipolar depression. J Clin Psychiatry 1997; 58: 104-7
69. Keller MB, Kocsis JH, Thase ME, et al., for the Sertraline Chronic Depression Study Group. Maintenance phase efficacy of sertraline for chronic depression. A randomized controlled trial. JAMA 1998; 280: 1665-72
70. Franchini L, Gasperini M, Perez J, et al. Dose-response efficacy of paroxetine in preventing depressive recurrences: a randomized, double-blind study. J Clin Psychiatry 1998; 59: 229-32
71. Georgotas A, McCue RE, Cooper TB. A placebo-controlled comparison of nortriptyline and phenelzine in maintenance therapy of elderly depressed patients. Arch Gen Psychiatry 1989; 46: 783-6
72. Robinson DS, Lerfald SC, Bennett B, et al. Continuation and maintenance treatment of major depression with the monoamine oxidase inhibitor phenelzine: a double-blind placebo-controlled discontinuation study. Psychopharmacol Bull 1991; 27: 31-9
73. Quitkin FM, Harrison W, Stewart JM, et al. Response to phenelzine and imipramine in placebo non-responders with atypical depression. Arch Gen Psychiatry 1991; 48: 319-23
74. Himmelhoch JM, Thase ME, Mallinger AG, et al. Tranylcypromine versus imipramine in anergic bipolar depression. Am J Psychiatry 1991; 148: 910-6
75. Thase ME, Frank E, Mallinger A, et al. Treatment of imipramine-resistant recurrent depression: III. Efficacy of monoamine oxidase inhibitors. J Clin Psychiatry 1992; 53: 5-11
76. Thase ME, Mallinger AG, McKnight D, et al. Treatment of imipramine resistant recurrent depression: IV. A double-blind, crossover study of tranylcypromine in anergic bipolar depression. Am J Psychiatry 1992; 149: 195-8
77. Lonnqvist J, Sihvo S, Syvalahti E, et al. Moclobemide and fluoxetine in the prevention of relapses following acute treatment of depression. Acta Psychiatr Scand 1995; 91: 189-94
78. Moll E, Stabl M, Wegscheider R, et al. Long-term treatment with moclobemide. An open-label, non-comparative, multiple-distributed study in patients with a major depressive episode as defined by DSM-III. Psychopharmacology (Berl) 1992; 106 Suppl.: 120-2
79. Peselow ED, Difiglia C, Fieve RR. Relationship of dose to antidepressant prophylactic efficacy. Acta Psychiatr Scand 1991; 84: 571-4
80. Rouillon F, Serrurier D, Miller HD, et al. Prophylactic efficacy of maprotiline on unipolar depression relapse. J Clin Psychiatry 1991; 52: 423-31
81. Frank E, Kupfer DJ, Perel JM, et al. Comparison of full dose versus half dose pharmacotherapy in the maintenance treatment of recurrent depression. J Affect Disord 1993; 27: 139-45
82. Agosti V, Stewart JW, Quitkin FM, et al. Factors associated with premature medication discontinuation among responders to an MAOI or a tricyclic antidepressant. J Clin Psychiatry 1988; 49: 196-8
83. Schou M. Effects of long-term lithium treatment on kidney function: an overview. J Psychiatr Res 1988; 22: 287-96
84. Coppen A, Montgomery SA, Gupta RK, et al. A double-blind comparison of lithium carbonate and maprotiline in the prophylaxis of the affective disorders. Br J Psychiatry 1976; 128: 479-85
85. Mason BJ, Kocsis JH, Frances AJ, et al. Amoxapine versus amitriptyline for continuation therapy of depression. J Clin Psychopharmacol 1990; 10: 338-43
86. Fabre Jr LF, Feighner JP. Long-term therapy for depression with trazodone. J Clin Psychiatry 1983; 44: 17-21
87. Gardner EA. Long-term preventative care in depression: the use of bupropion in patient intolerant of other antidepressants. J Clin Psychiatry 1983; 44 (5, sec 2): 157-62
88. Kupfer DJ, Frank E, Perel JM, et al. Five-year outcome for maintenance therapies in recurrent depression. Arch Gen Psychiatry 1993; 50: 24-30
89. Fava GA. Do antidepressant and antianxiety drugs increase chronicity in affective disorders? Psychother Psychosom 1994; 61: 125-31
90. Conte HR, Plutchik R, Wild KV, et al. Combined psychotherapy and pharmacotherapy for depression. Arch Gen Psychiatry 1986; 43: 471-9
91. Klerman GL, DiMascio A, Weissman M, et al. Treatment of depression by drugs and psychotherapy. Am J Psychiatry 1974; 131: 186-91
92. Reynolds III CF, Frank E, Perel JM, et al. Nortriptyline and interpersonal psychotherapy as maintenance therapies for recurrent major depression. A randomized controlled trial in patients older than 59 years. JAMA 1999; 281: 39-45
93. Weissman MM, Klerman GL, Paykel ES, et al. Treatment effects on the social adjustment of depressed patients. Arch Gen Psychiatry 1974; 30: 771-8
94. Frank E, Kupfer DJ, Wagner EF, et al. Efficacy of interpersonal psychotherapy as a maintenance treatment of recurrent depression: contributing factors. Arch Gen Psychiatry 1991; 48: 1053-9
95. Spanier C, Frank E, McEachran AB, et al. The prophylaxis of depressive episodes in recurrent depression following discontinuation of drug therapy: integrating psychological and biological factors. Psychol Med 1996; 26: 461-75

96. Blackburn IM, Eunson KM, Bishop S. A two-year naturalistic follow-up of depressed patients treated with cognitive therapy, pharmacotherapy and a combination of both. J Affect Disord 1986; 10: 67-75
97. Kovacs M, Rush AJ, Beck AT, et al. Depressed outpatients treated with cognitive therapy of pharmacotherapy: a one-year follow-up. Arch Gen Psychiatry 1981; 39: 33-9
98. Simons AD, Murphy GE, Levine JL, et al. Cognitive therapy and pharmacotherapy for depression: sustained improvement over one year. Arch Gen Psychiatry 1986; 43: 43-8
99. Fava GA, Rafanelli C, Grandi S, et al. Prevention of recurrent depression with cognitive behavioral therapy. Preliminary findings. Arch Gen Psychiatry 1998; 55: 816-20
100. Paykel ES, Scott J, Teasdale JD, et al. Prevention of relapse in residual depression by cognitive therapy. Arch Gen Psychiatry 1999; 56: 829-35
101. Thase ME. Maintenance treatments of recurrent affective disorders. Curr Opin Psychiatry 1993; 6: 16-21
102. Kupfer DJ, Perel JM, Frank E. Adequate treatment with imipramine in continuation treatment. J Clin Psychiatry 1989; 50: 250-5
103. Fava M, Rappe SM, Pava J, et al. Relapse in patients on long-term fluoxetine treatment: response to increased fluoxetine dose. J Clin Psychiatry 1995; 56: 52-5
104. Vaughn CE, Leff JP. The influence of family and social factors on the course of psychiatric illness: a comparison of schizophrenic and depressed neurotic patients. Br J Psychiatry 1976; 129: 125-37
105. Hooley JM, Orley J, Teasdale JD. Levels of expressed emotion and relapse in depressed patients. Br J Psychiatry 1986; 148: 642-7
106. Frank E. Interpersonal psychotherapy as a maintenance treatment for recurrent depression. Psychotherapy 1991; 28: 259-66
107. Post RM, Weiss SB. Sensitization, kindling, and carbamazepine: an update on their implications for the course of affective illness. Pharmacopsychiatry 1992; 25: 41-3
108. Schatzberg AF, Rothschild AJ. Psychotic (delusional) major depression: should it be included as a distinct syndrome in DSM-IV? Am J Psychiatry 1992; 149: 733-45
109. Robinson DG, Spiker DG. Delusional depression: a one-year follow-up. J Affect Disord 1985; 9: 79-83
110. McElroy SL, Dessain EC, Pope Jr HG, et al. Clozapine in the treatment of psychotic mood disorders, schizoaffective disorder, and schizophrenia. J Clin Psychiatry 1991; 52: 411-4
111. Kay DWK, Fahy T, Garside RF. A seven-month double-blind trial of amitriptyline and diazepam in ECT-treated depressed patients. Br J Psychiatry 1970; 117: 556-71
112. Seager CP, Bird RL. Imipramine with electrical treatment in depression: a controlled trial. J Ment Sci 1962; 108: 704-7
113. Prudic J, Sackeim HA, Devanand DP. Medication resistance and clinical response to electroconvulsive therapy. Psychiatry Res 1989; 31: 287-96
114. Sackheim HA, Prudic J, Devanand DP, et al. The impact of medication resistance and continuation pharmacotherapy on relapse following response to electroconvulsive therapy in major depression. J Clin Psychopharmacol 1990; 10: 96-104
115. Thase ME, Rush AJ. Treatment resistant depression. In: Bloom FE, Kupfer DJ, editors. Psychopharmacology: a fourth generation of progress. New York: Raven Press, 1995: 1081-97
116. Kramer BA. Maintenance ECT: a survey of practice. Convulsive Ther 1987; 3: 260-8
117. Meader-Woodruff JH, Gurguis G, Grunhaus L, et al. Multiple depressive episodes and plasma postdexamethasone cortisol levels. Biol Psychiatry 1987; 22: 583-92
118. Thase ME, Kupfer DJ, Buysse DJ, et al. Electroencephalographic sleep profiles in single-episode and recurrent unipolar forms of major depression: 1. Comparison during acute depressive states. Biol Psychiatry 1995; 38: 506-15
119. Thase ME, Simons AD, Reynolds III CF. Abnormal electroencephalographic sleep profiles in major depression. Association with response to cognitive behavior therapy. Arch Gen Psychiatry 1996; 53: 99-108

Correspondence: Dr *Michael E. Thase,* Western Psychiatric Institute and Clinic, Department of Psychiatry, University of Pittsburgh School of Medicine, 3811 O'Hara Street, Pittsburgh, PA 15213, USA.

Substitution Therapy in Patients with Major Depression

Russell T. Joffe

Regional Mood Disorders Program, McMaster University, Hamilton, Canada

It is now generally accepted that unipolar major depressive disorders may have a chronic or recurrent course of illness with a generally poor prognosis.[1-3] Evidence from large naturalistic studies suggest that approximately 1 in 5 patients with a major depressive disorder treated by usual clinical treatment will develop a chronic course of illness with a limited remission of symptomatology.[1,2] Moreover, in those who recover, approximately two-thirds will have a recurrence of major depression within 5 years of follow-up and, at 10 years of follow-up, as many as 80% may have a recurrence.[3,4] Data from these studies also suggest that depression which has not resolved within 6 months of presentation is much more likely to run a chronic and recurrent course.[2,5] If these findings are directly applied to the clinical situation, then it would be important to institute effective antidepressant treatment very early on in the patient's episode so as to enhance the likelihood of response and potentially reduce the risk of chronicity.

Even when antidepressant therapy is optimum, a substantial proportion of patients still do not respond to prescribed antidepressant agents.[6] Fava and Davidson[7] reported that approximately 46% of depressed patients will have no response or only a partial response when given optimal antidepressant therapy. They observed that about 12 to 15% of patients would have only a partial response to antidepressant treatment whereas about one-third would have a complete nonresponse.[7] Their data indicate that even if patients receive effective antidepressant therapy, approximately 1 in 2 will require further intervention to achieve a complete antidepressant response and thereby reduce the long term risks of a chronic and recurrent disorder.[2]

For patients who do not respond to initial antidepressant therapy, there are three broad options available: (i) optimisation; (ii) augmentation/combination treatment; and (iii) substitution. Optimisation and augmentation/combination are considered briefly in section 1 and substitution is discussed in some detail in section 2.

1. Approaches to Treatment-Resistant Depression

1.1 Optimisation

Optimisation refers to providing the patient with optimum antidepressant therapy to ensure that the correct drug is given at the right dosage for the appropriate duration of treatment.[8]

Optimum dosages vary with the different classes of antidepressants. In general, the dosage should be increased to the maximum recommended dose or the highest tolerated dose below that. This is more completely reviewed elsewhere.[8,9]

Regarding the correct duration of antidepressant therapy, it has been suggested that an adequate trial of an antidepressant agent should last ≈12 weeks.[10] However, this duration of trial is often regarded as impractical given that some depressed patients are seriously ill and, therefore, it is generally agreed that a trial of ≥4 weeks and preferably 6 weeks is reasonable.[9] It is important that the trial is of adequate duration to allow for a therapeutic response and, therefore, it is better to err on the side of a longer trial.

To achieve optimum treatment, drug selection should take into account the particular subtype of depression. Certain subtypes of depression may be preferentially responsive to different classes of antidepressants. For example, atypical depression may be more responsive to monoamine oxidase inhibitors (MAOIs)[11,12] or to selective serotonin (5-hydroxytryptamine; 5-HT) reuptake inhibitors (SSRIs)[13] than to other agents. Patients with comorbid anxiety disorders may also be more likely to respond to either MAOIs[14,15] or SSRIs than other agents. Patients with psychotic depression may be more likely to respond either to antidepressants in combination with antipsychotic agents[16] or to electroconvulsive therapy.[17,18] It is likely that in the future, further, more specific, subtypes of depression may be defined which will help to guide antidepressant choice.

1.2 Augmentation/Combination

Augmentation/combination refers to the addition of a second compound to the first antidepressant agent in the hope of boosting therapeutic response. In general, augmentation refers to the addition of a second compound which is not usually regarded as an antidepressant. Such compounds would include lithium, the thyroid hormone triiodothyronine, buspirone, pindolol and the psychostimulants such as methylphenidate.[9] Combination therapy refers to the addition of a second antidepressant agent.[9] Augmentation and combination strategies have been discussed in detail elsewhere.[8,9] In general, they tend to be effective in about 50 to 60% of cases, although the evidence for the efficacy of each strategy varies. There are considerable data to support the efficacy of lithium augmentation.[19] However, for other augmentation and combination strategies, there are fewer studies involving smaller numbers of patients, and these appear to have several methodological limitations.

2. Substitution

Substitution refers to stopping the initial antidepressant agent that failed to elicit a response and starting a trial of a second antidepressant agent. After optimisation, substitution is the most commonly applied approach to treatment-resistant depression. Depending on the initial antidepressant class used, substitution may involve delays in initiation of the second trial owing, in some instances, to the need for dosage tapering before discontinuation and, in other cases, to the need for a period of withholding of therapy in order to achieve a complete washout of the initial agent. Response rates will vary depending on which is the initial and which is the substituting antidepressant. In general, changing to an antidepressant of a different class for the second antidepressant trial yields an enhanced rate of therapeutic response.

If the initial unsuccessful antidepressant is a tricyclic antidepressant (TCA), studies indicate that substitution with a second TCA generally results in a clinical response in 20 to 30% of patients.[13] Substitution with other classes of antidepressants will lead to substantially higher rates of response, approximately 50 to 60%, for example after switches to an SSRI,[20] MAOI,[18,21] or to novel agents such as amfebutamone (bupropion).[22]

If the initial antidepressant used is an SSRI, then there is the option of a second trial with another SSRI. Three studies[23-25] have now examined responses to a second SSRI after a lack of response to a first SSRI in patients with major depression. First, Zarate et al.[25] showed that 42% (13 of 31) of inpatients who had not responded to fluoxetine had a subsequent response to sertraline. In 2 outpatient populations, Joffe et al.,[24] and Thase et al.,[23] observed response rates of 51 and 63%, respectively, when a second SSRI was tried after a first SSRI failed to elicit adequate responses. In a related study, Brown and Harrison,[26] reported a 71% response rate to sertraline in a group of outpatients who had been intolerant but not treatment resistant with a trial of fluoxetine.

Taken together, these data suggest that the overall response rate to a second SSRI after the first has failed to elicit a response is approximately the same as that which would be expected 4 to 6 weeks after substitution with an alternative class of antidepressant. Thus, it is reasonable to expect similar response rates of about 50 to 60% when an SSRI is substituted with a TCA, amfebutamone, or the newer agents venlafaxine or nefazodone.[27] Although it is reasonable to expect that with the switches to alternative classes of antidepressant drugs, response rates would be enhanced, there are limited data on which to base these assumptions. However, anecdotal evidence from clinical practice suggests that response rates of 50 to 60% are expected when newer antidepressants such as amfebutamone and venlafaxine are substituted after failure of an initial SSRI.

When switching from a TCA to an MAOI, response rates of 57 to 65% have been reported.[20,22] While there are limited data on switches between MAOIs and other classes of antidepressants or on success rates with TCAs after failure of an MAOI, anecdotal evidence from clinical practice suggests that the response rates would be similar to those of other substitution strategies, in the range of 50 to 60%.

Thase and Rush[27] have defined the advantages of substitution with monotherapy as compared with the use of augmentation strategies. These include that fewer dose-limiting adverse events may occur during monotherapy than during augmentation therapy, a possible different mechanism of action, less expense in administering the regimens and lower risks of drug-drug interactions. Substitution may involve the complete discontinuation of the initial drug, the use of a washout period where appropriate and then initiation of the second compound. Often, this unnecessarily prolongs the time to the onset of therapeutic response, such that an overlap of treatment with the first and substituting antidepressant may be help to speed up the onset of a treatment response. Of course, the appropriateness of use of a period of overlap of two drugs depends on which specific antidepressants are being discontinued and initiated.

With a switch between SSRIs and TCAs, attention must be paid to the pharmacokinetic interaction between these two drug classes.[28] SSRIs are potent inhibitors of the cytochrome P450 (CYP) hepatic microsomal enzyme system. These enzymes are responsible for the metabolism of a broad range of drugs, including the TCAs. Various SSRIs will differentially affect enzymes of this microsomal system, in particular CYP2D6 and CYP3A4 enzymes. As a result, coadministration of an SSRI with a TCA will lead to inhibition of metabolism of the TCA, resulting in elevated blood concentrations of the tricyclic agent and its metabolites.[28] Consequently, if dosages of TCAs are not adjusted downwards before the addition of the SSRI, toxicity may supervene.

When switching from a TCA to an SSRI, it is appropriate to lower the TCA dose by at least 50% for a period of 1 week before introducing the SSRI. Once the SSRI is introduced, it is best to wait for 5 days while obtaining steady-state concentrations and closely monitoring the clinical status of the patient one can obtain a plasma concentration of the TCA to determine that toxic concentrations have not been reached if the clinical situation demands. Thereafter, the TCA can be tapered and discontinued and the remainder of the SSRI trial can proceed.

If a patients is switched from an SSRI to a TCA, the TCA should be initiated slowly so as to ensure that toxic concentrations are not reached before the SSRI is discontinued and eliminated from the body. This may take longer with fluoxetine, which has a substantially longer half-life than other SSRIs. In this regard, it is very helpful to use the secondary amine TCAs, e.g. nortriptyline or desipramine, both of which can be reliably measured in plasma to ensure appropriate and clinically well tolerated plasma concentrations are achieved.

In the event of a switch in either direction between SSRIs and first generation MAOIs, serious pharmacodynamic interactions can result in the serotonin syndrome.[29] This syndrome, caused by the accumulation of serotonin in the CNS, leads to a heterogeneous group of symptoms, most commonly fever as well as neurological and gastrointestinal symptoms. The serotonin syndrome is commonly fatal. To ensure that the patient is not at risk, there should be an adequate washout between the first and second drug. In the case of switching from an MAOI to an SSRI, a minimum of 2 weeks' washout is required. In the other direction, switching from an SSRI to an MAOI, a 2-week washout should occur after discontinuation of the SSRI before the start of MAOI use, except when the SSRI is fluoxetine. Because of the longer half-life of fluoxetine, a longer washout of at least 5 weeks should be undertaken before the MAOI can be introduced.

Caution is also needed when switching between MAOIs and TCAs, to ensure that the serotonin syndrome does not occur.[30] It is generally clinically accepted that a greater danger exists when switching from an MAOI to a TCA, so that a period of 2 weeks' washout is required when this change occurs. In the opposite direction, washout is generally recommended, although in some cases, the MAOI can be introduced more quickly and MAOIs have also been used in combination with TCAs in patients who are refractory to monotherapy. It is important that when using TCAs that are more serotonergic, such as clomipramine, that the full 2-week washout period be carefully observed.[30]

It has been conventional clinical practice that, when switching between two SSRIs, a 2-week washout be observed with all the SSRIs except for fluoxetine (for which a 5-week washout should occur). In fact, clinical experience suggests otherwise. It appears that an immediate switch from one SSRI to another can occur with relative safety, although there may be temporary, usually benign, exacerbations of serotonergic symptoms.

Much less is known about switches between the newer types of antidepressants, particularly venlafaxine and nefazodone. In general, pharmacokinetic interactions between venlafaxine and other antidepressants, particularly the TCAs, are less common than with other agents because venlafaxine is not a potent an inhibitor of hepatic microsomal enzymes as are the SSRIs.[31]

3. Conclusion

Substitution is an alternative when a patient does not respond to the first antidepressant that is tried. Substitution is certainly comparable in efficacy to other strategies such as augmentation or combination therapies, although optimisation of antidepressant treatment is always the first approach that should be carefully exercised.

There are few trials that have systematically evaluated the various substitution options after failure of the first antidepressant trial with various classes of antidepressants. Further studies of this nature are urgently needed. Furthermore, there are few studies directly comparing substitution with augmentation or combination treatments. Randomised controlled trials of this nature are urgently required to assist development of a rational treatment algorithm for refractory depression.

Substitution of drugs from one antidepressant class for another is generally well tolerated, even in the absence of a complete washout. However, if first generation MAOIs are involved, then extreme caution must be exercised because of potentially fatal drug interactions between these agents and either the TCAs or the SSRIs. When switching between other classes of antidepressants, temporary exacerbation of adverse effects may occur. Also, discontinuation symptoms from the first antidepressant may occur, especially if it is rapidly withdrawn. Those symptoms may be mistaken for adverse effects of the substituting agent. However, with careful attention to potential drug interactions, the patient is usually not endangered by drug substitution, although they may experience the inconvenience of a temporary exacerbation of symptoms.

References

1. Keller MB, Lavori PW, Wright J, et al. The persistent risk of chronicity in recurrent episodes of non-bipolar major depressive disorder: a prospective follow-up. Am J Psychiatry 1986; 143: 24-8
2. Keller MB, Lavori PW, Mueller TI, et al. Time to recovery, chronicity and level of psychopathology in major depression: a five year prospective follow-up of 431 subjects. Arch Gen Psychiatry 1992; 49: 809-16
3. Keller MB. Depression: a long-term illness. Br J Psychiatry 1994; 165 Suppl. 26: 9-15
4. Mueller TI, Keller MB, Leon AC, et al. Recovery after five years of unremitting major depressive disorder. Arch Gen Psychiatry 1996; 53: 794-9
5. Kupfer DJ, Frank E, Perel JN. The advantage of early treatment intervention in recurrent depression. Arch Gen Psychiatry 1989; 46: 771-5
6. Joffe RT, Levitt AJ. Antidepressant failure: augmentation or substitution? J Psychiatr Neurosci 1995; 15: 7-9
7. Fava M, Davidson KG. Definition and epidemiology of treatment-resistant depression. Psychiatr Clin North Am 1996; 2: 179-98
8. Phillips KA, Nierenberg AA. The assessment treatment of refractory depression. J Clin Psychiatry 1994; 55: 20-6
9. Sokolov STH, Joffe RT. Practical guidelines for combination drug therapy of treatment-resistant depression. CNS Drugs 1995; 4: 341-50
10. Minter RE, Mandel M. The treatment of psychotic major depressive disorder with drugs and electroconvulsive therapy. J Nerv Ment Dis 1979; 167 (12): 726-33
11. Liebowitz MR, Quitkin FM, Stewart JW, et al. Antidepressant specificity in atypical depression. Arch Gen Psychiatry 1988; 45 (2): 129-237
12. Quitkin FM, McGrath PJ, Stewart JW, et al. Atypical depression, panic attacks and response to imipramine and phenelzine: a replication. Arch Gen Psychiatry 1990; 47: 935-41
13. Reimherr SW, Wood DR, Beasley D, et al. Characteristics of responders to fluoxetine. Psychopharmacol Bull 1984; 21: 70-2
14. Nies A, Robertson DS, Lambon KR, et al. The efficacy of the monoamine oxidase inhibitor phenelzine: dose effect and predictions of response. In: Boissier JR, Hippius A, Bichop P, editors. Neuropsychopharmacology. Amsterdam: Excerpta Medica, 1975: 765-70
15. Robinson DS, Kayser A, Corcella J, et al. Panic attacks in outpatients with depression: response to antidepressant treatment. Psychopharmacol Bull 1985; 21: 562-7
16. Kaskey GB, Nasr S, Meltzer HY. Drug treatment in delusional depression. Psychiatry Res 1980; 2 (3): 267-77
17. Minter RE, Mandel MR. A prospective study of the treatment of psychotic depression. Am J Psychiatry 1979; 136 (11): 1470-2
18. McGrath PJ, Stewart JM, Harrison W, et al. Treatment of tricyclic refractory depression with a monoamine oxidase inhibitor antidepressant. Psychopharmacol 1987; 23: 169-72
19. Price LH. Pharmacological strategies in refractory depression. In: Post R, editor. Treatment of refractory mood disorders. APA Review of Psychiatry. Vol. 9. Washington, DC: Am Psychiatry Assoc Press, 1990; 116-31
20. Beasley CM, Sayler NE, Cunningham GE, et al. Fluoxetine in tricyclic refractory major depressive disorder. J Aff Disord 1990; 20: 193-200
21. Thase ME, Frank E, Mallinger A, et al. Treatment of imipramine-resistant recurrent depression. III. Efficacy of monoamine oxidase inhibitors. J Clin Psychiatry 1992; 53 (1): 5-11
22. Stern WC, Harto-Truax N, Bauer N. Efficacy of bupropion in tricyclic-resistant or intolerant patients. J Clin Psychiatry 1983; 44: 5 (2): 148-52
23. Thase ME, Blongren SL, Birkett MA, et al. Fluoxetine treatment of patients of major depressive disorder who failed initial treatment with sertraline. J Clin Psychiatry 1997; 58: 16-21

24. Joffe RT, Levitt AJ, Sokolov STH, et al. Response to an open trial of a second SSRI in major depression. J Clin Psychiatry 1996; 57: 114-5
25. Zarate CA Jr, Kando JC, Tohen M, et al. Does intolerance or lack of response with fluoxetine predict the same will happen with sertraline? J Clin Psychiatry 1996; 57: 67-71
26. Brown WA, Harrison W. Are patients who are intolerant to one serotonin selective reuptake inhibitor intolerant to another? J Clin Psychiatry 1995; 56: 30-4
27. Thase ME, Rush AJ. When at first you don't succeed: sequential strategies for antidepressant non-responders. J Clin Psychiatry 1997; 58 Suppl. 13: 23-9
28. Otton SV, Wu D, Joffe RT, et al. Inhibition by fluoxetine of cytochrome P450 2D6 activity. Clin Pharmacol Ther 1993; 53: 401-9
29. Sternbach H. The serotonin syndrome. Am J Psychiatry 1991; 148: 705-13
30. White K, Simpson G. The combined use of MAOIs and tricyclics. J Clin Psychiatry 1984; 45 (7 Pt 2): 67-9
31. Ereshefsky L. Drug-drug interactions involving antidepressants: focus on venlafaxine. J Clin Psychopharmacol 1996; 16 Suppl. 2: 37S-53

Correspondence: Dr *Russell T. Joffe*, McMaster University, 1200 Main St W, Room 2E1, Hamilton, Ontario L8N 3Z5, Canada.
E-mail: joffe@fhs.csu.mcmaster.ca

Risk of Adverse Events with the Use of Augmentation Therapy for the Treatment of Resistant Depression

Isaac Schweitzer and *Virginia Tuckwell*

University of Melbourne and Professorial Unit, The Melbourne Clinic, Richmond, Victoria, Australia

The addition of a second agent to an existing antidepressant regimen, with the aim of achieving an improved clinical response, is referred to as augmentation therapy. This should be distinguished from combination therapy where 2 or more medications are used together to effect a synergistic response and adjunctive therapy where a second agent is added to reduce associated symptoms such as anxiety or insomnia. Augmentation therapy is considered for those situations where depression is either treatment-resistant, or partially and/or insufficiently, responsive to treatment. It may also occur in an attempt to accelerate treatment response.

Augmenting antidepressant response has proven to be an increasingly popular clinical strategy and there are now claims for many drugs to have such an effect. The principle reason for the rise in augmentation therapy is the continuing failure of existing antidepressant treatments to successfully treat all depressed patients. Between 10 and 30% of depressed patients are classified as treatment-resistant and another 12 to 15% are only partial responders to adequate therapy.[1-3]

The clinical effect of augmentation may be through a synergistic effect or via different neurotransmitter and second messenger systems. The actual mechanisms of action are not known but are hypothesised with varying amounts of evidence. However, combinations of drugs may also increase the risk of adverse effects, either through interference with the efficacy of the primary drug, potentiation of existing adverse effects, or large alterations in plasma concentrations of either drug. It is important that clinicians are aware of potential risks of augmentation therapy.

This review critically assesses current scientific evidence pertaining to the tolerabilities of augmentation therapies. A large proportion of current data supporting a variety of augmentation strategies is either anecdotal or derived from case reports. There are few controlled studies; hence, data regarding drug tolerability as well as response are scarce, and the frequency of adverse effects cannot be calculated. Data from controlled studies, where available, have been emphasised.

1. Lithium Augmentation

The most intensively studied augmentation strategy is the addition of lithium to currently existing tricyclic antidepressant therapy. Studies, both open and controlled, have demonstrated consistent and significant responses to lithium augmentation of antidepressant treatment.[4-7] The dosage of lithium carbonate used has usually been between 500 to 1200 mg/day, subsequently adjusted to achieve adequate plasma lithium concentrations if considered necessary.

Published data concerning lithium augmentation of monoamine oxidase inhibitor (MAOI) therapy are limited. There are no placebo-controlled studies, although clinical perception through open trials and case reports is of similar response rates to the tricyclic antidepressants.[8,9]

Serious adverse reactions have been reported rarely in the extensive investigation of lithium augmentation of tricyclic antidepressants. Adverse effects are those that would be expected with the individual drugs – the anticholinergic and cardiovascular adverse effects of the tricyclic antidepressants, and nausea, diarrhoea, abdominal pain, muscle weakness and fine tremor with lithium. To date, there have been reports of mood elevation after the addition of lithium to a cyclic antidepressant in 6 patients: 2 (in a study of 9) with a history of bipolar disorder;[10] 2 patients with unipolar disorder who experienced a hypomanic episode when on the tricyclic antidepressant alone;[11] a patient with a history of psychosis and bipolar disorder;[12] and 1 patient (unipolar/bipolar not specified) in a study of 51 elderly people.[13] The plasma concentrations of the tricyclic antidepressants were not reported. Mood elevation has also been seen following discontinuation of lithium augmentation of desipramine and nortriptyline.[14] We can therefore conclude that lithium augmentation is relatively well tolerated and the dangers are no greater than using these medications on their own.

There are also no reports of serious adverse events when lithium has been added to MAOI therapy. There is no indication that the risks of hypertensive crises are greater when lithium is added.

Response to lithium augmentation of selective serotonin (5-hydroxytryptamine; 5-HT) reuptake inhibitor (SSRI) therapy in case reports and open treatment trials has been reported by a number of groups.[15-18] In 1 of 2 published, double-blind, placebo-controlled trials of lithium augmentation of SSRIs, lithium was found to be superior to placebo in 62 patients: there were no withdrawals in the fluoxetine-lithium group due to adverse effects.[19] This positive finding was replicated by the second study using citalopram in 69 patients: the authors reported no evidence of accentuation or aggravation of adverse events.[20]

With lithium augmentation of SSRIs there are reports of occasional but significant complications involving a central serotonin syndrome, i.e. a toxic serotonergic hypersensitivity, marked by confusion, restlessness, myoclonus, hyperreflexia, diaphoresis, shivering, tremor, hypomania, diarrhoea and possibly death.[21-23] There are 2 reported cases of lithium augmentation inducing mania or hypomania.[24] One case of absence seizures,[25] and 1 of delirium[26] have also been reported. These reactions have occurred both with therapeutic plasma concentrations and when plasma lithium has risen to toxic concentrations (without physical symptoms) with fluoxetine. Clinicians must be mindful that, although a serotonin syndrome is rare and the risks with the other SSRIs and venlafaxine and nefazodone may not be comparable to that of fluoxetine, any combination of drugs which together increase serotonin neurotransmission via different mechanisms of action theoretically has the potential to cause a serotonin syndrome.[23]

CNS adverse effects occur more frequently in elderly patients using lithium (tremor and delirium). In addition, renal as well as thyroid abnormalities and dose-limiting adverse effects (neuromuscular or neurological) have been reported when lithium carbonate was added to existing antidepressant treatment in elderly participants, even at therapeutic concentrations of lithium.[13,27] In 1 of these studies, 50% of patients experienced adverse effects, and they were older than those not experiencing adverse effects.[27] In the other study, 11% of patients experienced neurotoxicity.[13] There appears to be a risk of recurrence of depression and subsequent lithium resistance in the elderly when lithium augmentation is discontinued.[28]

Studies that have shown positive effects of lithium augmentation have generally achieved plasma concentrations of lithium within the normal range (0.4 to 1 mmol/L). However, there appears to be no correlation of response to lithium concentrations:[5,6,18,29] there are reports of a small number of patients responding to lower concentrations of lithium, such as 0.3 and 0.54 mmol/L.[5,17,18,27] de Montigny[30] suggests there may be a plateau effect and titrating concentrations up may only increase the risk of adverse effects.

The site of pharmacological response produced by lithium augmentation remains unclear, mainly because of the multiple effects of lithium. Lithium carbonate has been shown not to modify antidepressant plasma concentrations.[5,29,31,32] It is postulated that the rapid response to lithium augmentation is due to presynaptic serotonergic enhancement of antidepressant-induced sensitisation of postsynaptic serotonin receptors.[5] Other neurotransmitter systems, particularly noradrenergic transmission and second messenger systems have also been implicated.[6,33-36]

2. Thyroid Hormone Augmentation

Tri-iodothyronine (T_3) added to imipramine was found to enhance and accelerate recovery in patients described as experiencing retarded depression.[37] As cited in a review of thyroid hormones in the treatment of affective disorders, a number of studies replicated this work, most of them substantiating it.[38] Other studies have yielded mixed results: some have found a lack of efficacy of T_3,[39,40] 1 suggested particular efficacy in subclinical hypothyroidism[41] and another indicated that T_3 was equally effective as lithium.[42]

Plasma concentrations of tricyclic antidepressants are not altered by T_3.[38,43] Desipramine was found to have no significant effect on thyroid indices.[44,45] Therapeutic dosages of T_3 (25 to 50 μg/day) or thyroxine (T_4) [100 μg/day] appear well tolerated with standard doses of tricyclic antidepressants.[38] The combination does not increase the adverse effects of either drug or cause additive effects; the most common adverse effects reported have been drowsiness, dizziness, dry mouth, tremor, anxiety, agitation and insomnia, but are usually mild or absent.[37,38,46] Cardiotoxicity, known to be an effect of both thyroid hormones and tricyclic antidepressants, has not been reported with T_3 or T_4 augmentation.[38,43] However, caution is advised in prescribing thyroid hormones for elderly patients or those with cardiac insufficiency.[46]

There is a paucity of controlled studies of MAOIs and thyroid hormones. A single case study reported clinical improvement when T_3 was added to phenelzine with no significant adverse effects.[47] MAOIs and thyroid hormones affect the adrenergic system, but no adverse effects are found in the literature.[38]

Case studies of T_3 augmentation of fluoxetine suggest it may be effective.[48,49] Double-blind studies are still required with each of the SSRIs before any conclusions can be drawn regarding tolerability or efficacy.

A number of hypotheses regarding the mechanisms underlying thyroid hormone potentiation of tricyclic antidepressants have been postulated as follows:

- in patients who are euthyroid, the addition of T_3 may bring them to a previously not attained optimal state[43]
- T_3 enhances receptor response synergistically with increased neurotransmitter concentrations induced by the antidepressant[37]
- there is evidence that thyroid hormones enhance central β-adrenergic receptor function.[50]

No consistent effect on adrenergic receptor number and function has been demonstrated, but this does not exclude the possible potentiation of adrenergic receptors by T_3.[51]

The evidence to date of the tolerability and efficacy of thyroid hormone augmentation of antidepressant treatment is encouraging. Routine monitoring of thyroid indices and low dosages (25 to 50 μg/day) of T_3 augmentation in euthyroid patients for 2 to 3 weeks are recommended. Such an approach reduces the risk of inducing hypothyroidism via a negative feedback effect on the thyroid axis.[1] Others advocate maintaining the T_3 for longer periods, including continuing for 60 days if the depression responds.[52] Long term studies are not available.

3. Tricyclic Augmentation of Specific Serotonin Reuptake Inhibitors

Tricyclic augmentation of SSRIs has become a popular approach amongst clinicians despite limited research. The catalyst was a finding of an improvement in 87% of patients when fluoxetine was added to ongoing non–MAOI antidepressant treatment in a retrospective study.[53] This was substantiated in the open addition of a tricyclic antidepressant to fluoxetine[54] and a combination of nortriptyline and either sertraline or fluoxetine, with or without concurrent lithium.[55] No adverse effects were reported in these studies. Low doses of tricyclic antidepressants were used because of the possibility of elevation of serum tricyclic antidepressant concentrations and subsequent toxicity. However, in another study, of 12 patients taking a combination of fluoxetine and desipramine, 2 were removed from study because of adverse effects: agitation, blurred vision, panic attacks and micropsia.[16]

In a single case report, a 60% increase in steady-state desipramine concentrations was measured after the addition of sertraline 50 mg/day.[56] The patient experienced no adverse effects and felt more motivated than on previous successful therapy.

A serious concern with using a tricyclic antidepressant to augment an SSRI is the effect of the SSRI on the cytochrome P450 (CYP) isoenzyme system and the resulting significant increase in tricyclic antidepressant blood concentrations. All SSRIs potentially inhibit the CYP2D6 isoenzyme, and thus the metabolism of other drugs, including tricyclic antidepressants, which are cleared by this system. The SSRIs differ in their effects on specific CYP enzymes. Paroxetine and fluoxetine are potent inhibitors of CYP2D6, whereas sertraline, citalopram and fluoxetine have a weaker effect (and nefazodone and venlafaxine weaker still).[57]

Coadministration of SSRIs and tricyclic antidepressants can lead to potentially toxic plasma concentrations of the tricyclic antidepressant with significant clinical consequences, such as delirium and grand mal seizures,[58] and psychomotor retardation, decreased energy and drowsiness.[59] Weilburg et al.[54] reported that toxic plasma tricyclic antidepressant concentrations were not observed in patients taking low doses of tricyclic antidepressants, although the plasma concentrations were higher than expected. They did however recommend initiation of tricyclic antidepressant augmentation (desipramine or nortriptyline) at low dosages (25 to 50 mg/day), with plasma monitoring.

These cases have all been with fluoxetine and it is likely that those SSRIs with weaker inhibition of CYP2D6 will not raise tricyclic antidepressant concentrations to the degree that fluoxetine does.[60] There is also the potential for drug-drug interactions with other CYP isoenzymes. For example, nefazodone and fluvoxamine are potent inhibitors of CYP3A4 and fluvoxamine also of CYP1A2; the other SSRIs have moderate to minimal effects and venlafaxine has minimal effects on these two systems.[57,60,61]

The reported enhancement of antidepressant response by SSRI and tricyclic antidepressant augmentation of TCA and SSRI therapy, respectively, may be due to an interaction between the serotonergic and adrenergic systems. There may be a synergistic effect of acceleration of ß-adrenoceptor down-regulation and enhancement of serotonergic activity.[55,62,63] Elevated plasma tricyclic antidepressant concentrations were not considered to be causal in effect by these investigators.

4. Pindolol Augmentation

Interest has been generated recently by reports of rapid potentiation of the SSRI antidepressant effect when pindolol has been added to therapy. Based on preclinical evidence that blocking serotonin 5-HT_{1A} somatodendritic receptors might augment the efficacy of serotonin uptake blockers, Artigas and colleagues[64] augmented SSRI or MAOI treatment with pindolol, a β-blocker which shows strong antagonist activity at 5-HT_{1A} receptors. In their open study, 7.5mg pindolol daily was added to a regimen of paroxetine, phenelzine, fluvoxamine or imipramine. The results showed a rapid, full recovery in 5 of 8 patients whose mood disorder had shown a partial or no response previously.

Further studies of concurrent treatment substantiated these results.[65,66] However, patients taking sertraline in one study did not show the same response.[65] It was postulated that as sertraline has a lesser affinity for the CYP2D6 isoenzymes than do fluoxetine and paroxetine, plasma concentrations of pindolol may have been lower in this group. Two double-blind, placebo controlled, studies of fluoxetine plus pindolol found neither any difference in the rate of response between the groups[67] nor in differences in average time to remission and overall disease response between groups.[68]

The investigators have noted that the general tolerability of these combinations was good, although 1 patient (of 9 taking paroxetine in a total of 19 taking SSRIs plus pindolol) became manic.[65] In a double-blind placebo controlled study with fluoxetine, adverse events were reported in 9.1% of patients, mainly nausea and diarrhoea; heart rate reduction was between 3 to 8 beats/min and there was no change in blood pressure.[66]

The most recent studies in this area have reported positive results with combinations (not augmentation) of pindolol and paroxetine,[69] fluoxetine,[70] buspirone and fluvoxamine,[71] and nefazodone.[72] Two placebo-controlled studies of pindolol with paroxetine and with fluoxetine, reported no differences in the incidence or severity of adverse effects between active and placebo groups. A small number of participants were withdrawn due to adverse effects: 2 of 40 in each of the active and the placebo groups in the paroxetine study; 5 of 56 taking pindolol plus fluoxetine; and 1 of 56 in the comparison placebo group in the second study.[69,70] Nausea, diarrhoea and headache were the most common adverse effects and tended to be transient.[69]

The SSRIs are believed to desensitise 5-HT_{1A} autoreceptors which control cell firing and terminal serotonin release by a negative feedback mechanism.[64] Tolerance develops, which pindolol may hasten and increase by blocking 5-HT_{1A} autoreceptors and preventing the inhibitory action.[64] This hypothesis is still under discussion. β-Blockers have been implicated in causing depression and, while a recent review of the literature indicates there is inadequate evidence to support this, the authors also believe it cannot be discounted.[73] The benefits of pindolol augmentation, its tolerability and any mechanism of action are still to be elucidated.

5. Carbamazepine and Valproic Acid (Valproate Sodium) Augmentation

The usefulness of the addition of the mood stabilisers carbamazepine and valproic acid (valproate sodium) to antidepressant therapy has not been well studied and there are no controlled studies to support these combinations. Case reports indicate marked improvement after the addition of carbamazepine to clomipramine[74] and valproic acid to fluoxetine or fluvoxamine (both in elderly patients).[75] The addition of phenelzine or tranylcypromine to carbamazepine, with or without lithium, resulted in substantial improvement in 4 of 10 patients, despite having failed to respond to the same MAOI without carbamazepine previously.[76]

The literature suggests caution when using either carbamazepine or valproic acid in combination with a tricyclic antidepressant with regard to pharmacokinetic interactions.[32,76,77] Carbamazepine is a potent enzyme inducer whereas valproic acid is an enzyme inhibitor. The former lowers tricyclic antidepressant concentrations and the latter probably raises antidepressant concentrations.[32] Carbamazepine may increase hydroxy-tricyclic antidepressant metabolites and thus may be cardiotoxic.[77]

6. Augmentation with the Psychostimulants

Methylphenidate has been reported to be useful in refractory depression, although there have been no controlled studies.[32] A small early study described the successful addition of methylphenidate 20mg to imipramine in psychotic depression. Methylphenidate increased plasma tricyclic antidepressant concentrations and the authors hypothesised a mechanism of action involving enzymatic inhibition by methylphenidate.[78]

A retrospective study showed 1 of 5 patients' depression responded when methylphenidate or dextroamphetamine was added to MAOIs alone, and 5 of 8 patients' depression responded when added methylphenidate or dextroamphetamine was to a combination of MAOI and tricyclic antidepressants.[79] The most frequent adverse effect was orthostatic hypotension. In a complex study of the effects of the addition of a stimulant, either dextroamphetamine or pemoline, to an MAOI, 25 (78%) of 32 patients' condition responded for at least 6 months, with 31% of patients reporting a maintained improvement. No hypertensive crises were reported, although the authors warned of the need to take precautions in using this combination.[80]

An open trial of methylphenidate augmentation of paroxetine and fluoxetine proved to be efficacious, rapid and well tolerated.[81] The investigators noted that the improvement could be due to increased plasma concentrations of the SSRIs, treatment of unrecognised asthenia or even a placebo effect. Methylphenidate has a number of neurochemical actions, including influencing dopaminergic and noradrenergic transmission.

Methylphenidate elevates mood by releasing catecholamines and blocking their reuptake. Stimulants may increase blood concentrations of other drugs and risk hypertensive crises in combination with MAOIs. However, data are not available or are limited on drug interactions.

The adverse effects of these stimulants, including hypertensive and hyperthermic crises[79] and the risks of abuse and dependence potential and withdrawal reactions are an additional consideration, particularly in combination with other antidepressants.[46]

7. Buspirone

Open studies suggest buspirone augmentation of SSRIs may be useful in treatment-resistant depression, but again the data are limited. A full or partial recovery was demonstrated after the open addition of buspirone to fluoxetine,[82,83] to fluoxetine or fluvoxamine,[84] and to trazodone in 2 geriatric patients.[85] The adverse effects in these trials were reported to be minimal and included dizziness, nervousness, restlessness, nausea and headache.[86] However, buspirone has been reported to induce mania,[86] euphoria[85] and a serotonin syndrome after ingestion of higher than prescribed doses of citalopram and buspirone.[87]

Buspirone is a partial 5-HT_{1A} agonist and with an SSRI would enhance serotonin transmission at several points.[84] This could potentiate SSRI adverse effects such as apathy or sexual dysfunction. Howland[88] has proposed a possible role for the buspirone metabolite 1-(2-pyrimidinyl)-piperazine, which is an α_2-adrenergic antagonist enhancing the release of noradrenaline (norepinephrine).

8. Discussion

Most of the evidence supporting augmentation agents is anecdotal and in the form of case reports. Few well performed double-blind placebo controlled studies of augmentation therapy have been carried out to determine tolerability as well as efficacy. There is a body of scientific evidence supporting lithium and T_3 as well tolerated and effective augmentation agents.

Case reports and open studies indicate augmentation with buspirone, carbamazepine, valproic acid, methylphenidate and amphetamine may be effective and cause minimal adverse effects. However, there is no empirical evidence supporting this. There is also no empirical evidence for the tolerability and efficacy of the addition of a tricyclic to an SSRI. Recent work is finding evidence supporting a role for pindolol combination with regard to tolerability and efficacy.[69-71]

Because of possible complex pharmacodynamic and pharmacokinetic interactions, augmentation therapy is not without its potential complications, although reports have been relatively uncommon. Lithium toxicity and the serotonergic syndrome have been reported to occur when lithium has been added to an SSRI. It is therefore advisable to add lithium to an SSRI with caution, commencing with low doses and careful monitoring of serum concentrations and clinical state of the patient. Lithium augmentation requires the usual follow-up testing of plasma concentrations every 3 or 4 months, and yearly checks of thyroid and renal function.

An SSRI and tricyclic antidepressant combination can result in toxic concentrations of the tricyclic and there are several reports of serious complications, such as delirium and convulsions. Close plasma monitoring of the tricyclic together with administration of low doses of tricyclic antidepressants is essential if this strategy is embarked upon. Electrocardiographic monitoring is also advised as tricyclic toxicity will result in cardiac abnormalities.

Data are not available to indicate whether adverse effects are related to faster rather than slower augmentation. Augmentation agents tend to be initiated at relatively low doses. The potential for drug-drug interactions occurs when a new drug is initiated, when the dose of any drug is altered, or when a drug is ceased. Adverse events that have been reported have appeared anytime from between a couple of days and a few weeks, sometimes months, after initiation of the augmentation therapy; however, they have not always been documented.

There is evidence that there are neither differences between men and women in the development of adverse events, nor between unipolar and unipolar patients; however, adverse effects may limit the usefulness of some augmentation strategies in the elderly.[89] There is an even greater paucity of work in augmentation therapy in geriatric patients (who are considered to be at greater risk of interactions) than in younger age groups, so it is not possible to make any firm conclusions, but caution is advisable.

Unfortunately, the topic of augmentation therapy is permeated with more mythology than scientific data. Considerable caution should be exercised when considering embarking upon psychotropic drug combinations, and it should be done with the full knowledge of the compounds involved and their pharmacological properties. The clinician should also avoid 'researching' the effects of drug combinations on his patients in the clinical setting and should apply well established and proven approaches which are known to be relatively well tolerated.

If an augmentation strategy which is not well established for efficacy and/or tolerability is used, informed consent should be obtained from the patient after discussing risks, benefits and possible adverse effects of this strategy. When appropriate, clinicians should obtain a second opinion from a senior colleague. Such procedures can also be monitored more easily if in-patients are involved.

References

1. Nierenberg AA, Amsterdam JD. Treatment-resistant depression: definition and treatment approaches. J Clin Psychiatry 1990; 51: 39-47
2. Burrows GD, Norman TR, Judd FK. Definition and differential diagnosis of treatment-resistant depression. Int Clin Psychopharmacol 1994; 9: 5-10
3. Fava M, Davidson KG. Definition and epidemiology of treatment-resistant depression. Psych Clin North Am 1996; 19: 179-200
4. Lingjaerde O, Edlund AH, Gormsen CA, et al. The effect of lithium carbonate in combination with tricyclic antidepressants in endogenous depression. Acta Psychiatr Scand 1974; 50: 233-42
5. de Montigny C, Grunberg F, Mayer A, et al. Lithium induces rapid relief of depression in tricyclic antidepressant drug non-responders. Br J Psychiatry 1981; 138: 252-6
6. Heninger GR, Charney DS, Sternberg DE. Lithium carbonate augmentation of antidepressant treatment. Arch Gen Psychiatry 1983; 40: 1335-42
7. Austin M-PV, Souza FGM, Goodwin GM. Lithium augmentation in antidepressant-resistant patients: a quantitative analysis. Br J Psychiatry 1991; 159: 510-4
8. Nelson JC, Byck R. Rapid response to lithium in phenelzine non-responders. Br J Psychiatry 1982; 141: 85-6
9. Price LH, Charney DS, Heninger GR. Efficacy of lithium-tranylcypromine treatment in refractory depression. Am J Psychiatry 1985; 142: 619-23
10. Louie AK, Meltzer HY. Lithium potentiation of antidepressant treatment. J Clin Psychopharmacol 1984; 4: 316-21
11. Price LH, Charney DS, Heninger GR. Manic symptoms following addition of lithium to antidepressant treatment. J Clin Psychopharmacol 1984; 4: 361-2
12. DeLisle JD. Rapid switch in a bipolar patient during lithium-tricyclic therapy. Am J Psychiatry 1986 Oct; 143 (10): 1326-7
13. van Marwijk HWJ, Bekker FM, Nolen WA, et al. Lithium augmentation in geriatric depression. J Affective Dis 1990; 20: 217-23
14. Hoaken PCS, Hoaken P. Undue mood elevation in unipolar patients following cessation of lithium augmentation treatment: implications for the understanding of mood disorders. Can J Psychiatry 1996; 46-8
15. Pope HG, McElroy SL, Nixon RA. Possible synergism between fluoxetine and lithium in refractory depression. Am J Psychiatry 1988; 145: 1292-4
16. Fava M, Rosenbaum JF, McGrath PJ, et al. Lithium and tricyclic augmentation of fluoxetine treatment for resistant major depression: a double-blind, controlled study. Am J Psychiatry 1994; 151: 1372-4
17. Ontiveros A, Fontaine R, Elie R. The combination treatment was more effective than individual therapies alone: refractory depression - the addition of lithium to fluoxetine or desipramine. Acta Psychiatr Scand 1991; 83: 188-92
18. Dinan TG. Lithium augmentation in sertraline-resistant depression: a preliminary dose-response study. Acta Psychiatr Scand 1993; 88 (4): 300-1
19. Katona CLE, Abou-Saleh MT, Harrison DA, et al. Placebo-controlled trial of lithium augmentation of fluoxetine and lofepramine. Br J Psychiatry 1995; 166: 80-6

20. Baumann P, Nil R, Souche A, et al. A double-blind, placebo-controlled study of citalopram with and without lithium in the treatment of therapy-resistant depressive patients: a clinical, pharmacokinetic, and pharmacogenetic investigation. J Clin Psychopharmacol 1996; 16: 307-14
21. Sternbach H. The serotonin syndrome. Am J Psychiatry 1991; 148: 705-13
22. Muly EC, McDonald W, Steffens D, et al. Serotonin syndrome produced by a combination of fluoxetine and lithium [letter]. Am J Psychiatry 1993; 150: 1565
23. Lane R, Baldwin D. Selective serotonin reuptake inhibitor-induced serotonin syndrome. J Clin Psychopharmacol 1997; 17: 208-21
24. Hadley A, Cason MP. Mania resulting from lithium-fluoxetine combination [letter]. Am J Psychiatry 1989; 146: 1637-8
25. Sacristan JA, Iglesias C, Arellano F, et al. Absence seizures induced by lithium: possible interaction with fluoxetine [letter]. Am J Psychiatry 1991; 148: 146-7
26. Noveske FG, Hahn KR, Flynn RJ. Possible toxicity of combined fluoxetine and lithium [letter]. Am J Psychiatry 1989; 146: 1515
27. Flint AJ, Rifat SL. A prospective study of lithium augmentation in antidepressant-resistant geriatric depression. J Clin Psychopharmacol 1994; 14: 353-6
28. Hardy BG, Shulman KI, Zucchero C. Gradual discontinuation of lithium augmentation in elderly patients with unipolar depression. J Clin Psychopharmacol 1997; 17: 22-6
29. de Montigny C, Cournoyer G, Motisette R, et al. Lithium carbonate addition in tricyclic antidepressant-resistant unipolar depression. Arch Gen Psychiatry 1983; 40: 1327-34
30. de Montigny C. Lithium addition in treatment-resistant depression. Int Clin Psychopharmacol 1994; 9: 31-5
31. Dinan TG, Barry S. A comparison of electroconvulsive therapy with a combined lithium and tricyclic combination among depressed tricyclic non-responders. Acta Psychiatr Scand 1989; 80: 97-100
32. Nelson CJ. Combined treatment strategies in psychiatry. J Clin Psychiatry 1993; 54: 42-9
33. Price LH, Charney DS, Delgado PL, et al. Lithium treatment and serotonergic function. Arch Gen Psychiatry 1989; 46: 13-9
34. Cowen PJ, McCance SL, Ware CJ, et al. Lithium in tricyclic-resistant depression: correlation of increased brain 5-HT function with clinical outcome. Br J Psychiatry 1991; 159: 341-6
35. Hyman SE, Nestler EJ. Initiation and adaptation: a paradigm for understanding psychotropic drug action. Am J Psychiatry 1996; 153: 151-62
36. Bitran JA, Manji HK, Potter WZ, et al. Down regulation of PKC alpha by lithium *in vitro*. Psychopharmacol Bull 1995; 31 (2): 449-52
37. Prange AJ, Wilson IC, Rabon AM, et al. Enhancement of imipramine antidepressant activity by thyroid hormone. Am J Psychiatry 1969; 126: 457-69
38. Stein D, Avni J. Thyroid hormones in the treatment of affective disorders. Acta Psychiatr Scand 1988; 7: 623-36
39. Gitlin MJ, Weiner H, Fairbanks L, et al. Failure of T_3 to potentiate tricyclic antidepressant response. J Affective Dis 1987; 13: 267-72
40. Thase ME, Kupfer DJ, Jarrett DB. Treatment of imipramine-resistant recurrent depression: I: an open clinical trial of adjunctive L-triiodothyronine. J Clin Psychiatry 1989; 50: 385-8
41. Targum SD, Greenberg RD, Harmon RL, et al. Thyroid hormone and the TRH stimulation test in refractory depression. J Clin Psychiatry 1984; 45: 345-6
42. Joffe RT, Singer W, Levitt AJ, et al. A placebo-controlled comparison of lithium and triiodothyronine augmentation of tricyclic antidepressants in unipolar refractory depression. Arch Gen Psychiatry 1993; 50: 387-93
43. Goodwin FK, Range AJ, Post RM, et al. Potentiation of antidepressant effects by L-triiodothyronine in tricyclic non-responders. Am J Psychiatry 1982; 139: 34-8
44. Schwarcz G, Halaris A, Baxter L, et al. Normal thyroid function in desipramine non-responders converted to responders by the addition of L-triiodothyronine. Am J Psychiatry 1984; 141: 1614-6
45. Joffe RT, Singer W. A comparison of triiodothyronine and thyroxine in the potentiation of tricyclic antidepressants. Psychiatry Res 1990; 32: 241-51
46. Rosenbaum JF, Fava M, Nierenberg AA, et al. Treatment-resistant mood disorders. In: Gabbard GO, editor. Treatments of psychiatric disorders. 2nd ed. Washington DC: American Psychiatric Press, 1995: 1276-94
47. Hullet FJ, Bidder TG. Phenelzine plus triiodothyronine combination in a case of refractory depression. J Nerv Ment Dis 1983; 171: 318-20
48. Gupta S, Masand P, Tanquary JF. Thyroid hormone supplementation of fluoxetine in the treatment of major depression. Br J Psychiatry 1991; 159: 866-7
49. Joffe RT. T_3 potentiation of fluoxetine. Can J Psychiatry 1992; 37: 48-50
50. Whybrow PC, Prange AJ. A hypothesis of thyroid-catecholamine-receptor interaction. Arch Gen Psychiatry 1981; 38: 106-13
51. Norman TR, Sartor DM, McIntyre IM. Clinical and experimental studies on the potentiation of antidepressant drugs by thyroid hormones. Med Sci Res 1988; 16: 545-50
52. Schatzberg AF, Cole JO. Combination and adjunctive treatments. In: Gabbard GO, editor. Manual of clinical psychopharmacology. 2nd ed. Washington DC: American Psychiatric Press, 1991: 263-79
53. Weilburg JB Rosenbaum JF, Biederman J, et al. Fluoxetine added to non-MAOI antidepressants converts nonresponders to responders: A preliminary report. J Clin Psychiatry 1989; 50: 447-9
54. Weilburg JB, Rosenbaum JF, Meltzer-Brody S, et al. Tricyclic augmentation of fluoxetine. Annals Clin Psychiatry 1991; 3: 209-13
55. Seth R, Jennings AL, Bindman J, et al. Combination treatment with noradrenaline and serotonin reuptake inhibitors in resistant depression. Br J Psychiatry 1992; 161: 562-5
56. Lydiard RB, Anton RF, Cunningham T. Interactions between sertraline and tricyclic antidepressants. Am J Psychiatry 1993; 150: 1125-6

57. Ereshefsky L. Drug-drug interactions involving antidepressants: focus on venlafaxine. J Clin Psychopharmacol 1996; 16: 37S-53S
58. Preskorn SH, Beber JH, Faul JC, et al. Serious adverse effects of combining fluoxetine and tricyclic antidepressants [letter]. Am J Psychiatry 1990; 147: 532
59. Vaughan DA. Interaction of fluoxetine with tricyclic antidepressants [letter]. Am J Psychiatry 1988; 145: 1478
60. Preskorn SH. Clinically relevant pharmacology of selective serotonin reuptake inhibitors: an overview with emphasis on pharmacokinetics and effects on oxidative drug metabolism. Clin Pharmacokinet 1997; 32: 1-21
61. Sussman N, Stahl S. Update in the pharmacotherapy of depression. Am J Med 1996; 101 Suppl 6A: 6A26S-6A36S
62. Nelson JC, Mazure CM, Bowers MB, et al. A preliminary, open study of the combination of fluoxetine and desipramine for rapid treatment of major depression. Arch Gen Psychiatry 1991; 48: 303-7
63. Baron BM, Ogden A-M, Siegel BW et al. Rapid down regulation of β-adrenoreceptors by co-administration of desipramine and fluoxetine. Eur J Pharmacol 1988; 154: 125-34
64. Artigas F, Perez V, Alvarez E. Pindolol induces a rapid improvement of depressed patients treated with serotonin reuptake inhibitors. Arch Gen Psychiatry 1994; 51: 248-51
65. Blier P, Bergeron R. Effectiveness of pindolol with selected antidepressant drugs in the treatment of major depression. J Clin Psychopharmacol 1995; 15: 217-22
66. Artigas F, Romero L, Perez V, et al. Augmentation of antidepressant effects with $5HT_{1A}$ antagonists: basic and clinical studies [abstract]. Eur Neuropsychopharmacol 1996; 6: 16
67. Charney D. Double-blind study on the effect of pindolol addition to accelerate the antidepressant response [abstract]. Eur Neuropsychopharmacol 1996; 6: 17
68. Berman RL, Darnell AM, Miller HL, et al. Effect of pindolol in hastening response to fluoxetine in the treatment of major depression: a double-blind, placebo-controlled trial. Am J Psychiatry 1997; 154: 37-3
69. Tome MB, Isaac MT, Harte R, et al. Paroxetine and pindolol: a randomized trial of serotonergic autoreceptor blockade in the reduction of antidepressant latency. Int Clin Psychopharmacol 1997; 12: 81-9
70. Perez V, Gilaberte I, Faries D, et al. Randomised, double-blind, placebo-controlled trial of pindolol in combination with fluoxetine antidepressant treatment. Lancet 1997 May 31; 349 (9065): 1594-7
71. Blier P, Bergeron R, de Montigny C. Selective activation of postsynaptic $5\text{-}HT_{1A}$ receptors induces rapid antidepressant response. Neuropsychopharmacol 1997 May; 16: 333-8
72. Bakish D, Hooper CL, Thornton MD, et al. Fast onset: an open study of the treatment of major depressive disorder with nefazodone and pindolol combination therapy. Int Clin Psychopharmacol 1997 Mar; 12: 91-7
73. Patten SB, Love EJ. Drug-induced depression. Psychother Psychosom 1997; 66: 63-73
74. De la Fuente JM, Mendlewicz J. Carbamazepine addition in tricyclic antidepressant-resistant unipolar depression. Biol Psychiatry 1992; 32: 369-74
75. Corrigan FM. Sodium valproate augmentation of fluoxetine or fluvoxamine effects. Biol Psychiatry 1992; 31: 1178-9
76. Ketter TA, Post RM, Parekh PI, et al. Addition of monoamine oxidase inhibitors to carbamazepine: preliminary evidence of safety and antidepressant efficacy in treatment-resistant depression. J Clin Psychiatry 1995; 56: 471-5
77. Baldessarini RJ, Teicher MH, Cassidy JW. Anticonvulsant co-treatment may increase toxic metabolites of antidepressants and other psychotropic drugs [letter]. J Clin Psychopharmacol 1988; 8: 381
78. Wharton RN, Perel JM, Dayton PG, et al. A potential clinical use for methylphenidate with tricyclic antidepressants. Am J Psychiatry 1971; 127: 1619-25
79. Feighner JP, Herbstein J, Damlouji N. Combined MAOI, TCA, and direct stimulant therapy of treatment-resistant depression. J Clin Psychiatry 1985; 46: 206-9
80. Fawcett J, Kravitz HM, Zajecka JM, et al. CNS stimulant potentiation of monoamine oxidase inhibitors in treatment-refractory depression. J Clin Psychopharmacol 1991; 11: 127-32
81. Stoll AL, Pillay SS, Diamond L, et al. Methylphenidate augmentation of serotonin selective reuptake inhibitors: a case series. J Clin Psychiatry 1996; 57: 72-6
82. Jacobsen FM. Possible augmentation of antidepressant response by buspirone. J Clin Psychiatry 1991; 52: 217-20
83. Bakish D. Fluoxetine potentiation by buspirone: three case histories. Can J Psychiatry 1991; 36: 749-50
84. Joffe RT, Schuller DR. An open study of buspirone augmentation of serotonin reuptake inhibitors in refractory depression. J Clin Psychiatry 1993; 54: 269-71
85. Robillard M, Lieff S. Augmentation of antidepressant therapy by buspirone: three geriatric case histories. Can J Psychiatry 1995; 40: 639-40
86. Harvey KV, Balon R. Augmentation with buspirone: a review. Ann Clin Psychiatry 1995; 7: 143-7
87. Spigset O, Adielsson G. Combined serotonin syndrome and hyponatraemia caused by a citalopram-buspirone interaction. Int Clin Psychopharmacol 1997; 12: 61-3
88. Howland RH. Biochemical and clinical effects of buspirone augmentation. J Clin Psychiatry 1994; 55: 264
89. Flint AJ. Augmentation strategies in geriatric depression. Int J Ger Psychiatry 1995; 10: 137-46

Correspondence: Assoc. Prof. *Isaac Schweitzer*, Professorial Unit, The Melbourne Clinic, 130 Church Street, Richmond, Victoria 3121, Australia.
E-mail: i.schweitzer@medicine.unimelb.edu.au

Risks and Benefits of Selective Serotonin Reuptake Inhibitors in the Treatment of Depression

Patricia Mourilhe and *Peter E. Stokes*

The New York Hospital-Cornell Medical Center, White Plains, New York, USA

Nearly four decades ago, investigators noticed that iproniazid caused elevation of mood in some patients being treated for tuberculosis. That discovery led to a major breakthrough in the way major depressive disorder was regarded and treated: it gave great impetus to the concept of depression as a biochemical disturbance of the CNS and provided the basis for the first effective pharmacotherapy of depression.

Recent research has shown depression to be a chronic condition with a lifetime risk of approximately 20% for women and 10% for men.[1-5] However, despite the availability of effective pharmacological treatment for nearly 40 years, it is estimated that only about 2.5% of people who meet the criteria for major depression ultimately receive appropriate treatment.[1-7] Patients who respond to treatment gradually return to euthymia during several weeks to a few months of adequate antidepressant pharmacotherapy.[8]

However, the overall clinical efficacy of past available antidepressants used in clinical practice has been significantly hampered by the frequency of untoward treatment-emergent events, intolerable adverse effects, and difficulty in adjusting the dosage. Together, these three factors have contributed significantly to decreased compliance, subtherapeutic dosages, or premature discontinuation of treatment. This in turn is associated with incomplete remission and/or more frequent relapse, all of which leave patients open to the morbidity of major depressive disorder, including suicide. The need for improvement over available agents led researchers to seek drugs with more advantageous tolerability profiles.

In the past 20 years,[9] drug development has shifted from the discovery of compounds by chance to rationally targeting specific mechanisms of action believed to be important in the pathophysiology of psychiatric syndromes.[10] Selective serotonin (5-hydroxytryptamine, 5-HT) reuptake inhibitors (SSRIs) were the first class of psychiatric medications to be developed based on molecular targeting. A major consequence of the introduction of such agents has been greater compliance among patients, as a result of fewer adverse effects and less complicated dosage schedules.

Easier management is also expected to enhance physician attention to diagnosis, and increase the likelihood of using adequate dosages and adequate durations of antidepressant pharmacotherapy. Depression is a common chronic disorder that frequently presents in non-psychiatric practice (e.g. primary care), where it is often underdiagnosed and undertreated.[11] In addition, the high morbidity and mortality associated with this disorder[12,13] may well be decreased. According to Nemeroff,[14] antidepressants are more efficacious than most classes of drugs, with the exception of antimicrobial agents and a few other drug classes.

Nearly 3 out of every 4 outpatients being treated for depression with antidepressants will respond successfully during this treatment,[3,5,6,15] and individual patients who do not respond to one antidepressant sometimes respond to another.[3] However, as many as 1 of 3 outpatient responders may in fact be placebo or spontaneous responders,[3,14] so *specific* drug responders could number as low as 50% of those treated. However, this is of little importance to the clinician faced with the decision of whether or not to treat since there is no reliable manner to identify the potential placebo or spontaneous responder *before* treatment.

Apart from efficacy, which is about the same for all antidepressants, drug choice is, by and large, based on tolerability and ease of administration because these factors relate so strongly to compliance. Since the advent of SSRIs, safety has become another factor in drug choice, since the SSRIs are better tolerated in overdose than any of the tricyclic antidepressants (TCAs), heterocyclic antidepressants (HCAs) or older monoamine oxidase inhibitors (MAOIs).[3,14,16,17] Drug acquisition costs, once thought to be of major importance, are now being shown to be less important in the context of the overall cost effectiveness of antidepressant treatment.[18-20]

In this review, we discuss the tolerability profiles and efficacy of the currently used SSRIs: fluoxetine, paroxetine, sertraline, fluvoxamine and citalopram. Most attention is given to the first three agents, which are the most widely used.

1. Epidemiology of Depression

In weighing up the advantages and disadvantages of a specific drug, it is crucial for the clinician to bear in mind some data on the epidemiology of depression. The disorder is associated with high mortality, morbidity and economic cost.[21] Depression is more common than hypertension in primary care practice.[22] It occurs from childhood to senescence, but most patients are initially affected during early adulthood and their most productive later adult years, between 20 and 50 years of age. 15% of patients with (especially recurrent) major depression ultimately commit suicide.[23] Moreover, 45 to 70% of all people who commit suicide have an affective disorder.[6,23,24] In addition, 19 to 42% of those who commit suicide have previously attempted suicide, and 10% of those who attempt suicide will eventually succeed within 10 years.[25] Although probably underestimated, suicide ranks as the eighth leading cause of death in the US, higher than AIDS.[26,27] Depression can affect the outcome of other clinical entities. For example, it increases mortality among patients following myocardial infarction.[12]

The costs of depression, not only to individuals and their families, but also the indirect costs to the healthcare system, employers and society, are enormous.[28] These costs may be substantially diminished by successful diagnosis and antidepressant treatment, especially if accomplished early in the course of the disease[21,29-32] and if compliance is maintained at adequate dosage for adequate time.[18]

2. Pharmacotherapy in Depression

Pharmacotherapy has been shown by Elkin et al.[15] to be the most effective treatment for moderate to severe depression. Prior to the advent of focused systems of psychotherapy, no evidence existed for efficacy of dynamic psychotherapeutic approaches in the treatment of depression. Pharmacotherapy and focused structured psychotherapy (e.g. cognitive behavioural or interpersonal therapy) are perhaps equally effective in the management of mild depression, but recovery is more rapid with pharmacotherapy.[15] Where indicated, psychotherapy may assist in the resolution of other psychological problems as patients recover from their depression with the assistance of pharmacotherapy. In some cases, concomitant psychotherapy may also assist in inducing remission from depression[33] and contribute to a decreased relapse rate.

3. Place of Selective Serotonin Reuptake Inhibitors

The major drawbacks in the use of older agents for treating depression are the poor tolerability and safety profiles as well as the multiple daily doses that are often required, all of which decrease compliance and lead to suboptimal dosage and premature discontinuation of treatment.[19,20,31]

SSRIs possess four major advances over the older antidepressants:

1) A more benign tolerability profile with fewer adverse events; most of those which do occur are mild and transient in nature.[34,35] It is estimated that only 20 to 25% of patients taking TCAs receive adequate therapeutic dosages,[36-38] because of the desire to avoid the associated adverse effects.

2) Easier administration. Fluoxetine often requires no titration, and can be administered once daily.[39] Other SSRIs require minimal titration compared with older antidepressant drugs and can also be routinely given once daily.[34]

3) SSRIs have been shown to be involved in far fewer drug interactions, especially those of a serious nature (e.g. involving sedatives, sympathomimetics, alcohol, antiarrhythmics), compared with older antidepressants.[14,40] This has proven true in clinical practice even though, as a class, the SSRIs inhibit at least one of the cytochrome P450 (CYP) isoenzymes, which results in the *potential* to enhance (sometimes beyond the appropriate therapeutic range) the effects of other concomitant drugs that are metabolised by these enzymes.

4) The SSRIs are better tolerated in overdose than the irreversible MAOIs, TCAs, HCAs and amfebutamone (bupropion).[35] The safety of SSRIs in overdose contrasts with that of the still widely used TCAs, which cause more deaths from overdose than any other prescription drug category (table I).[16] This safety in overdose occurs despite the fact that antidepressant drugs are prescribed for patients who have an illness in which suicide is a recognised risk. The increased safety of SSRIs compared to older drugs is true even though, in a mixed overdose situation, all SSRIs can potentially increase the plasma and tissue concentrations of a number of co-ingested drugs by inhibiting the hepatic CYP enzyme metabolism of those drugs.[41]

The utility of an antidepressant with a more benign tolerability profile becomes even greater, since emerging data point to the fact that for most patients, depression is a recurrent disorder with episodes increasing in frequency throughout life,[42-47] and many patients require long term maintenance treatment with

Table I. Fatal toxicity index of antidepressant drugs (reproduced from Tollefson,[35] with permission)

Drug	No. of fatal poisonings per million prescriptions
Amitriptyline	166
Maprotiline	115
Imipramine	105
Doxepin	99
Trimipramine	93
Clomipramine	34
Fluoxetine	10[a]

a Extrapolated from one reported fatal overdose in 100 000 patients.

antidepressants. Recent data show that at least 50% of patients who have had a single episode of depression will experience recurrence.[48,49] Therefore, one goal of management is to identify those in need of long term pharmacotherapy and enhance their compliance during continuation therapy after the initial period of acute recovery. In many cases, very long or lifetime prophylactic therapy will then be appropriate.

In this regard, SSRIs have been shown to be efficacious in reducing relapse and recurrence rates by more than 50% when compared with placebo.[50-52] Furthermore, SSRIs have proven extremely useful in the management of depression in patients with concomitant medical conditions such as cardiac disease and stroke, because of their improved tolerability.[3,53,54] Over 35 million patients have been treated with SSRIs since they were first used in Europe in the mid-1980s.[40]

4. Comparisons With Older Antidepressants

Nemeroff[14] has stated that the ideal antidepressant for elderly patients should have no clinically significant cardiotoxic or orthostatic effects, cause little sedation and no impairment of memory, and not impair physical ability. In our opinion, based on an extensive review of the literature, SSRIs can be considered to be the first-line agent for all depressed patients including elderly patients, and we shall review some of the data to support this assertion. Due to the higher selectivity of drug effect with SSRIs, as exemplified by the absence of unwanted CNS and peripheral receptor blockade, which occurs with older antidepressants, SSRIs tend to be better tolerated in patients with comorbid medical conditions.[55,56] In addition, as has been pointed out,[10] drugs that are rationally developed to affect only the mechanism mediating a desired response tend to have a wider therapeutic index than drugs discovered by chance. The latter drugs frequently have either multiple mechanisms of action (e.g. TCAs) or such a basic mechanism of action that they have an impact on a wide variety of systems (e.g. MAOIs). Patients receiving drugs like TCAs, with multiple mechanisms of action occurring over a relatively narrow concentration range, are likely to experience multiple effects, both desired and undesired.

SSRIs have high specificity for serotonin uptake blockade and do not cause unwanted blockade of peripheral and central adrenergic, cholinergic and histaminergic receptors, which is characteristic of the TCAs and MAOIs. TCAs are associated with a wide range of adverse effects resulting from unwanted receptor blockade. Muscarinic blockade produces effects such as dry mouth, blurred vision, memory impairment, constipation, urinary retention and sinus tachycardia. These drugs also block α_1-adrenergic receptors, which may cause orthostatic hypotension and tachycardia, as well as histaminergic blockade, which may cause sedation and bodyweight gain. These adverse effects are shared by HCAs to various degrees.

In addition to their unwanted receptor blockade, TCAs have a direct dose-related quinidine-like effect on the myocardium that can induce potentially life-threatening cardiac conduction disturbances, especially in patients with pre-existing, even subclinical, cardiac disease.[57-59] This effect is thought to be mediated through the inhibition of sodium fast channels and occurs at concentrations only one order of magnitude higher than the concentration needed to inhibit the neuronal uptake pump for norepinephrine (noradrenaline) and serotonin, the putative mechanism of action mediating their antidepressant effect. In susceptible individuals, these effects can occur at usual full therapeutic doses of TCAs.

The efficacy of SSRIs in major depression has now been established in numerous controlled double-blind studies and through vast clinical experience.[60] Tollefson,[17] commenting on the use of SSRIs for the treatment of depression, mentioned that the efficacy of these agents is similar to (or perhaps slightly better than) that of TCAs, a view supported by others;[61-63] however, these findings have not been universally reported.[64,65]

Boyer and Feighner[66] reviewed comparative efficacy studies of SSRIs and older antidepressants (mainly secondary and tertiary amine TCAs) and found that of 25 comparisons with fluoxetine, no differences were found in 23, and fluoxetine was significantly superior in two of them. For fluvoxamine, no significant differences were found, with the exception of one study, which found fluvoxamine to be superior to the 'gold standard' TCAs. Among nine studies of paroxetine, seven found no significant differences, one found imipramine to be superior to paroxetine, and one found the opposite. Of eight studies on citalopram, six found no significant differences between this drug and the TCA comparator, one showed citalopram to be superior, and one found that clomipramine was superior to citalopram. There were three studies on sertraline, of which one showed amitriptyline to be superior to sertraline and two showed no significant differences between the two agents. Overall, these findings[66] support the conclusion that there is no clearly definable superiority in efficacy for any one class of antidepressants over another.

In some studies, in which there was overall superior efficacy of SSRIs as compared to TCAs, this was clearly related to the more benign adverse event profile of these drugs.[66,67] Better tolerability, combined with ease of administration, compared with TCAs, MAOIs and some HCAs, increases compliance in patients being treated for depression, particularly patients being treated over long periods of time,[68] and the elderly and patients with comorbid medical conditions.[69]

The high specificity of SSRIs translates into a unique and relatively benign adverse-effect profile with superior patient acceptance and compliance, which in clinical trials, results in greatly diminished withdrawal rates in SSRI-treated groups, compared with TCA- and MAOI-treated patients. For example, Boyer and Feighner[66] and others[67,70] compared short term withdrawal rates during tertiary or secondary amine TCA and SSRI treatment, and showed SSRI compliance to be significantly superior (10 to 20% dropout in SSRI group, as opposed to 30 to 35% in TCA group and 5 to 10% in the placebo group).

Besides sharing many similar adverse effects with TCAs, the older MAOIs are associated with potentially life-threatening interactions with dietary tyramine, or proximal (within 2 weeks for paroxetine, sertraline, clomipramine and citalopram, and 4 weeks for fluoxetine) or concurrent administration of serotonergic agents. This can be a problem in the long term management of patients who might be compliant with the drug regimen, but not adequately compliant with dietary restrictions or who inadvertently ingest tyramine-containing foods. MAOIs are also associated with greater risk in overdose compared with SSRIs.

In summary, the SSRIs, being more pharmacologically selective than the older agents such as TCAs, HCAs and MAOIs, have better tolerability and are safer in overdose than these older agents. They have been shown to be at least as clinically efficacious as these agents and to have improved compliance and lower dropout rates in a number of clinical studies. It is worth mentioning that the clinical premise that patients who do not respond to one antidepressant class can become responders when switched to an agent of another drug group remains true for SSRIs, which are reported to be effective among a significant percentage of TCA-resistant patients with depression.[71,72]

5. Pharmacology

In order to attain the most benefit from available agents, clinicians need to be familiar with the specific characteristics of individual agents which can vary within each class. The structure of the individual SSRIs varies. The activity patterns of these drugs can have class similarities with some between-drug differences in activity which can be helpful as guidelines provided one is careful in considering that *in vitro* receptor-specific metabolic and *in vivo* pharmacokinetic data do not precisely predict clinical response or adverse effects.

5.1 Receptor Activity

An overview of receptor activity of SSRIs is useful in understanding the behaviour and advantages of these compounds and as an additional guide in their clinical use. Some of the most important findings from receptor studies with SSRIs are that: (i) clinically, all SSRIs have negligible activity at muscarinic and histaminergic receptors;[9,14,40,53] (ii) although relative differences in weak adrenoceptor affinity exist across the class, they do not appear to be of clinical significance;[53] (iii) no significant dopaminergic receptor activity has been demonstrated;[53] (iv) the clinical relevance of *in vitro* γ-aminobutyric acid (GABA)ergic activity is unclear;[53,73] and (v) corticotrophin-releasing factor antagonism, which would reduce the elevated discharge rates in the locus coeruleus of depressed patients, has been hypothesised as a mechanism of action for antidepressant activity – such a role has not been established for SSRIs.

In vitro studies of paroxetine have reported some activity at muscarinic cholinergic receptors, suggesting an increased chance of anticholinergic activity, compared with other SSRIs.[66] However, even paroxetine does not clearly display clinically significant anticholinergic activity, and the blurred vision and constipation seen occasionally with this agent are most probably related to the serotonergic innervation of the pupil and gut, rather than 'true' anticholinergic effects.[53] For sertraline, characteristics include more potent inhibition activity at adrenergic receptor sites than other SSRIs (which nevertheless is also very low and unlikely to be clinically meaningful) and higher (but apparently not clinically significant) *in vitro* affinity for the σ receptor binding site (this receptor has been implicated in psychotic symptomatology). Finally, there are differences in patterns of hepatic enzyme inhibition between the various SSRIs (section 6).

Despite some individual variability, SSRIs have a favourable tolerability profile. This generally derives from their lack of unwanted receptor blockade (α_1-adrenergic, muscarinic, cholinergic, histaminergic) [table II].[3,79] The main established action of the SSRIs, thought to be related to their therapeutic effect, is to increase synaptic serotonin transmission through inhibition of synaptic serotonin reuptake and consequent metabolism.

Different hypotheses have been raised regarding postsynaptic serotonin 5-HT_{1A} and 5-HT_2 receptor binding in explaining serotonergic-related antidepressant activity and an interaction between these two sites has been advocated. Additionally, the role of somatodendritic 5-HT_{1A} and hetero receptors as feedback inhibitors of synaptic serotonin release, as serotonin 'leaks' from the adjacent serotonin synthesising cell body, is still incompletely understood. These somatodendritic receptors may be functionally downregulated in the face of continued

Table II. Receptor binding affinities of selective serotonin (5-hydroxytryptamine; 5-HT) reuptake inhibitors.[74-78] None of these agents has significant affinity for dopamine D_2 receptors

Drug	Reuptake blockade			Receptor blockade			
	serotonin	noradrenaline (norepinephrine)	dopamine	histamine H_1	muscarine	serotonin 5-HT_2	α-adrenergic
Paroxetine	++	–	–	–	+	–	–
Fluoxetine	++	–	–	–	±	–	–
Sertraline	++	–	±	–	±	–	–
Fluvoxamine	++	–	–	–	±	–	–
Citalopram	++	–	–	–	±	–	–
Desipramine	–	++	–	+	+	–	++
Imipramine	+	+	–	+	++	+	+

++ = pronounced; + = mild; ± = probably not clinically significant; – = nil.

increased serotonin concentration secondary to ongoing SSRI action, and this could permit continued serotonin synthesis, release and trans-synaptic transmission during long term SSRI treatment.[80] One theory for the potential augmenting effect of the 5-HT_{1A} blocker pindolol is via its purported inhibition (blockade) of somatodendritic 5-HT_{1A} receptors.[81]

5.2 Pharmacokinetics

The metabolism and associated pharmacokinetics of SSRIs varies between drugs. *In vivo*, fluoxetine has an extended half-life of 3 days and a highly active metabolite (norfluoxetine), which has a half-life of about 1 week,[3] while other pure SSRIs or TCAs and HCAs generally have half-lives of 1 day or less. This provides a clear advantage for fluoxetine over these drugs, regarding missed doses over intervals of a few days, since plasma fluoxetine and norfluoxetine concentrations remain in the therapeutic range.

Continued experience with fluoxetine has revealed other advantages stemming from its extended half-life. For example, patients are very unlikely to experience withdrawal symptoms or relapse in situations of inadvertent occasional noncompliance or abrupt discontinuation of drug. Withdrawal syndromes, sometimes severe, have been documented with abrupt discontinuation of TCAs[82] and, more recently, with the other SSRIs,[83] all of which have comparatively short half-lives, similar to most TCAs. Patients suddenly discontinuing these shorter half-life drugs[82] (with the possible exception of sertraline[81,83]) may experience symptoms ranging from sleep disturbance, gastrointestinal upset, headache and fatigue to depression or mania. On the other hand, the extended half-life of fluoxetine requires a longer waiting period (4 to 5 weeks *vs* 2 to 3 weeks for other SSRIs) following discontinuation if standard MAOIs are being considered as alternative drugs because of the risk of an interaction between the drugs. However, this particular medication shift is becoming very infrequent. Progressive accumulation resulting from the extended half-life of fluoxetine and its metabolite does not occur. At constant dosages, steady state is reached after 5 or 6 weeks, even if hepatic metabolism by usual CYP isoenzymes is inhibited, presumably because of alternative metabolic pathways.[84]

Experience with more than 25 million patients treated with fluoxetine, and many millions more with other SSRIs, has shown that clinically important adverse effects secondary to drug

Table III. Agent-specific pharmacokinetic considerations for the selective serotonin (5-hydroxytryptamine; 5-HT) reuptake inhibitors (SSRIs)[40,50,73,85]

Drug	Active metabolites	Half-life of parent (metabolite)[a]	Comments
Fluoxetine	Norfluoxetine	++++ (++++++)	Metabolite has a half-life of about 1 week; it possesses both serotonin and (to a lesser extent) noradrenaline (norepinephrine) reuptake-blocking selectivity;[80] racemic compound (pharmacokinetic differences in enantiomers and their metabolites not clinically significant)
Sertraline	Demethyl-sertraline	+ (++++)	Extended half-life of metabolite is of little clinical significance, since the ability of the metabolite to inhibit serotonin reuptake is much weaker than that of the parent compound[73]
Paroxetine	None	+	Paroxetine has a slightly shorter half-life than the other short half-life SSRIs, which may contribute to its pronounced tendency to withdrawal or breakthrough depression when doses are missed[81,86]
Fluvoxamine	None	+	Pharmacology suggests tendency to induce withdrawal symptoms, as with other short half-life compounds, but no controlled data are available
Citalopram	Demethyl-citalopram	+ (+++)	Racemic compound (differences in pharmacokinetics and metabolism of the enantiomers and their metabolites not clinically important)

a The more '+'s, the longer the half-life.

interactions with SSRIs are rare (with the exception of the interactions with MAOIs, particularly the older (nonselective irreversible) ones. Nevertheless, physicians must remain aware of these possibilities, which are discussed in section 6.

Agent-specific pharmacokinetic considerations are shown in table III.

An important consideration regarding the metabolism of all these drugs is that pharmacokinetic studies in the elderly[73] reveal that, although pharmacokinetic behaviour is not remarkably changed, potentially the drugs are more slowly metabolised (especially paroxetine and citalopram), and therefore, lower initial dosages may be appropriate in elderly patients. In general, elderly patients should be started on lower dosages of SSRIs. Age-related pharmacokinetic changes with paroxetine are significant enough to cause the manufacturer to advise a lower starting dose in elderly patients (10 mg/day, with gradual upward titration to a maximum of 40mg instead of the usual maximum dose of 50mg).[87]

All of the SSRIs are well absorbed after oral administration, and this is not diminished by concomitant food intake, thus providing excellent bioavailability.[73] The absorption of sertraline is enhanced when taken with meals, compared with between meals,[73] and it is possibly best administered in this manner.

The metabolic elimination of SSRIs is delayed by hepatic or severe renal disease, in the presence of which dosages should be lowered or administered less frequently.[73]

There is no therapeutic window for SSRIs. No relationship has been found between plasma concentrations of the parent drug, metabolites or 'ratios' of drug/metabolite to therapeutic efficacy or toxic concentrations.[88]

5.3 Tolerability

SSRIs are associated with their own specific adverse effect profile, which tends to be milder than those of older antidepressant agents, and contributes to the documented higher compliance rates across studies.[35,89,90]

5.3.1 Gastrointestinal

The most common adverse effect associated with SSRIs is nausea, which, we believe is generally better described as 'mild dyspepsia'; vomiting has been reported, but only rarely, with all drugs in this class. Nausea occurs in up to 20% of patients receiving fluoxetine; this adverse effect is typically mild and transient, and usually dosage related.[91] In a 1985 review of comparative studies, the 3% discontinuation rate of fluoxetine due to nausea was similar to that observed for imipramine.[91]

Loss of appetite can occur transiently and may be associated with some bodyweight loss. Although it is good clinical practice to monitor bodyweight in severely underweight patients, the evidence shows that bodyweight loss associated with SSRI therapy (which may particularly occur with fluoxetine) is more pronounced in overweight patients and in those with carbohydrate craving.[92,93] The bodyweight loss associated with SSRIs, if present, is generally mild (2kg) and self limited.[92,94] This tendency to slight bodyweight reduction can be beneficial to many depressed patients (some of whom may have increased bodyweight secondary to treatment with older antidepressants), especially those who are already overweight or fall into the category of hyperphagic depression. However, the clinician must be aware of the (rarely observed) potential for abuse in patients presenting with symptoms of anorexia nervosa or bulimia nervosa, who may erroneously believe that SSRIs will produce progressive bodyweight loss. The latter has not been observed in our experience or reported in the literature. In fact, fluoxetine-induced bodyweight loss in long term animal and human obesity studies has been non-progressive, with bodyweight gradually returning to pretreatment levels.[92] A tendency to develop diarrhoea can occur with SSRIs and is also generally transient and dosage related.[40]

5.3.2 Neurological

Although having an overall more favourable profile of behavioural toxicity than conventional antidepressants, SSRIs have also been associated with increased anxiety, nervousness and insomnia in a minority of patients.[40,53] These tend to occur early in treatment and may appear *de novo* or temporarily enhance pre-existing anxiety symptoms. However, the presence of anxiety in depression may in fact be a predictor of high likelihood of response to fluoxetine or other SSRIs.[95] Dosage reduction or the introduction of a benzodiazepine during the first few weeks of therapy can help such patients. Experience with SSRIs has shown that anxiety decreases, as measured by anxiety factors in the Hamilton Depression Rating Scale (HDRS) scores, in depressed patients.[91,96] Paroxetine may be associated with unwanted daytime somnolence in perhaps 20% of patients, while fluoxetine may be most likely to induce, initially at least, emergent symptoms of anxiety, nervousness and restlessness, which are transient; sertraline is associated with a higher incidence of sexual dysfunction and gastrointestinal problems.[53,97] Rarely, tremor can occur in association with SSRI use, and may respond to dosage reduction or the addition of a β-blocker or a benzodiazepine if it persists.[98,99]

5.3.3 Sexual Dysfunction

TCAs and MAOIs reduce erectile function and are contraindicated in patients with erectile impotence. These drugs and, to an even greater degree, the SSRIs have also been associated with inability to ejaculate, delayed ejaculation and anorgasmia.[100,101] There is no reliable, safe or easy solution to overcoming these adverse effects, although dosage reduction or switching to another SSRI may help.[102] Some patients have found relief over the weekend by stopping the shorter half-life compounds on Friday and resuming them on Sunday.[103]

In view of the dissociation often observed between relatively rapid (2 to 3 days) subsidence of emerging adverse events related to fluoxetine and its known extended half-life, it is possible that interruption of therapy for a few days could diminish or abolish complaints of sexual dysfunction in patients receiving this drug. A technique that we have used, which requires confirmation in a prospective controlled study, is to prescribe the entire week's dosage of fluoxetine spread over a few days (e.g. starting Sunday night or Monday through to Wednesday or Thursday morning).

Finally, it is sometimes possible to produce a significant degree of amelioration of this adverse effect by treating with gradually increasing doses of cyproheptadine (a serotonin and histamine antagonist) up to as high as 32 mg/day, as needed, or amantadine in usual clinical dosages, until symptoms abate.[104,105] In patients with bronchial asthma or glaucoma, cyproheptadine should be used with caution because of its atropine-like effects. As with all antihistamines, daytime drowsiness may occur, and may be dosage-related.

5.3.4 Other

The currently used SSRIs have not been implicated in causing allergic reactions, such as were observed with zimeldine, an early SSRI, which is no longer available. In fact, there have been reports of patients who had an allergic reaction with zimeldine, but who have been treated with currently available SSRIs with no such complications.[66] Nevertheless, in the event of any pruritic rash occurring, discontinuation of the current SSRI is advisable.

An extremely rare, but serious, central serotonin syndrome has been reported during SSRI therapy.[106] The risk of this idiosyncratic event increases markedly with concomitant or proximal administration of a serotonin-enhancing agent, such as a MAOI or precursor agent such as tryptophan, to an SSRI regimen. Consequently, SSRIs should never be used proximal to or concomitant with one of these agents. The syndrome can present as abdominal pain, diarrhoea, sweating, fever, arthralgia, tachycardia, elevated blood pressure, delirium, myoclonus, increased motor activity, irritability, hostility and mood change. It can lead to hyperpyrexia, shock or death in severe cases.[107] Tollefson[17] recommends waiting at least five half-lives of the parent SSRI or of its active metabolite (if longer) before starting MAOI therapy. Consistent with this advice, Ciraulo and Shader[108] recommend waiting for 5 weeks after stopping fluoxetine and 2 weeks after stopping one of the other SSRIs.

6. Drug Interactions

6.1 Benzodiazepines

Data point to the fact that SSRIs are relatively free of cumulative CNS depression in combination with benzodiazepines.[98,99] This represents an advance over TCAs, HCAs and MAOIs, which have cumulative depressant effects with CNS sedatives, anticholinergic agents or histaminergic compounds. However, it has been reported that fluvoxamine and, to a lesser extent, the other SSRIs, which inhibit one or more hepatic CYP isoenzymes, increase plasma diazepam and alprazolam concentrations. However, when these anxiolytics are used appropriately, this does not present a clinically significant problem because benzodiazepines should be started at low dosages and increased only as needed to obtain anxiolytic effects while observing for unwanted effects (e.g. excessive sedation, increased agitation, disorientation).

It must be kept in mind that since benzodiazepines do not treat depression, their indiscriminate use in patients with depression should be strongly discouraged. Nevertheless, the fact that SSRIs do not significantly increase sedation when used with such agents make SSRIs a valuable tool for physicians treating depression in patients who have a clear clinical indication for short-term concomitant benzodiazepine administration. Benzodiazepines may be indicated temporarily in a minority of depressed patients presenting with pronounced anxiety or in those who develop anxiety when SSRI therapy is initiated.

6.2 Drugs Metabolised by Cytochrome P450 Enzymes

Other drugs that may interact with SSRIs are those that are metabolised by or affect the function of the same hepatic enzymes that metabolise the SSRIs, especially certain CYP enzymes. Within the CYP enzyme group, some 3 dozen different isoenzymes have been identified, with the 2D6, 3A3, 3A4 and 2C isoenzymes being the most relevant to our consideration of drug-drug interactions with SSRI antidepressants. For extensive reviews of CYP enzyme activity and drug-drug interactions see Nemeroff et al.[41]

Since all SSRIs inhibit some of the CYP isoenzymes to a degree, plasma and tissue drug concentrations of other concomitantly administered compounds normally metabolised by these isoenzymes might be increased during SSRI administration. This inhibition has been observed in the approximately 90% of Caucasian, Mexican American, African American and Asian individuals who are extensive metabolisers (EM) with regard to the activity of CYP2D6.[109] Individuals with this EM CYP2D6 genotype can be transformed into 'apparent' (phenotypic) poor metaboliser (PM) types in the presence of the CYP2D6 isoenzyme inhibitor SSRI compounds. This could produce increases in plasma and tissue concentrations of concomitantly administered drugs normally metabolised by the CYP isoenzyme (table IV). Those individuals genetically endowed with low activity (amount) of CYP2D6 isoenzyme will already be phenotypic PM types and will be unable to process much of any compound that requires metabolic action by that isoenzyme. Administration of SSRIs to these patients will produce little change in the metabolism of xenobiotics processed by the 2D6 isoenzyme. No genetic polymorphism has yet been identified for CYP3A3 or CYP3A4 isoenzymes and all individuals so far studied are EM regarding this isoenzyme, but activity can be inhibited by some SSRIs.[41,109]

Table IV. Newer antidepressants and potentially important drug interactions (adapted from Nemeroff et al.,[41] with permission)

Antidepressant	Cytochrome P450 enzyme system inhibited	Drugs that may be affected
Fluoxetine	2D6	Secondary amine TCAs, haloperidol, class 1C antiarrythmics
	2C	Phenytoin, diazepam
Sertraline	2D6	Secondary amine TCAs, antipsychotics, class 1C antiarrythmics
	2C	Tolbutamide, diazepam
Paroxetine	2D6	Secondary amine TCAs, antipsychotics, class 1C antiarrythmics, trazodone
Fluvoxamine	1A2	Theophylline, clozapine, haloperidol, amitriptyline, clomipramine, imipramine
	2C	Diazepam, warfarin
	3A4	Carbamazepine, alprazolam, terfenadine, astemizole
Citalopram	2D6 (? other isoenzymes)	Desipramine, imipramine (? all TCAs); further studies needed with other combinations[a]

a Serotonin syndrome, seizures and death reported in at least 3 patients treated with citalopram combined with reversible monoamine oxidase inhibitors, moclobemide plus benzodiazepines, or alcohol (ethanol).

TCAs = tricyclic antidepressants.

Concomitant administration of SSRIs and drugs with a narrow therapeutic index normally metabolised by CYP isoenzymes, such as TCAs, has the potential to increase plasma and tissue concentrations of the latter compounds, with subsequent emergence of adverse events, or (in this case) the emergence of therapeutically planned and desirable events (remission of depression) when these drugs are combined as an adjuvant treatment in patients not responsive to either drug alone.

Dosage adjustments are often necessary for drugs with a narrow therapeutic index when combined with SSRIs. Inhibition of CYP2D6, CYP3A3, CYP3A4 or CYP2C by various SSRIs can raise plasma and tissue concentrations of TCAs,[110] warfarin (coumadin), anticonvulsants [valproic acid (sodium valproate), carbamazepine], certain antipsychotics (including clozapine), quinidine and some other antiarrhythmic drugs, β-blockers and some opioids.[41,109] Therefore, dosage adjustment of these compounds may be required in patients receiving SSRIs. For example, a recent report documented increased warfarin concentrations and prothrombin time in a patient receiving warfarin and fluoxetine.[111]

SSRI-induced enzyme inhibition is dosage related and has been reported with all SSRIs, although the particular isoenzymes involved vary with the particular SSRI and concomitant drug administered.[112] Crewe et al.[112] ranked a number of antidepressants according to their *in vitro* ability to inhibit CYP2D6 in the following order: paroxetine > fluoxetine (norfluoxetine) > sertraline > citalopram > fluvoxamine > clomipramine and amitriptyline. However, the relative *in vitro* inhibition is not remarkably different between the three most widely used and most potent inhibitors of the isoenzyme, paroxetine, fluoxetine and sertraline, and the latter two are closest together (table V).[112] Citalopram inhibits CYP2D6 far more weakly than any of the three most widely used SSRIs (fluoxetine, sertraline and paroxetine), but it does inhibit other isoenzymes.[112]

In vivo studies of fluoxetine and paroxetine (at full therapeutic dosages) found them to be equal in inhibiting CYP2D6, as revealed by decrease in desipramine metabolism with resultant increased plasma concentrations.[109] In the same report, low doses of sertraline (50mg) produced less interference with desipramine metabolism (less increase in steady-state desipramine concentrations, compared with other SSRIs).[109] However, the dose of sertraline studied was often a clinically subtherapeutic dose,[113] and higher doses would be expected to proportionately increase drug concentrations.[114] This would cause greater inhibition of CYP2D6 and further elevate plasma and tissue concentrations of desipramine.[114]

When using compounds with a narrow therapeutic index in conjunction with SSRIs, monitoring of plasma concentrations of these compounds and/or their active metabolites, or measuring their physiological effects, is advisable (e.g. ECG during concomitant TCA administration or prothrombin levels during warfarin administration), and clinical monitoring of individual patients is mandatory.

Table V. Inhibition constants (K_i) for cytochrome P450 2D6–mediated inhibition of 2-dehydrosparteine metabolism in human liver microsomes (reproduced from Crewe et al.,[112] with permission)

Drug (and major metabolites)	K_i (μmol/L)
Paroxetine	0.15
(M-1 glucuronide)	>200
(M-1 sulphate)	120
Fluoxetine	0.60
(norfluoxetine)	0.43
Sertraline	0.70
Citalopram	5.1
Fluvoxamine	8.2
Clomipramine	2.2
Desipramine	2.3
Amitriptyline	4.0
Quinidine	0.03

Nevertheless, despite clear *in vitro* and more recent *in vivo* evidence of the inhibiting effects of all SSRIs on various isoenzymes of the CYP enzyme system, and reported increases in TCA plasma concentrations during concomitant SSRI administration, it is reassuring that the adverse events related to this form of enzyme inhibition have proven to be rarely of clinical importance. This conclusion is similar to that expressed by Nemeroff et al.[41] Our search of the literature revealed only rare reports of significant drug-drug interactions with SSRIs, even after 10 years of extensive post-marketing use.

Physicians must keep the possibility of potential drug-drug interactions clearly in mind. A further caveat of caution is appropriate here because it is not currently possible to accurately predict in which patients, and to what degree, plasma concentrations of TCAs or other drugs may be enhanced in the presence of concomitant SSRI administration. It is useful for clinicians to refer to a table of potential drug-drug interactions that can possibly complicate concomitant drug administration with SSRIs so that appropriate monitoring can be pursued (table IV).

6.3 Highly Protein-Bound Drugs

SSRIs tend to be highly protein bound (especially sertraline, paroxetine and fluoxetine),[3,53,73,85] and may displace other drugs bound to plasma proteins (e.g. warfarin and digitalis), thereby increasing the concentration of the free (non–protein-bound) and generally 'active' fraction of these compounds. This propensity of SSRIs to displace compounds bound to plasma proteins may work in conjunction with SSRI inhibition of CYP metabolism to further elevate levels and enhance the activity of co-administered compounds. Although clinical experience to date has not revealed frequent or severe problems with these combinations, awareness of this potential is appropriate.

7. Intentional Overdose

Patients with depression are at high risk of suicide attempts. The older antidepressant drugs are among the most commonly used agents in suicide, in part because patients with depression have access to these prescription drugs. One of the major advantages of SSRIs is their safety in overdose, in contrast with TCAs, HCAs and MAOIs.[53] Overall, TCAs cause more deaths from overdose than any other prescription drug. Our own extensive experience with suicidal patients corresponds with that of Tollefson's[17] recommendation that SSRIs are first-line therapy for patients at risk of drug overdose.

In a review of the number of deaths per million prescriptions, Leonard reported,[53] consistent with the findings of others in the United States and Europe,[35,79] that the number of suicides per million prescriptions of SSRIs is orders of magnitude lower than that reported for TCAs and MAOIs (table I). The few deaths observed in clinical trials with many thousands of depressed patients were usually limited to situations in which patients overdosed with a combination of SSRIs and other drugs.[96,115-118] Worldwide post-marketing experience with these compounds confirms the finding that there is little documentation of deaths in suicide attempts using SSRIs alone,[119] although there have been several case reports of suicide with citalopram alone.[120]

Symptoms of SSRI overdose include tachycardia, sedation, tremor, nausea and emesis. Aggressive supportive measures are recommended as sufficient therapy. There is little risk of serious cardiovascular or neurological complications, and patients have recovered without lasting harm from overdoses of up to 3000mg of fluoxetine, over 37 times the usual recommended daily dose.[115]

Experience with sertraline up to January 1997 (over 10 million patients have been exposed to the drug) revealed 16 accidental overdoses and 190 intentional overdoses (personal communication, Pfizer Inc.); few of these were fatal when sertraline alone was ingested.

During worldwide clinical trials with paroxetine in more than 4000 patients, 28 cases of overdose were reported, of which 9 were overdoses with paroxetine alone; there were no deaths (personal communication, SmithKline Beecham). Postmarketing experience with paroxetine up to December 1995, with over 7.5 million patients treated, revealed 135 validated overdoses and 19 fatalities. However, all but two fatalities involved other drugs and/or alcohol (ethanol), or external factors (e.g. hypothermia secondary to exposure). Over a 2-year period, overdoses with paroxetine in 28 children were reported to the Pittsburgh Poison Control Center, Pittburgh, USA (dose 10 to 800mg); no case had a fatal outcome (personal communication, SmithKline Beecham).

We have been unsuccessful in obtaining similar data on citalopram and fluvoxamine. However, of the 354 cases of deliberate or accidental overdose of fluvoxamine reported up to 1992,[85] there were 19 fatalities, only 2 of which were associated with the ingestion of fluvoxamine alone; an estimated 4.5 million patients had been exposed by that time.

It must be borne in mind that 20 to 40% of patients with affective disorders show suicidal behaviour.[115] Some studies have found decreased tritiated imipramine binding sites (serotonin uptake pump) in the frontal cortex of individuals who have committed suicide,[121] compared with the frontal cortex of individuals killed suddenly in accidents. Findings of low CSF 5-hydroxyindole acetic acid (5-HIAA) levels,[122] a serotonin metabolite, also contribute to the current concepts of psychobiology of suicide impulsivity and aggression.[123]

Although suicidal ideation and behaviour can emerge at any point during the course of antidepressant treatment of depressive illness, untreated patients are at a greater risk of attempting suicide. Episodes of anger attacks and aggressive behaviour may occur in patients with untreated depression, and contribute to impulsive suicidal acts.[124] Since SSRIs are safer in overdose than older antidepressants, SSRIs can be recommended as first-line agents for patients at risk of overdose or those manifesting suicidal thinking or with a history of suicidal behaviour. Obviously, non-responsive patients (for any reason) remain at risk, similar to their pre-treatment state, and a re-evaluation of their diagnosis and therapy is indicated.

Although questions have been raised about the association between SSRIs and the emergence of suicidal ideation, several studies have concluded from all the data available that suicidal ideation may emerge during treatment with all types of antidepressants, but that a causal relationship to antidepressants has not been established.[24,116] Retrospective postmarketing studies[117] and evaluation of premarketing clinical study data in thousands of fluoxetine-treated patients[96] have revealed no evidence of a relationship between fluoxetine therapy and suicide. On the contrary, there is evidence for an apparent decrease in suicidal ideation as measured by the HDRS.[24,96,117,125] The same conclusion has been drawn in relation to paroxetine,[118,125] and extensive clinical experience to date supports this with all SSRIs and TCAs,[96] and implies the same for all antidepressants.

A review of eight recently completed drug comparator and/or placebo-controlled, double-blind trials of depressed outpatients receiving one of six drugs (etoperidone, fluparoxan, nefazodone, adinazolam, dothiepin, fluoxetine) confirm the decrease in suicidal ideation observed in responders during treatment, and this correlated with overall treatment response.[119]

8. Uses in Medical Illnesses

There are a variety of medical conditions that can cause or worsen depression or make the management of this disorder a further challenge to the clinician. SSRIs play an important role in the treatment of depression in these settings.

8.1 Cardiovascular Disease

Depression is commonly seen (20 to 25%) in patients following an acute myocardial infarction, in cardiac patients with poor prognosis and hospitalised patients with coronary artery disease (CAD).[54] It is notable that depression is the strongest independent predictor (apart from the CAD itself) of negative outcome in patients with CAD.[126,127] Because of the absence of significant effects on heart rate and rhythm or on blood pressure, SSRIs are the drugs of choice to treat depression in patients with heart conduction disease, orthostatic hypotension, ventricular arrhythmias, ischaemic heart disease or past acute myocardial infarction.[40]

TCAs have quinidine-like effects and slow intraventricular conduction and should be avoided in patients with heart block and those maintained on other drugs (e.g. procainamide, flecainide and other group 1A antiarrhythmics) that slow intraventricular impulse conduction. TCAs also produce orthostatic hypotension and rebound tachycardia, posing a risk to patients with coronary artery disease or with congestive heart failure, especially those with left ventricular impairment, and patients taking drugs such as diuretics or vasodilators which may exacerbate TCA-induced hypotension.[128] Therefore, although TCAs have been used safely in patients with cardiac conditions, it is appropriate that these drugs should be used with caution in such patients, if at all. In our own clinical experience, we have used SSRIs almost exclusively as first-line drugs in patients with the above cardiovascular problems over the past 10 years, without significant drug-induced untoward effects.

MAOIs share some of the same adverse effects as TCAs, in particular, induction of hypotension and enhancement of sympathomimetic agents.[3] For these reasons, and considering that a 'safer' option is available, all of the older agents should be reserved as second-line alternatives in patients with cardiac disease, and prescribed only for those whose symptoms of depression fail to respond to SSRIs.

8.2 Neurological Disease

SSRIs are among the drugs preferred for patients at higher risk of seizures, since they reduce the seizure threshold much less than older antidepressants.[40] The combination of older antidepressants and antipsychotics can further reduce the seizure threshold. Therefore, SSRIs are useful in patients with depression and epilepsy as well as in patients with factors predisposing to seizure activity such as head trauma, medications that reduce the seizure threshold, and substance abuse.[40]

Depressed patients with organic brain syndrome benefit from SSRIs and experience essentially no cholinergic effects.[129] The same can be said for the elderly or patients with stroke up to 30% of whom are reported to have depressive symptomatology.[130] The anticholinergic effects of the TCAs and HCAs can increase the chance of confusional states developing in these populations. Stroke patients also benefit from the lower incidence of cardiovascular adverse effects of SSRIs compared to older drugs that might precipitate hypotension or cardiac arrhythmias, and all the SSRIs have been used successfully and with better tolerability in such patients.[8,40]

Various reports reveal that up to 50% of patients with Parkinson's disease have depression.[131] The anticholinergic effects of some older antidepressants may, in some cases, contribute to improved motor performance in these patients. Long term administration of SSRIs can, secondary to enhanced serotonergic transmission, inhibit dopamine neuron activity and, theoretically, could worsen Parkinson's disease. However, a single prospective study of the use of fluoxetine in Parkinson's disease did not find clinical worsening of extrapyramidal symptoms.[131] Evidence that a deficient serotonin system might play a role in Parkinson's disease[132] and could be helped by SSRIs awaits further study and clarification.

8.3 Cancer

Up to 25% of patients with cancer report clinically significant depressive symptoms, and this is especially true in those with an uncertain or poor prognosis, chronic pain or physical impairment. In patients for whom the anticholinergic activity of TCAs can be detrimental (e.g. post abdominal surgery, patients with stomatitis), SSRIs are particularly preferred.[40] TCAs, when tolerated in fully effective antidepressant dosages, may be useful in patients with severe bodyweight loss because of the tendency of these drugs to increase appetite and induce bodyweight gain when taken long term. However, the anticholinergic effects of these drugs could produce significant constipation and gastrointestinal problems as well as other adverse effects (hypotension, falls and fractures), particularly in patients who are partially bedridden or inactive.

It is possible to hypothesise, based on the known adverse effects of SSRIs, that these drugs might decrease appetite and exacerbate bodyweight loss in patients with cancer, depressed anorectic medically ill patients or patients with anorexia nervosa. However, we have been unable to find reports in the literature supporting this, and we are unaware of any prospective controlled studies in this regard. The tendency of SSRIs to produce mild to moderate bodyweight loss appears to be restricted to patients who are overweight at the beginning of treatment. Progressive continued bodyweight loss does not persist, even in these patients, unless other measures to reduce caloric intake below expenditure are involved.[133]

8.4 Gastrointestinal Disease

SSRIs can be useful in depressed patients with chronic constipation, a condition that could be worsened by TCAs because of their anticholinergic effects, especially in the elderly and postoperative or chronically ill patients. By the same token, we have seen patients with diarrhoea and irritable bowel syndrome benefit from this effect of TCAs.

9. Use in the Elderly

Depression in the elderly is frequently underdiagnosed and undertreated.[6,134] An analysis of symptoms of depression in hospitalised older persons identified a vulnerable group more likely to have a subsequent negative health outcome.[135] This is in part caused by the fact that symptoms of depression such as changes in appetite and sleep, complaints of anergia, and evidence of social withdrawal may erroneously be regarded as related to the aging process. Managing depression in the elderly is further complicated by the fact that this population is more likely to have concomitant medical disorders, to be taking other medications that may interact with antidepressants, and to excrete and metabolise drugs less efficiently than the younger population. The elderly are particularly vulnerable to the orthostatic hypotensive effect of older antidepressants which may cause postural hypotension, dizziness and fainting.[3] These factors, and also the blurred vision associated with anticholinergic blockade, may cause elderly patients to be more susceptible to falls.[76]

The ideal antidepressant for use in the elderly population should have no cardiotoxic or orthostatic effects, little sedative potential, and should not impair memory or produce physical disability.[14] Therefore, the SSRIs may be particularly effective for elderly patients because of the virtual absence of cardiovascular and anticholinergic adverse effects.

Doxepin, one of the most frequently prescribed older antidepressants in geriatric patients, has been compared with fluoxetine[136] and paroxetine.[137] After 6 weeks, the SSRIs were shown to be as efficacious as doxepin. The lower incidence of serious adverse events (dizziness, drowsiness, confusion) and anticholinergic-related adverse effects led to a lower discontinuation rate among the SSRI-treated groups. Sertraline has been compared with amitriptyline in elderly patients with depression and was found to be as effective as, and to have a more acceptable tolerability profile than, the TCA.[138]

A recent publication[139] underscored the need for frequent long term full-dosage maintenance antidepressant therapy in the elderly population. This is especially true in those whose first episode occurs over the age of 50 years and in those with delayed treatment or slow response to treatment in the index episode. SSRIs lend themselves to successful long term maintenance therapy because of their benign, generally transient adverse-effect profile, safety in overdose and ease of administration.

Individual pharmacokinetic characteristics of the SSRIs must be taken into account when they are used in the treatment of older patients. Fluoxetine pharmacokinetics are reported to be basically unchanged in this population,[129,140] but changes have been noted in studies of sertraline and paroxetine.[73] These changes are significant enough with paroxetine to recommend lower starting dosages (10 mg/day instead of the usual 20 mg/day), with a gradual upward titration to a maximum of 40 mg/day (instead of the usual 50 mg/day).

Besides being effective antidepressants, the virtual absence of cardiovascular and anticholinergic effects with SSRIs is especially useful in the elderly population in which events such as orthostatic hypotension or confusion can be more common and conditions such as glaucoma and prostate disease more prevalent than in the younger population. All these events and conditions may be worsened by the older antidepressant drugs because of their known pharmacological actions.[8-10,18,41]

10. Depression and Childbearing

One problem faced by physicians is counselling a patient with a history of depression who wants to become pregnant. The general guideline that applies to these patients and those who become depressed during pregnancy is to try to avoid any agents that have not been widely proven to be harmless to the fetus. In the case of mild depression, alternative approaches to medication, e.g. interpersonal or cognitive behavioural therapy, may be helpful until pregnancy is over or at least until past the first trimester when organogenesis has progressed and medications can be used with less concern regarding adverse events if they are still necessary. If nonpharmacological approaches are used, close clinical monitoring is essential and consideration should be given to promptly adding pharmacotherapy or electroconvulsive therapy (ECT) if clinical deterioration occurs or the patient fails to respond.

In patients with more severe depression, the risk to the fetus must be weighed against symptoms of depression that could potentially jeopardise both the mother and the fetus. Some factors to be considered include severity of depression, risk of potentially harmful behaviour such as suicidality and other forms of impulsiveness and aggressive behaviour, and inability to maintain reasonable bodyweight gain during pregnancy. In these situations, the possibility of fetal harm secondary to antidepressants, now recognised as very unlikely, support the priority of the pregnant woman's need for treatment.[141-143] There is no evidence to suggest that any antidepressant (with the probable exception of lithium) is teratogenic. The long clinical experience with TCAs largely substantiates their safety, and recent studies with fluoxetine and the extensive post-marketing experience with this drug support its safety.[142]

Based on preclinical studies,[40] extensive personal experience, review of case reports to date and (most importantly) recent prospective studies in pregnancy,[141,142,144,145] it appears that fluoxetine is as 'safe' as the TCAs when used during pregnancy. One study[144] reported an increased risk of perinatal complications in mothers taking fluoxetine, although another[145] found no such relationship. Overall, these controlled data strongly suggest that fluoxetine is probably the antidepressant of choice when pharmacotherapy is indicated for the treatment of depression in pregnancy or in patients with a high likelihood of becoming pregnant during antidepressant treatment. A recent study involving about 750 women exposed to fluoxetine in the first trimester of pregnancy, and followed prospectively, found no increase in congenital malformations above that seen in the general (unmedicated) population (i.e. 3 to 4%).[146] One prospective study[142] found no abnormalities in developmental milestones up to age 7 years in children whose mothers received fluoxetine during pregnancy. Since the incidence of depression is high among young women of childbearing age and many pregnancies are unplanned, the data on fluoxetine are very reassuring for individuals who are already receiving this antidepressant drug when they conceive.

Although fewer data are available regarding the use of other SSRIs during pregnancy, their lack of teratogenicity in animal studies is supported by the absence of post-marketing data suggesting teratogenicity.

All SSRIs can be excreted in breast milk; however, the limited data available to date have not included reports of adverse events in breastfeeding infants of mothers receiving treatment with SSRIs.[147] The American Academy of Paediatrics does not advise against breastfeeding during SSRI therapy.[148]

11. Use in Depressive Subtypes and Comorbid Psychiatric Conditions

To date, no single antidepressant stands out as having superior efficacy (i.e. greater frequency of acute remission) for all kinds or any one subtype of major depression. The choice of a specific agent must be based on tolerability and specific patient-related characteristics, especially medication acceptance and compliance, consideration of comorbid medical and psychiatric conditions and, since the advent of the SSRIs, safety in overdose.

A particularly important consideration in choosing a specific antidepressant is the need for relatively long term treatment; a minimum of 4 to 6 months continuation therapy after full remission is required, with subsequent gradual antidepressant discontinuation.[149] It may be appropriate to continue antidepressant treatment for many years or even permanently as prophylaxis, since depression is a chronic relapsing illness.[150] Patients with early onset of depression (before age 20 years), with their first episode occurring after age 50 years, or those with multiple episodes (especially 2 or more episodes in the previous 5 years) are candidates for full-dosage prophylactic therapy.[150] When this is the case, SSRIs are the antidepressant of choice, particularly fluoxetine, as its long half-life assists in preventing withdrawal symptoms, relapse or recurrence (this can occur with short half-life antidepressants when a few doses or several days of missed medication occurs) [see section 5.2].

The Danish University Antidepressant Group has raised the question of whether citalopram or paroxetine are as effective as older antidepressants in the treatment of severe depression.[151,152] However, we have found fluoxetine to be as effective as full-dose imipramine in hospitalised severely depressed patients.[153]

11.1 Anxious Agitated Depression

One of the early observations regarding the use of SSRIs was the lack of sedating properties compared with older TCAs.[40] Some clinicians have postulated that this might be disadvantageous for patients with features such as anxiety or agitation, which are common in depression. Several retrospective analyses of therapeutic trials and new prospective studies have shown that fluoxetine is indeed efficacious in depression, regardless of baseline psychomotor activity or features such as anxiety or insomnia.[154-156]

In fact, it appears that SSRIs may be particularly effective in treating depression presenting with anxiety.[95] This fact is noteworthy and consistent with many studies of SSRIs that have used the HDRS, which incorporates a significant emphasis on estimating anxiety, somatic symptoms and sleep disturbances.[157] Consequently, the favourable therapeutic comparison of SSRIs with sedating TCAs or other antidepressants in treating anxious depression as measured using the HDRS is even more significant.

Similar findings to those reported after fluoxetine treatment have been reported with paroxetine.[158] Trials with fluvoxamine have shown this agent to be as effective as benzodiazepines in treating anxiety in a general practice study of patients with mixed anxiety and depression,[159] but superior in the treatment of depression in these patients.[160]

As a comorbid feature of depression, anxiety tends to subside as the entire syndrome improves and has been shown to be one of the earliest symptoms to begin to improve during antidepressant therapy.[161] In choosing an antidepressant agent, the clinician must weigh the benefits of a rapid reduction in anxiety levels, which could be beneficial in some patients (e.g. when acute compliance is a management problem because of anxiety), against the detrimental factor of having to deal with sedation and impairment of psychomotor performance, which can lead to premature drug discontinuation – a particular problem in patients who need to continue to work during treatment and in the high percentage of patients who need long term prophylactic therapy. We believe that SSRIs are the best drugs available for long term maintenance prophylactic therapy because of their good tolerability, which contributes to long term compliance. The long half-life of fluoxetine is a further argument for the selection of this drug (see section 5.2).

The efficacy and tolerability of citalopram is similar to that of other SSRIs and the TCAs. More than a dozen controlled studies involving over 2500 depressed patients receiving citalopram, many with comorbid anxiety, have supported the clinical efficacy of the drug.[162] However, one report found clomipramine was perhaps more effective than imipramine or citalopram.[163] A controlled study of 217 depressed outpatients found citalopram to be better tolerated than fluvoxamine.[164] The SSRIs are also very useful in the treatment of patients with panic disorder,[165] as well as depressed patients with anxiety or panic attacks;[166] however, low dosages or increased dosage intervals are generally essential, at least initially to reduce the risk of precipitating panic attacks and/or increasing anxiety.[167]

In summary, it has been found that fluoxetine, paroxetine and sertraline decrease measured anxiety as promptly as the older sedating agents. Furthermore, data from the National Institute of Mental Health (NIMH) Collaborative Depression Study have clearly shown that improvement in sleep is *not* predictive of, or correlated with, global clinical improvement.[161] SSRIs are not only efficacious in reducing the anxiety, agitation and insomnia associated with depression, they generally have a more benign tolerability profile, and are associated with better acceptance resulting in higher compliance rates during maintenance therapy and long term prophylaxis. The SSRIs have proven to be first-line agents in patients with depression associated with anxiety features and in patients needing long term psychiatric pharmacological therapy.[149]

11.2 Delusional or Psychotic Major Depression

Some data[168] point to the possibility that delusional-psychotic depression is a separate entity, although this remains controversial. Response rates to antidepressants or antipsychotics alone are lower (perhaps by 30%) for delusional depression than for nonpsychotic depression,[151] and some delusional patients will eventually require ECT. About two-thirds of delusionally depressed patients achieve remission when antidepressant therapy is combined with antipsychotic agents,[168] but there is no evidence that one antidepressant works better than another.

A recent study of 30 patients with psychotic depression treated with combined therapy of fluoxetine and perphenazine showed a response rate of 73%, equivalent to the best response rates of patients with psychotic depression treated with older antidepressants plus an antipsychotic.[151]

11.3 Dysthymic Depression

Dysthymia tends to occur at an early age, and has an insidious onset and a chronic course. The biology of dysthymia is not well understood, and further research is needed on the aetiology and treatment of this illness.

The relevance of identifying and treating dysthymic patients cannot be overemphasised, since the condition is prevalent, disrupts quality of life, and is responsive to therapy with SSRIs as well as older antidepressants.[7] Dysthymia is underdiagnosed and undertreated.[7] Studies show that most of these patients go on to develop major depressive episodes superimposed on the dysthymia (so-called double depression).[169] These patients, even after recovering from the major depressive episode, are at a greater risk of relapse into major depression if they continue to experience dysthymic symptoms. This risk increases with the duration of the dysthymic episode.[170] Dysthymic patients are also at risk of suicide.[7]

The better tolerability profile of the SSRIs is especially helpful in increasing compliance among those patients who consider the less favourable tolerability profiles or dietary restrictions associated with older antidepressants unacceptable when weighed against the potential benefits of drug therapy. This is especially true with regard to long term 'continuation' treatment after recovery from acute depression, and even more so with those patients in need of longer term prophylactic therapy. The chronicity of dysthymia argues strongly for the use of SSRIs as first-line acute and prophylactic therapy, because of the safety of these drugs in overdose and generally better patient acceptance, reflected in increased long term compliance.[169]

11.4 Atypical Depression

Patients with atypical depression meet criteria for major depressive disorder, but are further characterised by having excessive mood reactivity (complete but transient remission from depressed mood in response to positive environmental factors) and one or more associated features of overeating, oversleeping (or extreme fatigue) or chronic hypersensitivity to rejection; some authors add complaints of 'leaden heaviness' of extremities.[171]

There is a considerable amount of data indicating that these patients respond better to MAOIs than to TCAs.[171-173] However, considering that many patients with atypical depression respond to SSRIs, some investigators have recommended that SSRIs be tried first because of their favourable tolerability profile.[174] There is some evidence to suggest that SSRIs are as effective as MAOIs in the treatment of patients with atypical depression, although the number of patients studied was relatively small.[7,175]

Therefore, it is reasonable to use SSRIs as first-line drugs in the treatment of patients with atypical depression.

12. Maintenance Therapy

Long term, double-blind, placebo-controlled studies of maintenance or 'prophylactic' treatment have demonstrated the ability of TCAs to maintain euthymia in most patients (>80%) with major depressive disorder for periods of up to 3 years;[149,176,177] in a small extension study, euthymia was maintained for up to 5 years[178] if full-dosage TCA therapy (e.g. imipramine 200 mg/day) could be tolerated and maintained.

More recently, fluoxetine,[52,169,179,180] sertraline[177] and paroxetine[181] (*vs* placebo) have been shown to be as effective as imipramine[176] (also *vs* placebo) in 1-year maintenance studies after recovery and completion of a 3- or 4-month euthymic continuation phase. Long term efficacy studies have shown the superiority of citalopram over placebo in preventing relapse when full therapeutic doses are continued, usually 20 to 40 mg/day.[162] The extended half-life of fluoxetine may provide increased protection against relapse as well as the already documented reduced likelihood of withdrawal symptoms, compared with shorter half-life SSRIs, when a few days of medication are missed.[182]

13. Conclusion

We have reviewed data comparing the individual SSRIs in the treatment of depression and we believe that, as a class, they are superior to TCAs and MAOIs. The SSRIs have numerous advantages over these older agents, such as comparable efficacy, a more benign adverse-effect profile that enhances patient compliance, a broader spectrum of activity – they are effective in various clinical subtypes of depression – markedly improved safety in overdose and an easier dosage schedule.

Treatment with the older antidepressants is often associated with adverse events such as sedation, bodyweight gain, dry mouth, constipation, urinary retention, cardiac effects (tachycardia, orthostatic hypotension, depression of cardiac conduction) and vision disturbances (blurred vision). These effects are particularly problematic in the elderly, those with comorbid medical illness and in the significant percentage of patients with depression who need long term prophylactic therapy. It is estimated that only 20 to 25% of patients taking TCAs receive adequate therapeutic dosages,[36-38] in an attempt to avoid the adverse effects of these drugs. Noncompliance and premature discontinuation of treatment result from these adverse effects and leave patients subject to the mortality, morbidity and economic burden that is associated with depression.

Although SSRIs present with their own unique spectrum of adverse effects, such as sexual dysfunction, dyspepsia, nausea, diarrhoea, insomnia, headaches, and mild nervousness or agitation, studies have shown TCAs to have the highest discontinuation rates resulting from adverse events; discontinuation because of adverse events with SSRIs was, in many instances, not significantly different from the rate with placebo.[10]

Clinicians may be wary of prescribing full dosages of TCAs because of their potential lethality in overdose and thus may see patients who do not respond, simply because they are taking subtherapeutic doses. SSRIs are more likely to be prescribed at full therapeutic dosages, thus providing an optimal chance of remission and minimising the risk of inadequate treatment, with a resultant effectively untreated depressive state with its continued morbidity and potential for suicide.

The easier dosage schedule of SSRIs allows for full therapeutic dosages from the beginning of treatment in almost all instances, with little requirement for titration compared with older antidepressants. These factors further increase acceptance and compliance, increasing the chance of successful treatment.

The costs of depression (e.g. hospitalisation, disruption of work and family) both for the individual and for society are high. The risk of not treating depression clearly outweighs the minimal risks of treating the disease. Pharmacotherapy is the primary treatment of this disorder, and this can shorten the duration of episodes. SSRIs have contributed remarkably to improving the risk-benefit ratio of the treatment of depression; improved compliance and easier management play a big role in this. Although TCAs are less expensive per tablet than other antidepressants, the need to closely and more extensively monitor patients during treatment significantly increases the cost of overall treatment.[13]

Withdrawal symptoms and possible relapse of depression can occur on cessation of therapy with SSRIs that have shorter half-lives. This does not occur with fluoxetine, probably because of its slow elimination secondary to its long half-life.

Effectively treating depression with a well-tolerated drug can not only alleviate the suffering of millions of patients, but decrease the cost of healthcare and the risk of disability for individuals who have affective disorders, a significant proportion of the work force in our society. Easier management, higher acceptance and effectiveness of SSRIs have turned these drugs into the most widely prescribed first-line agents for treatment of depression in the USA, and their continued increase in use suggests that they will generally supplant other drug classes worldwide.

Acknowledgements

The authors wish to thank Alexandra I. Barsdorf for library research, editing and comments about clarity; and Deidre Brown-Selvin and Herminia Ombid for manuscript preparation.

References

1. Katon W, Von Korff M, Lin E, et al. Adequacy and duration of antidepressant treatment in primary care. Med Care 1992; 30: 67-76
2. Wells KB, Katon W, Rogers B, Camp P. Use of minor tranquilizers and antidepressant medications by depressed outpatients: results from the medical outcomes study. Am J Psychiatry 1994; 151: 694-700
3. Stokes PE. Fluoxetine: a five year review. Clin Ther 1993; 15: 216-43
4. Thase ME, Kupfer DJ. Recent developments in the pharmacotherapy of mood disorders. J Consult Clin Psychol 1996; 64: 646-59
5. Regier DA, Hirschfeld RM, Goodwin FK, et al. The NIMH Depression Awareness, Recognition, and Treatment Program: structure, aims, and scientific basis. Am J Psychiatry 1988; 145: 1351-7
6. Hirschfeld RMA, Keller MB, Panico S, et al. The National Depressive and Manic-depressive Association consensus statement on the undertreatment of depression. JAMA 1997; 277 (4): 333-40
7. Shelton RC, Davidson J, Yonker KA, et al. The undertreatment of dysthymia. J Clin Psychiatry 1997; 58 (2): 59-65
8. Richelson E. Treatment of acute depression. Psych Clin North America 1993; 16 (3): 461-78
9. Wong DT, Bymaster FP, Horng JS, et al. A new selective inhibitor for uptake of serotonin into synaptosomes of rat brain: 3-(p-trifluoromethylphenoxy)-*N*-methyl- 3-phenylpropylamine. J Pharmacol Exp Ther 1975; 193: 804-11
10. Preskorn SH. Comparison of the tolerability of bupropion, fluoxetine, imipramine, nefazodone, paroxetine, sertraline, and venlafaxine. J Clin Psychiatry 1995; 56 Suppl. 6: 12-21
11. Kroenke K. Discovering depression in medical patients: reasonable expectations. Ann Intern Med 1997; 126 (6): 463-5
12. Frasure-Smith N, Lesperance F, Talajic M. Depression following myocardial infarction: impact on 6-month survival. JAMA 1993; 270: 1819-25
13. Wells KB, Stewart A, Hays RD, et al. The functioning and well-being of depressed patients: results from the Medical Outcomes Study. JAMA 1989; 262: 914-9
14. Nemeroff CB. Evolutionary trends in the pharmacotherapeutic management of depression. J Clin Psychiatry 1994; 55 Suppl. 12: 3-15
15. Elkin I, Shea MT, Watkins JT, et al. National Institute of Mental Health Treatment of Depression Collaborative Research Program: general effectiveness of treatments. Arch Gen Psychiatry 1989; 46: 971-83
16. Haddad LM. Managing tricyclic antidepressant overdose. Am Fam Phys 1992; 46: 153-9
17. Tollefson GD. Selective serotonin reuptake inhibitors. In: Schatzberg AF, Nemeroff B, editors. The American Psychiatric Press Textbook of Psychopharmacology. Washington, DC: American Psychiatric Press, Inc., 1995: 161-82
18. Simon GE, VonKorff M, Heiligenstein JH, et al. Initial antidepressant choice in primary care: effectiveness and cost of fluoxetine *vs* tricyclic antidepressants. JAMA 1996; 275: 1897-902
19. Sclar DA, Robinson LM, Skaer TL, et al. Antidepressant pharmacotherapy: economic outcomes in a health maintenance organization. Clin Ther 1994; 16 (4): 715-30
20. Sclar DA, Robinson LM, Skaer TL, et al. Antidepressant pharmacotherapy: economic evaluation of fluoxetine, paroxetine, and sertraline in a health maintenance organization. J Int Med Res 1995; 23: 395-412
21. Stoudemire A, Frank R, Hedemark N, et al. The economic burden of depression. Gen Hosp Psychiatry 1986; 8: 387-94
22. Katon W. The epidemiology of depression in medical care. Int J Psychiatry Med 1987; 17: 93-112
23. Guze SB, Robins E. Suicide and primary affective disorders. Br J Psychiatry 1970; 117: 437-8
24. Mann JJ, Kapur S. The emergence of suicidal ideation and behavior during antidepressant pharmacotherapy. Arch Gen Psychiatry 1991; 48: 1027-33
25. Avery D, Winokur G. Suicide, attempted suicide, and relapse rates in depression: occurrence after ECT and antidepressant therapy. Arch Gen Psychiatry 1978; 35: 749-53
26. Hagnell O, Lanke J, Rorsman B. Suicide rates in the Lundby study: Mental illness as a risk factor for suicide. Neuropsychobiology 1981; 7: 248-53
27. Tollefson GD, Fawcett J, Winokur G, et al. Evaluation of suicidality during pharmacologic treatment of mood and non-mood disorders. Ann Clin Psychiatry 1993; 5: 209-24
28. Greenberg PE, Stiglin LE, Finkelstein SN, et al. The economic burden of depression in 1990. J Clin Psychiatry 1993; 54 (11): 405-18
29. Katon W, Sullivan MD. Depression and chronic medical illness. J Clin Psychiatry 1990; 51 Suppl. 6: 3-11
30. Shapiro S, Skinner EA, Kessler LG, et al. Utilization of health and mental health services: three Epidemiologic Catchment Area sites. Arch Gen Psychiatry 1984; 41: 971-8
31. McCombs JS, Nichol MB, Stimmel GL, et al. The cost of antidepressant drug therapy failure: a study of antidepressant use patterns in a Medicaid population. J Clin Psychiatry 1990; 51 Suppl. 6: 60-71
32. Judd LL, Rapaport MH. Economics of depression and cost-benefit comparisons of selective serotonin reuptake inhibitors and tricyclic antidepressants. Depression 1995; 2: 173-7
33. Frank E, Kupfer DJ, Perel JM, et al. Three-year outcomes for maintenance therapies in recurrent depression. Arch Gen Psychiatry 1990; 47 (12): 1093-9
34. Donoghue JM. A comparison of prescribing patterns of selective serotonin reuptake inhibitors in the treatment of depression in primary care in the United Kingdom. J Serotonin Res 1995; 1: 47-51

35. Tollefson GD. Antidepressant treatment and side effect consideration. J Clin Psychiatry 1991; 52 Suppl.: 4-13
36. Gerber PD, Barrett J, Barrett J, et al. Recognition of depression by internists in primary care: a comparison of internist and "gold standard" psychiatric assessment. J Gen Intern Med 1989; 4: 7-13
37. Simon GE, Von Korff M. Recognition, management, and outcomes of depression in primary care. Arch Fam Med 1995; 4: 99-105
38. Lewis-Hall FC, Wilson MG, Tepner RG, Koke SC. Fluoxetine versus tricyclic antidepressants in women with major depressive disorder. J Womens Health 1997; 6: 337-343
39. Thompson D, Buesching D, Gregor KJ, et al. Patterns of antidepressant use and their relation to costs of care. AJMC 1996; 2 (9): 1239-46
40. Wong DT, Bymaster FP, Engleman EA. Minireview: Prozac (fluoxetine, Lilly 110140), the first selective serotonin uptake inhibitor and an antidepressant drug: twenty years since its first publication. Life Sci 1995; 57 (5): 411-41
41. Nemeroff CB, DeVane CL, Pollock BG. Newer antidepressants and the cytochrome P450 system. Am J Psychiatry 1996; 153 (3): 311-20
42. Keller MB. Diagnosis issues and clinical course of unipolar illness. Rev Psychiatry 1988; 7: 188-212
43. Thase ME. Relapse and recurrence in unipolar major depression: short term and long term approaches. J Clin Psychiatry 1990; 51 Suppl.: 51-9
44. Goodwin FK, Jamison KR. Course and outcome. In: Goodwin FK, Jamison KR, editors. Manic depressive illness. New York: Oxford University Press, 1990: 127-56
45. Grof P, Angst J, Haines T. The clinical course of depression: practical issues. In: Angst J, editor. Classification and prediction of outcome of depression. Symposium Schlob Reinhartshausen/Rhein; 1973 Sep 23-26. New York: FK Schattauer Verlag, 1973: 141-55
46. Consensus Development Panel. Mood disorders: pharmacologic prevention of recurrences. Am J Psychiatry 1985; 142: 469-76
47. Angst J, Bastrup P, Grof P, et al. The course of monopolar depression and bipolar psychoses. Psychiatr Neurol Neurochir (Amst) 1973; 76: 489-500
48. Angst J. Natural history and epidemiology of depression. In: Cobb J, Goeting N, editors. Results of community studies in prediction and treatment of recurrent depression. Southampton: Duphar Medical Relations, 1990
49. Lee AS, Murray AM. The long term outcome of Maudsley depressives. Br J Psychiatry 1988; 153: 741-51
50. Doogan DP, Caillard V. Sertraline in the prevention of depression. Br J Psychiatry 1992; 160: 217-22
51. Eric L. A prospective, double-blind, comparative, multicentre study of paroxetine and placebo in preventing recurrent major depressive episodes. Biol Psychiatry 1991; 29 Suppl. 11: 254S-5S
52. Montgomery SA, Dufour H, Brion S, et al. The prophylactic efficacy of fluoxetine in unipolar depression. Br J Psychiatry 1988; 153 Suppl. 3: 69-76
53. Leonard BE. Pharmacological differences of serotonin reuptake inhibitors and possible clinical relevance. Drugs 1992; 43 Suppl. 2: 3-10
54. Gonzalez MB, Snyderman TB, Colket JT, et al. Depression in patients with coronary artery disease. Depression 1996; 4 (4): 57-62
55. Nesse RE, Finlayson RE. Management of depression in patients with coexisting medical illness. Am Fam Phys 1996; 53: 2125-33
56. Stoudemire A. Expanding psychopharmacologic treatment options for the depressed medical patient. Psychosomatics 1995; 36: S19-26
57. Feighner JP, Cohn JB. Double-blind comparative trial of fluoxetine and doxepin in geriatric patients with major depressive disorder. J Clin Psychiatry 1985; 46: 20-5
58. Baldessarini RJ. Current status of antidepressants: clinical pharmacology and therapy. J Clin Psychiatry 1989; 50: 117-26
59. Haddad LM. Managing tricyclic antidepressant overdose. Am Fam Phys 1992; 46: 153-9
60. Kasper S, Fuger JD, Moller HJ. Comparative efficacy of antidepressants. Drugs 1992; 43 Suppl. 2: 11-23
61. Feighner JP, Boyer WF, Meredith CH, et al. A placebo-controlled inpatient comparison of fluvoxamine maleate and imipramine in major depression. Int Clin Psychopharmacol 1989; 4: 239-44
62. Guelfi JD, Dreyfus JF, Pichot P. Fluvoxamine and imipramine: results of a long-term controlled trial. Int Clin Psychopharmacol 1987; 2: 103-9
63. Wernicke JF, Bremner JD, Bosomworth J, et al. The efficacy and safety of fluoxetine in the long-term treatment of depression. International Fluoxetine Symposium: 1987 Oct 13-17; Tyrol, Austria
64. Peselow ED, Filippi AM, Goodnick P, et al. The short and long term efficacy of paroxetine HCl. B: data from a double-blind crossover study and from a year-long term trial *vs* imipramine and placebo. Psychopharmacol Bull 1989; 25 (2): 272-6
65. VanPraag HM, Kahn R, Asnis GM, et al. Therapeutic indications for serotonin-potentiating compounds: a hypothesis. Biol Psychiatry 1987; 22: 205-12
66. Boyer WF, Feighner JP. The efficacy of selective serotonin uptake inhibitors in depression. In: Feighner JP, Boyer WF, editors. Selective serotonin uptake inhibitors. Chichester, England: Wiley, 1991: 89-108
67. Lader M. Fluoxetine efficacy vs comparative drugs: an overview. Br J Psychiatry 1988; 153 Suppl. 3: 51-8
68. Tollefson GD. Adverse drug reactions/interactions in maintenance therapy. J Clin Psychiatry 1993; 54 Suppl.: 48-58
69. Fisch C. Effect of fluoxetine on the electrocardiogram. J Clin Psychiatry 1985; 46: 42-4
70. Fabre LF, Scharf MB, Itil TM. Comparative efficacy and safety of nortriptyline and fluoxetine in the treatment of major depression: a clinical study. J Clin Psychiatry 1991; 52 Suppl: 62-7
71. Beasley CM, Sayler ME, Cunningham GE, et al. Fluoxetine in tricyclic refractory major depressive disorder. J Affect Disord 1990; 20: 193-200

72. Delgado PL, Price LH, Charney DS, et al. Efficacy of fluvoxamine in treatment-refractory depression. J Affect Disord 1988; 15: 55-60
73. Leonard BE. SSRI differentiation: pharmacology and pharmacokinetics. Hum Psychopharmacol 1995; 10: S149-58
74. Baumann P. Clinical pharmacokinetics of citalopram and other serotonergic reuptake inhibitors (SSRI). Int Clin Psychopharmacol 1992; 6 Suppl. 5: 13-20
75. Koe BK, Weissman A, Welch WM, et al. Sertraline, 1S,4S-N-methyl-4-(3,4-dichlorophenyl)-1,2,3,4-tetrahydro-1-naphthylamine, a new uptake inhibitor with selectivity for serotonin. J Pharmacol Exp Ther 1983; 226: 686-700
76. Richelson E. Antidepressants and brain neurochemistry. Mayo Clin Proc 1990; 65: 1227-36
77. Thomas DR, Nelson DR, Johnson AM. Biochemical effects of the antidepressant paroxetine, a specific 5-hydroxytryptamine uptake inhibitor. Psychopharmacol Berl 1987; 93: 193-200
78. Bolden-Watson C, Richelson E. Blockade by newly developed antidepressants of biogenic amine uptake into rat brain synaptosomes. Life Sci 1993; 52: 1023-9
79. Tollefson GD, Rampey AH, Beasley CM, et al. Absence of a relationship between adverse events and suicidality during pharmacotherapy for depression. J Clin Psychopharmacol 1994; 14: 163-9
80. Wong DT, Reid LR, Bymaster FP, et al. Chronic effects of fluoxetine, a selective inhibitor of serotonin uptake, on neurotransmitter receptors. J Neural Transm 1985; 64: 251-69
81. Pérez V, Gilaberte I, Faries D, et al. Randomized, double-blind, placebo-controlled trial of pindolol in combination with fluoxetine antidepressant treatment. Lancet 1997; 349: 1594-7
82. Greden JF. Antidepressant maintenance medications: when to discontinue and how to stop. J Clin Psychiatry 1993; 54 Suppl.: 39-45
83. Fava G, Grandi S. Withdrawal syndromes after paroxetine and sertraline discontinuation. J Clin Psychopharmacol 1995; 15 (5): 374-5
84. Prozac (fluoxetine hydrochloride) Product Information. Indianapolis (IN): Dista Products Company, 1995 May 17
85. Physicians Desk Reference. 50th ed. Montvale, NJ: Medical Economics Company, Inc. 1996; 2544-8
86. Broadhead WE, Blazer DG, George LK, Tse CK. Depression, disability days, and days lost from work in a prospective epidemiologic survey. JAMA 1990; 264: 2524-8
87. Paxil® (brand of paroxetine HCL tablet) product information. SmithKline Beecham Pharmaceuticals. Philadelphia; May 1997
88. Baumann P. Pharmacokinetic-pharmacodynamic relationship of the selective serotonin reuptake inhibitors. Clin Pharmacokinet 1996; 31 (6): 444-69
89. Kulig K. Management of poisoning associated with 'newer' antidepressant agents. Ann Emerg Med 1986; 15: 1039-45
90. Montgomery SA. The benefits and risks of 5-HT uptake inhibitors in depression. Br J Psychiatry 1988; 153 (3 Suppl.): 7-10
91. Stark P, Hardison CD. A review of multicenter controlled studies of fluoxetine *vs* imipramine and placebo in outpatients with major depressive disorder. J Clin Psychiatry 1985; 45: 53-8
92. Goldstein DJ, Rampey AH Jr, Enas GG, et al. Fluoxetine: a randomized clinical trial in the treatment of obesity. Am J Clin Nutr 1992; 55: 181S-4S
93. Connolly VM, Gallagher A, Kesson CM. A study of fluoxetine in obese elderly patients with type 2 diabetes. Diabetic Med 1995; 12: 416-8
94. Kaye WH, Weltzin TE, Hsu LKG, et al. An open trial of fluoxetine in patients with anorexia nervosa. J Clin Psychiatry 1991; 52: 464-71
95. Filteau MJ, Baruch P, Lapierre YD, et al. SSRIs in anxious-agitated depression: a post-hoc analysis of 279 patients. Int Clin Psychopharmacol 1995; 10: 51-4
96. Beasley Jr CM, Dornseif BE, Bosomworth JC, et al. Fluoxetine and suicide: a meta-analysis of controlled trials of treatment for depression. BMJ 1991; 303: 685-92
97. DeVane CL. Comparative safety and tolerability of selective serotonin reuptake inhibitors. Hum Psychopharmacol 1995; 10: S185-93
98. Bannister SJ, Houser VP, Hulse JD, et al. Evaluation of the potential for interactions of paroxetine with diazepam, cimetidine, warfarin and digoxin. Acta Psychiatr Scand 1989; 80: 102-6
99. Lemberger L, Rowe H, Bosomworth JC, et al. The effect of fluoxetine on the pharmacokinetics and psychomotor responses of diazepam. Clin Pharmacol Ther 1988; 43: 412-9
100. Shen WW, Hsu JH. Female sexual side effects associated with selective serotonin reuptake inhibitors: A descriptive clinical study of 33 patients. Int J Psychiatry Med 1995; 25: 239-48
101. Hsu JH, Shen WW. Male sexual side effects associated with antidepressants: a descriptive clinical study of 32 patients. Int J Psychiatry Med 1995; 25: 191-205
102. Lane RM. A critical review of selective serotonin reuptake inhibitor-related sexual dysfunction; incidence, possible aetiology and implications for management. J Psychopharmacol 1997; 11: 72-82
103. Rothschild AJ. Selective serotonin reuptake inhibitor–induced sexual dysfunction: efficacy of a drug holiday. Am J Psychiatry 1995; 152: 1514-6
104. Harvey KV, Balon R. Clinical implications of antidepressant drug effects on sexual function. Ann Clin Psychiatry 1995; 7 (4): 189-201
105. Aizenberg D, Zemishlany Z, Weizman A. Cyproheptadine treatment of sexual dysfunction induced by serotonin reuptake inhibitors. Clin Neuropsychopharmacol 1995; 18 (4): 320-4
106. Steiner W, Fontaine R. Toxic reaction following the combined administration of fluoxetine and L-tryptophan: five case reports. Biol Psychiatry 1986; 21: 1067-71
107. Schatzberg AF. Dosing strategies for antidepressant agents. J Clin Psychiatry 1991; 52 (Suppl): 14-20

108. Ciraulo DA, Shader RI. Fluoxetine drug-drug interactions. I. Antidepressants and antipsychotics. J Clin Pharmacol 1983; 15: 349S-55S
109. Ereshefsky L, Riesenman C, Lam YWF. Antidepressant drug interactions and the cytochrome P450 system: the role of cytochrome P450 2D6. Clin Pharmacokinet 1995; 29 (4 Suppl. 1): 10-9
110. Rudorfer MV, Potter WZ. Antidepressants: a comparative review of the clinical pharmacology and therapeutic use of the 'newer' *vs* the 'older' drugs. Drugs 1989; 37: 713-38
111. Dent LA, Orrock MW. Warfarin-fluoxetine and diazepam-fluoxetine interaction. Pharmacotherapy 1997; 17 (1): 170-2
112. Crewe HK, Lennard MS, Tucker GT, et al. The effect of selective serotonin reuptake inhibitors on cytochrome P4502D6 (CYP2D6) activity in human liver microsomes. Br J Clin Pharmacol 1992; 34: 262-5
113. Gregor KJ, Overhage JM, Coons SJ, et al. Selective serotonin reuptake inhibitor dose titration in the naturalistic setting. Clin Ther 1994; 16 (2): 306-15
114. Preskorn SH, Magnus RD. Inhibition of hepatic P-450 isoenzymes by serotonin selective reuptake inhibitors: *in vitro* and *in vivo* findings and their implications for patient care. Psychopharmacol Bull 1994; 30 (2): 251-9
115. Cooper GL. The safety of fluoxetine: an update. Br J Psychiatry 1988; 153 (3 Suppl.): 77-86
116. Kapur S, Mieczkowski MA, Mann JJ. Antidepressant medications and the relative risk of suicide attempt and suicide. JAMA 1992; 268: 3441-5
117. Fava M, Rosenbaum JF. Suicidality and fluoxetine: is there a relationship? J Clin Psychiatry 1991; 52: 108-11
118. Jenner PN. Paroxetine: an overview of dosage, tolerability, and safety. Int Clin Psychopharmacology 1992; 4: 69-80
119. Tollefson GD, Tollefson SL, Sayler ME, et al. Absence of emergent suicidal ideation during treatment: a comparative, controlled, double-blind analysis employing several distinct antidepressants. Depression 1994; 2: 73-9
120. Grundemar L, Wohlfart B, Lagerstedt C, et al. Symptoms and signs of severe citalopram overdose [letter]. Lancet 1997; 349 (7065): 1602
121. Stanley M, Virgilio J, Gershon S. Tritiated imipramine binding sites are decreased in frontal cortex of suicides. Science 1982; 216: 1337-9
122. Åsberg M, Träskman L, Thorén P. 5-HIAA in cerebrospinal fluid – a biochemical suicide predictor? Arch Gen Psychiatry. 1976; 33: 1193-7
123. Åsberg M, Schalling D, Träskman-Bendz L, et al. Psychobiology of suicide, impulsivity, and related phenomena. In: Meltzer HY, editor. Psychopharmacology: the third generation of progress. New York: Raven Press, 1987: 655-68
124. Fava M, Rosenbaum JF, Pava JA, et al. Anger attacks in unipolar depression. Part I: clinical correlates and response to fluoxetine treatment. Am J Psychiatry 1993; 150: 1158-63
125. Montgomery SA, Dunner DL, Dunbar GC. Reduction of suicidal thoughts with paroxetine in comparison with reference antidepressants and placebo. Eur Neuropsychopharmacol 1995; 5 (1): 5-13
126. Dalack GW, Roose SP. Perspective on the relationship between cardiovascular disease and affective disorder. J Clin Psychiatry 1990; 51 Suppl.: 4-9
127. Gullette ECD, Blumenthal JA, Babyak M, et al. Effects of mental stress on myocardial ischemia during daily life. JAMA 1997; 277 (20): 1521-6
128. Glassman AH, Preud'homme XA. Review of the cardiovascular effects of heterocyclic antidepressants. J Clin Psychiatry 1993; 54 Suppl. 2: 16-22
129. Bergstrom RF, Lemberger L, Farid N, et al. Clinical pharmacology and pharmacokinetics of fluoxetine: a review. Br J Psychiatry 1988; 153 Suppl. 3: 47-50
130. Robinson RG, Price TR. Post-stroke depressive disorders: a follow-up study of 103 patients. Stroke 1982; 13: 635-41
131. Caley CF, Friedman JH. Does fluoxetine exacerbate Parkinson's disease? Clin Psychiatry 1992; 53 (8); 278-82
132. Mayeux R, Stern Y, Cote L, et al. Altered serotonin metabolism in depressed patients with Parkinson's disease. Neurology 1984; 34: 642-6
133. Goldstein DJ, Rampey Jr AH, Enas GG, et al. Fluoxetine: a randomized clinical trial in the treatment of obesity. Int J Obes 1994; 18: 129-35
134. NIH Consensus Development Panel on Depression in Late Life. Diagnosis and treatment of depression in late life. JAMA 1992; 268: 1018-24
135. Covinsky KE, Fortinsky RH, Palmer RM, et al. Relation between symptoms of depression and health status outcomes in acutely ill hospitalized older persons. Ann Intern Med 1995; 126 (6): 417-25
136. Feighner JP, Cohn JB. Double-blind comparative trials of fluoxetine and doxepin in geriatric patients with major depressive disorder. J Clin Psychiatry 1985; 46 (3): 20-5
137. Dunner DL, Cohn JB, Walshe T III, et al. Two combined, multicenter double-blind studies of paroxetine and doxepin in geriatric patients with major depression. J Clin Psychiatry 1992; 53 Suppl. 2: 57-60
138. Cohn CK, Shrivastava R, Mendels J, et al. Double-blind, multicenter comparison on sertraline and amitriptyline in elderly depressed patients. J Clin Psychiatry 1990; 51 Suppl. B: 28-33
139. Flint AJ, Rifat SL. The effect of treatment on the two-year course of late-life depression. Br J Psychiatry 1997; 170: 268-72
140. Feighner JP, Boyer WF, Meredith CH, et al. An overview of fluoxetine in geriatric depression. Br J Psychiatry 1988; 153 Suppl. 3: 105-8
141. Pastuszak A, Schick-Boschetto B, Zuber C, et al. Pregnancy outcome following first-trimester exposure to fluoxetine (Prozac). JAMA 1993; 269 (17): 2246-8
142. Nulman I, Rovet J, Stewart DE, et al. Neurodevelopment of children exposed *in utero* to antidepressant drugs. N Engl J Med 1997; 336: 258-62
143. Altshuler LL, Cohen L, Szuba MP, et al. Pharmacologic management of psychiatric illness druing pregnancy: dilemmas and guidelines. Am J Psychiatry 1996; 153: 592-606

144. Chambers CD, Johnson KA, Dick LM, et al. Birth outcomes in pregnant women taking fluoxetine. N Engl J Med 1996; 335 (14): 1010-5
145. Goldstein DJ. Effects of third trimester fluoxetine exposure on the newborn. J Clin Psychopharmacol 1995; 15 (6): 417-20
146. Goldstein D, Corbin L, Sundell K. Effects of first trimester fluoxetine exposure on the newborn. Am J Obs Gyn 1997; 89 (5): 713-8
147. Nulman I, Koren G. The safety of fluoxetine during pregnancy and lactation. Teratology 1996; 53: 304-8
148. Committee on Drugs, American Academy of Pediatrics. The transfer of drugs and other chemicals into human milk. Pediatrics 1994; 93: 137-50
149. Montgomery SA. Efficacy in long-term treatment of depression. J Clin Psychiatry 1996; 57 (2 Suppl.): 24-30
150. Stokes PE. A primary care perspective on management of acute and long-term depression. J Clin Psychiatry 1996; 54 (Suppl.): 74-84
151. Rothschild AJ, Samson JA, Bessette MP, et al. Efficacy of the combination of fluoxetine and perphenazine in the treatment of psychotic depression. J Clin Psychiatry 1993; 54: 338-42
152. Vestergaard P, Gram LF, Kragh-Sorensen P, et al. Therapeutic potentials of recently introduced antidepressants. Psychopharmacol Ser 1993; 10: 190-8
153. Hale AS, Stokes PE. The utility of serotonin reuptake inhibitors in endogenous and severe depression. In: Freeman HL, editor. The uses of fluoxetine in clinical practice. London: Royal Society of Medicine Services and International Congress and Symposium Series No. 183, 1991: 15-25
154. Montgomery SA. Fluoxetine in the treatment of anxiety, agitation and suicidal thoughts [abstract]. In: Stefanis CN, Soldatos CR, Rabavilas AD, editors. Psychiatry Today: VIII World Congress of Psychiatry Abstracts. New York: Elsevier, 1989: 335
155. Shaw DM, Crimmins R. A multicentre trial of citalopram and amitriptyline in major depressive illness. In: Montgomery SA, editor. Citalopram: the new antidepressant from Lundbeck Research. Amsterdam: Excerpta Medica 1989: 43-9
156. Beasley CM, Sayler ME, Bosomworth JC, et al. High-dose fluoxetine: efficacy and activating-sedating effects in agitated and retarded depression. J Clin Psychopharmacol 1991; 11: 166-74
157. Tollefson GD, Holman SL, Slayer ME, Potvin JH. Fluoxetine, placebo, and tricyclic antidepressants in major depression with and without anxious features. J Clin Psychiatry 1994; 55: 50-9
158. Dunbar GC, Cohn JB, Fabre LF, et al. A comparison of paroxetine, imipramine and placebo in depressed outpatients. Br J Psychiatry 1991; 159: 394-8
159. Laws D, Ashford JJ, Anstee JA. A multicentre double-blind comparative trial of fluvoxamine versus lorazepam in mixed anxiety and depression treated in general practice. Acta Psychiatr Scand 1990; 81: 185-9
160. Chabannes JP. Antidepressant and anxiety. Psychopharmacology 1988; 96 Suppl.: 272
161. Katz MM, Koslow SH, Maas JW, et al. The timing, specificity and clinical prediction of tricyclic drug effects in depression. Psychol Med 1987; 17: 297-309
162. Montgomery SA, Pedersen V, Tanghoj P, et al. The optimal dosing regimen for citalopram: a meta-analysis of nine placebo-controlled studies. Int Clin Psychopharmacol 1994; 9 Suppl. 1: 35-40
163. Fuglum E, Rosenberg C, Damsbo N, et al. Screening and treating depressed patients: a comparison of two controlled citalopram trials across treatment settings: hospitalized patients *vs* patients treated by their family doctors. Acta Psychiatr Scand 1996; 94 (1): 18-25
164. Haffmans PM, Timmerman L, Hoogduin CA. Efficacy and tolerability of citalopram in comparison with fluvoxamine in depressed outpatients: a double-blind, multicentre study. Int Clin Psychopharmacol 1996; 11 (3): 157-64
165. Sheehan DV, Harnett-Sheehan K. The role of SSRIs in panic disorder. J Clin Psychiatry 1996: 57 (Suppl.): 51-8
166. den Boer JA, Westenberg HGM. Serotonergic compounds in panic disorder, obsessive-compulsive disorder and anxious depression: a concise review. Hum Psychopharmacol 1995; 10: S173-83
167. Louie AK, Lewis TB, Lannon RA. Use of low-dose fluoxetine in major depression and panic disorder. J Clin Psychiatry 1993; 54: 435-8
168. Charney DS, Nelson JC. Delusional and nondelusional unipolar depression: further evidence for distinct subtypes. Am J Psychiatry 1981; 138: 328-33
169. Hellerstein DJ, Yanowitch P, Rosenthal J, et al. Long-term treatment of double depression: a preliminary study with serotonergic antidepressants. Prog Neuropsychopharmacol Biol Psychiatry 1994; 18: 139-47
170. Keller MB, Lavori PW, Mueller TI, et al. Time to recovery, chronicity, and levels of psychopathology in major depression: a 5-year prospective follow-up of 431 subjects. Arch Gen Psychiatry 1992; 49: 809-16
171. Quitken FM, Stewart JW, McGrath PJ, et al. Phenelzine versus imipramine in the treatment of probable atypical depression: defining syndrome boundaries of selective MAOI responders. Am J Psychiatry 1988; 145 (3): 306-11
172. Liebowitz MR, Quitkin FM, Stewart JW, et al. Antidepressant specificity in atypical depression. Arch Gen Psychiatry 1988; 45: 129-37
173. Quitkin FM, Stewart JW, McGrath PJ, et al. Columbia atypical depression: a subgroup of depressives with better response to MAOIs than to tricyclic antidepressants or placebo. Br J Psychiatry 1984; 41: 669-77
174. Charney DS, Miller HL, Licinio J, et al. Treatment of depression. In: Schatzberg AF, Nemeroff CB, editors. The American psychiatric press textbook of psychopharmacology. Washington, DC: American Psychiatric Press, Inc., 1995: 575-601
175. Reimherr FW, Wood DR, Byerly B, et al. Characteristics of responders to fluoxetine. Psychopharmacol Bull 1984; 20: 70-2
176. Frank E, Kupfer DJ, Perel JM, et al. Three-year outcomes for maintenance therapies in recurrent depression. Arch Gen Psychiatry 1990; 47 (12): 1093-9
177. Doogan DP, Caillard V. Sertraline in the prevention of depression. Br J Psychiatry 1992; 160: 217-22

178. Kupfer DJ, Frank E, Perel JM, et al. Five-year outcomes for maintenance therapies in recurrent depression. Arch Gen Psychiatry 1992; 49 (10): 769-73
179. Fava M, Rappe SM, Pava JA, et al. Relapse in patients on long-term fluoxetine treatment: response to increased fluoxetine dose. J Clin Psychiatry 1995; 56: 52-5
180. van Moffaert M, Bartholome F, Cosyns P, et al. A controlled comparison of sertraline and fluoxetine in acute and discontinuation treatment of major depression. Human Psychopharmacol 1995; 10: 393-405
181. Montgomery SA. The advantages of paroxetine in different subgroups of depression. Int Clin Psychopharmacol 1992; 6 Suppl. 4: 91-100
182. Price JS, Waller PC, Wood SM, et al. A comparison of the post-marketing safety of four selective serotonin re-uptake inhibitors including the investigation of symptoms occurring on withdrawal. Br J Clin Pharmacol 1996; 42: 757-63

Correspondence: Dr *Peter E. Stokes*, Laboratory of Psychobiology, New York Hospital-Cornell Medical Center, 21 Bloomingdale Road, White Plains, NY 10605, USA.

Antidepressant Metabolites
Therapeutic and Adverse Effects

Matthew V. Rudorfer[1] and *William Z. Potter*[2]

1 Division of Services and Intervention Research, National Institute of Mental Health, Bethesda, Maryland, USA
2 Eli Lilly & Company, Indianapolis, Indianapolis, USA

More than four decades have now passed since the serendipitous discovery of antidepressant medications.[1] During that time, even as additional drugs were being developed and brought to market, knowledge of the details of the pharmacokinetic and pharmacodynamic profiles of the antidepressants was yielding to scientific scrutiny. The complexity of antidepressant metabolism[2] was evident early on, with a wide variability in therapeutic dosages and adverse effects seen in patients treated with tricyclic antidepressants (TCAs). However, it was not until the development of valid and reliable laboratory assays[3] – a decade after introduction of the TCAs – permitting measurement of concentrations of antidepressants in biological fluids of patients and volunteers, that the metabolic pathways of tricyclic and other antidepressants could be fully delineated. Despite the considerable advances in assay methodology in the ensuing years, until recently the commonly used measures of antidepressant blood concentrations yielded an incomplete picture of the drug's fate in the body.[2]

A key mediating factor in antidepressant action – both therapeutic and adverse – is the production of active breakdown products during the normal hepatic metabolism of these medications.[2,4] Interindividual and interdrug variability are of paramount importance, permitting the presence of metabolites to be ignored under some circumstances (e.g. lithium, which is eliminated unchanged into the urine, possesses no metabolites) while overwhelming the role of the parent antidepressant in others. Among the antidepressants under consideration, all of which undergo liver metabolism, the absence of known pharmacological activity by the metabolites of a few, e.g. the selective serotonin (5-hydroxytryptamine; 5-HT) reuptake inhibitors (SSRIs) paroxetine and fluvoxamine, and the selective noradrenaline (norepinephrine) reuptake inhibitor, reboxetine, is the exception. At steady-state, the mean ratio of plasma concentrations of metabolite:parent antidepressant drug has been observed from well under 1 to >70 for well-characterised compounds,[5] with most at the lower end of the range.

The kinetic properties of antidepressant metabolites may differ from those of the parent compound. For instance, metabolites commonly possess a longer half-life, leading to a slow rise to steady-state, with a gradual accumulation during treatment even of metabolites present in only trace amounts after a single antidepressant dose.[5]

Antidepressant metabolites may act additively or synergistically with the parent drug in some cases, or in an opposite or totally unrelated fashion in others.[5,6-8] Although often not taken into account by clinicians or investigators, the actions of metabolites can have a profound influence on the antidepressant efficacy of an administered compound, as well as contribute to the adverse effect burden of the patient.

In this review we will endeavour to describe the current state of knowledge regarding the role of active metabolites of the tricyclics and other classes of medications used in the treatment of depression. Areas where knowledge of metabolite activity has been shown to play a substantive role in understanding the clinical and adverse responses to medications will be highlighted, as will gaps in the present database. Additionally, patient and illness factors that contribute to the presence, or extent, of various active antidepressant metabolites will be discussed.

1. Tricyclic Antidepressants

Although newer antidepressants have supplanted the classical tricyclic compounds in routine practice, the TCAs remain the 'gold standard' treatment for severe melancholic depression.[9] Moreover, the understanding of the formation, disposition, and activity of the metabolites of these prototype antidepressants is most complete and offers insight into the situation with less well-studied newer agents.[6,8] While often considered as a homogeneous class of drugs, there are important differences among the TCAs.[10] The most useful subdivision of these medications is by chemical structure, into *tertiary amines*, such as amitriptyline, dothiepin, imipramine, and clomipramine, and *secondary amine* tricyclics, including nortriptyline, desipramine, and protriptyline. In some cases, secondary amines are in fact active metabolites themselves, having originally been identified as the demethylation products (e.g. nortriptyline, desipramine) of their parent tertiary amines (amitriptyline and imipramine, respectively). The tricyclic compound, lofepramine, may be a prodrug. Its therapeutic ingredient (with steady-state plasma concentrations 3 times higher than those of the parent drug) is apparently its major demethyl-metabolite, desipramine.[5,6] The 24-hour plasma elimination half-life of desipramine is 4 to 6 times longer than that of lofepramine.[11] With administration of lofepramine, the demethyl-metabolites of both the parent drug and of desipramine also appear to possess antidepressant activity.[12]

The next several sections of this article will review the *pharmacokinetic* aspects of TCA metabolites, focusing on their production and elimination. This will be followed by consideration of the metabolites' preclinical and clinical *pharmacodynamic* activities, both therapeutic and toxic. A similar format will be used in presenting data on other classes of antidepressants.

1.1 Pharmacokinetic Aspects

1.1.1 Formation of TCA Metabolites

As highly lipophilic compounds, all antidepressants undergo multiple biotransformation reactions in the liver, producing progressively more polar metabolites which can then be readily excreted by the kidneys.[2,13] Less than 5% of a dose of a tricyclic antidepressant is eliminated unchanged. Formation of active metabolites occurs primarily through the hepatic mixed function P450 oxidases, through two major pathways.[14] Tertiary amine TCAs are *N*-demethylated to secondary amine forms. Both tertiary and secondary amine tricyclics undergo aromatic hydroxylation, with the location of this biotransformation on the drug varying for different compounds.[15,16] Thus, hydroxylation occurs at ring position 2 on imipramine (and desipramine)[4,17] and at ring position 8 on clomipramine and its demethyl-metabolite.[18-20] Although there is more interindividual variability in demethylation than in hydroxylation,[2,19] of these two pathways the hydroxylation route represents more of a functional 'rate-limiting' step for the TCAs, as it is needed prior to conjugation and to produce sufficient polarity to permit renal excretion.[2]

The metabolism of amitriptyline is more complicated, entailing demethylation to nortriptyline and 10-hydroxylation of both amitriptyline and nortriptyline, each of these hydroxy-metabolites existing in two isomers: *E* (*trans*) and *Z* (*cis*).[21,22] In turn, each 10-hydroxy(OH)-metabolite in the amitriptyline series can have 2 enantiomers: (+) and (–). Minor metabolites identified for the secondary amine TCAs include demethylated and hydroxylated products;

hydroxy-metabolites of the iminodibenzyl derivatives of the tertiary and secondary amine tricyclics have also been identified.[2,13]

Structurally related to amitriptyline, dothiepin undergoes demethylation and *S*-oxidation, with the biochemically active metabolites predominating after dosing.[23] In particular, a therapeutic role for the demethyl-metabolite of dothiepin (northiaden) is suggested by the longer elimination half-life of the metabolite (36 to 46 hours) compared with the parent drug (14 to 24 hours).[11] Mianserin, a racemic tetracyclic compound, similarly to amitriptyline is demethylated and hydroxylated to (*S*)- and (*R*)-demethyl-mianserin and (*S*)- and (*R*)-8-hydroxy-mianserin.[24]

The extremely high affinity of the hepatic P450 enzymes for these drugs as they flow through the liver via the portal vein to the hepatic vein prior to entering the systemic circulation produces a marked 'first-pass' metabolism for TCAs taken orally.[2,25] Parenteral administration of tricyclics delays[26] or reduces[27] the appearance of TCA metabolites in plasma. Neither the demethylation nor the hydroxylation of amitriptyline or nortriptyline is consistently affected by food intake.[28]

Glucuronide conjugation of TCA hydroxy-metabolites contributes the most to rendering the lipophilic tricyclics water-soluble and thereby subject to more efficient renal excretion,[29] although a significant fraction of hydroxy-metabolites are cleared into urine in their unconjugated form.[2,10] The glucuronide metabolites, which do not cross the blood-brain barrier, are considered inactive.[10] Direct glucuronidation of tricyclics constitutes a minor metabolic pathway for these compounds.[30]

During treatment of depression with either amitriptyline or nortriptyline, *E*-10-OH-nortriptyline predominates over parent drug or other metabolite concentrations in both plasma[31-35] and CSF.[22,35] In geriatric depressed patients treated with nortriptyline, *Z*-10-OH-nortriptyline plasma concentrations averaged only 14% those of the *E*-10-OH metabolite.[21] Metabolism of TCAs may differ in other conditions, such as eating disorders.[36] The ratio of mean plasma concentrations of total unconjugated hydroxy-nortriptyline metabolites to nortriptyline with repeated dosing of nortriptyline is approximately 1.2:1.4.[32,34,35]

Well-documented pharmacokinetic and pharmacodynamic data on antidepressant metabolites are limited by the lack of availability of many such metabolites in pure form. In a key exception, the Karolinska group has reported interesting hydroxy-nortriptyline pharmacokinetic data derived from the direct oral administration of the metabolite itself.[37-40] With a half-life of 8 hours, half of a single oral dose of *E*-10-OH-nortriptyline was excreted conjugated, via a metabolic pathway with less interindividual variability than hydroxylation.[37] However, plasma concentrations of unconjugated (–)*E*-10-OH-nortriptyline were 2 to 5 times higher than those of the (+)enantiomer following single doses of racemic *E*-10-OH-nortriptyline, and were unaffected by genetic hydroxylation status (see below).[39] A similar ratio in the plasma concentrations of the two enantiomers, which was ascribed to more efficient hepatic glucuronidation of the (+)enantiomer, was seen during a preliminary 3-week treatment trial of *E*-10-OH-nortriptyline in depressed patients.[40]

In contrast, when desipramine is administered, the parent drug's plasma concentration is generally twice that of its 2-hydroxy-metabolite,[4,41] with the two concentrations highly correlated. Collating all pharmacokinetic studies of desipramine treatment reported in the literature between 1982 and 1991, totalling 395 patients across a wide age range, Wilens et al.[42] reported a mean hydroxy-desipramine:desipramine plasma concentration ratio of 0.442. Hydroxy-desipramine, like its nortriptyline counterpart[35] easily enters the CSF.[4] When imipramine is the administered medication, its own 2-hydroxy form represents only a quarter of the total metabolism, analogous to amitriptyline.[4,43-45] Some investigators have observed apparent saturation of hydroxylation (or perhaps of an alternative metabolic pathway)[46] of imipramine and desipramine, with dose-dependent kinetics at high doses (including overdose) of imipramine[43,44,47,48] or desipramine,[46,49] but this has not been reported consistently at therapeutic tricyclic doses.[2,4,46,50] Perhaps as a result of the recruitment of alternative metabolic pathways, in the case of TCA overdose, unusual metabolites may be observed, e.g. imipramine-*N*-oxide and didesipramine following imipramine overdose.[43]

In general, the hydroxy-metabolites of TCAs, the best characterised, exhibit shorter half-lives and smaller volumes of distribution than their parent compounds.[22,51,52] With a larger ratio of CSF:plasma concentrations, in an animal model 2-OH-imipramine appears to penetrate the central nervous system to a greater extent than does imipramine itself,[52] perhaps related to the lower plasma protein binding seen for the metabolite. Similar results were seen for nortriptyline and its *E*-, but not *Z*-, 10-hydroxy-metabolite in this animal model;[52,53] in humans, the predominance of 10-OH-nortriptyline over other forms of the drug in CSF during nortriptyline treatment has been noted.[22]

Steady-state metabolite data are more limited for the less commonly prescribed TCAs. In the case of dothiepin,[23] the two most common metabolites with repeated dosing are the *S*-oxide byproducts of northiaden (demethyldothiepin) and of the parent drug itself, together accounting for >22% of an administered dose. Demethyl-clomipramine steady-state plasma concentrations are more than twice those of clomipramine,[18-20,54] while 8-hydroxy-clomipramine concentrations are nearly half and 8-OH-demethyl-clomipramine plasma concentrations approximately equal to those of clomipramine.[19,20,54] Slightly higher relative concentrations of the hydroxy-metabolites of clomipramine and demethyl-clomipramine were reported in the largest published samples of depressed patients treated with this tricyclic (table I).[20,50,55]

In summary, the key step in the formation of the active metabolites of TCAs is the action of a few members of the hepatic cytochrome P450 oxidative enzyme system. The activity of these oxidases is under genetic control, but is also subject to alteration from a variety of exogenous factors. Once formed, clearance of the metabolites is dependent on renal function. Tricyclic metabolism is similar after single or repeated dosing.[41] These aspects of the pharmacokinetics of TCA metabolites will next be considered.

1.1.1a Genetic Factors

Clinical reports of widespread variability in therapeutic doses and sensitivity to the antidepressant and adverse effects of TCAs in various countries and cultures have spurred detailed study of these phenomena.[15,17,56-58] Pharmacogenetic data have begun to link these clinical observations with analysis of the genetic basis of antidepressant metabolism.[58,59] With increasing understanding of the role of the specific isoenzymes of the hepatic P450 microsomal oxidase system, in recent years it has become possible to characterise their influence on antidepressant metabolism across individuals and populations.[14]

Several P450 isoenzymes are responsible for the metabolism of antidepressants.[16,59,60] In particular, the highly polymorphic CYP2D6 catalyses most hydroxylation reactions among these compounds, whereas CYP2C19 activity is associated with *N*-demethylation.[10,58,61-64] The biotransformation steps controlled by these enzymes are quite specific, e.g. CYP2D6 appears to regulate 10-hydroxylation of amitriptyline and nortriptyline in the (–)*E*- but not the (+)*E*- or the *Z*-position.[22,62,65] Other P450 isoenzymes, such as 1A2 and 3A3/4, play a more minor role in tricyclic demethylation.[59,66,67] Using a human cytochrome *in vitro* model, Venkatakrishnan et al.[64] demonstrated the dose-dependent nature of amitriptyline *N*-demethylation as being under the control of CYP2C19 at low, therapeutically relevant doses; at higher doses of the tricyclic, CYP3A4 assumes a greater role as amitriptyline *N*-demethylase.

Genetically based differences in activity of these enzymes account in large part for the very wide interindividual variability in metabolism and steady-state plasma concentrations of

Table I. Active metabolites of representative tricyclic antidepressants (TCAs). For references to the information in this table, see section 1 of the main text

Parent drug	Active metabolites	Mean elimination half-life (h)	Special characteristics
Nortriptyline		28	Both OH-metabolites exist in (+) and (–) enantiomers. The metabolites are noradrenaline (norepinephrine) reuptake inhibitors with half the potency of the parent compound. They contribute to the antidepressant efficacy of nortriptyline at low and moderate doses. Formation of the predominant *E*-10-OH-, but not *Z*-10-OH-, metabolite correlates with debrisoquine hydroxylation. The metabolites are dependent on elimination by the kidney, and as a result clearance slows with aging, possibly adding to the cardiovascular toxicity of the drug
	E-10-OH-nortriptyline	8	
	Z-10-OH-nortriptyline	NA	
Clomipramine		24	Parent TCA and OH-metabolites primarily inhibit serotonin (5-hydroxytryptamine; 5-HT) reuptake. The demethyl-metabolite blocks noradrenaline reuptake
	Demethyl-clomipramine	65.5	
	8-OH-clomipramine	NA	
	8-OH-demethly-clomipramine	NA	
Amoxapine		10	Metabolites share the noradrenaline reuptake inhibiting properties of the parent drug. The 7-OH-metabolite is a more potent dopamine receptor antagonist than the parent compound, an action which is associated with clinical antipsychotic activity (and toxicity)
	7-OH-amoxapine	4	
	8-OH-amoxapine	30	

NA = data not available.

TCAs.[2] Patients with genetically slow TCA clearance ('poor metabolisers') may generate plasma total drug concentrations several-fold higher than unaffected individuals during routine dosing, with associated toxicity;[68] metabolite concentrations will be low, because of the impaired rate of formation.[69]

Conversely, attention has subsequently focused on the phenomenon of ultrarapid metabolism of TCAs and similar medications, which can necessitate the use of unusually high daily doses to achieve therapeutic plasma drug concentrations.[70] Inherited gene amplification and duplication have been identified as the molecular basis for the extremely rapid breakdown of TCAs, debrisoquine, and other CYP2D6-metabolised drugs in some individuals.[71,72] Detailed reviews of the genetically determined differences in the cytochrome P450 system and their pharmacokinetic and therapeutic implications have been published.[60,73]

Another physiological parameter of interest in the study of TCA pharmacokinetics is *age*. Although early reports described elevated tricyclic plasma concentrations in older patients, later controlled studies were not consistent.[2,36] Of relevance to the consideration of antidepressant metabolites, Pollock et al.[53,74] have found both CYP2D6 and mephenytoin hydroxylase activity to lack correlation with age, suggesting that the production of TCA hydroxy- and demethyl-metabolites should be unaffected by advancing age. Instead, the influence of age on tricyclic metabolite concentrations appears to mediated by changes in renal clearance of the metabolites, as will be discussed below. In one study[63,74] elderly African-Americans demonstrated a significantly higher rate of slow mephenytoin metabolism than their Caucasian counterparts, but this observation awaits replication. Other factors contributing to age effects on TCA metabolite kinetics are reviewed below.

A still-understudied area of pharmacokinetic variability is *gender*. As reviewed by Dawkins and Potter[75] no consistent differences between men and women in TCA metabolism have been identified. Among modern studies, one report[76] cited lower hydroxylation clearance of clomipramine in young women treated for depression. Furthermore, the disposition of tricyclic hydroxy-metabolites, which are more polar than their parent compounds, may differ in male and female depressed patients. Nordin[77] found, only in men, a curvilinear relationship between body height and the CSF/plasma ratio of 10-OH-nortriptyline (not nortriptyline) during nortriptyline treatment, possibly accounted for by disparate mechanisms of clearance from the CSF of the OH-metabolite and its less polar parent TCA.

One area in need of controlled trials relates to anecdotal findings of varying antidepressant kinetics in association with changes in phase of the menstrual cycle.[2] Issues dealing with altered antidepressant metabolite formation during pregnancy and lactation are also coming under scrutiny. Clomipramine treatment throughout pregnancy, with its consequent significant neonatal plasma concentrations of parent drug and metabolites,[78,79] is associated with neurological symptoms, including hypotonia and tremor in the newborn, given the shared circulation between fetus and mother and the immature liver in the former.[80,81]

With the recognition of the postpartum period as a high-risk time for mood disorders, and the renewed popularity of breast-feeding among new mothers, the transfer of psychotropic drugs and metabolites from mother to nursing infant has assumed significant practical as well as theoretical importance. The reduced plasma protein binding of some active TCA metabolites, such as *E*-10-hydroxy-nortriptyline,[82] compared with the parent drug also suggests the likelihood that tricyclic metabolites will easily distribute into breast milk. In the above case of the neonate whose mother was treated with clomipramine during and following gestation,[79] clomipramine concentrations in maternal milk approximated those in her plasma during the first month after delivery; the infant, who began breast-feeding on day 7, demonstrated falling plasma clomipramine concentrations during that time and was reported to be developing normally. A more recent series of 4 clomipramine-treated nursing mothers accounted for the demethyl-, hydroxy-, and hydroxy-demethyl-metabolite as well as clomipramine concentrations in plasma of both mothers and infants;[83] despite therapeutic plasma drug concentrations in at least 3 of the women, clomipramine and metabolite concentrations in the all infant serum samples were zero-to-trace.

These investigators have found similar results for 7 breast-feeding infants of mothers taking nortriptyline,[84] with no detectable plasma nortriptyline in any infant and low concentrations of *E*- and *Z*-10-OH-nortriptyline in 2 of the 4 infants in whom these metabolites were measured; breast milk TCA concentrations were not assayed. Subsequently replicating their findings in an additional 7 young infants, Wisner et al.[85] were able to quantify very low serum concentrations of nortriptyline in one infant and hydroxy-metabolites in another, with no observable adverse effects. A similar lack of measurable TCAs or metabolites in nursing infants' serum, and absence of tricyclic-related toxicity, despite appreciable medication concentrations in their mothers' breast milk, has been reported for amitriptyline.[86-88] One detailed analysis of a nursing woman treated with amitriptyline 175 mg/day[88] compared TCA and hydroxy-metabolite concentrations in the mother's milk with those in a simultaneously collected blood sample. Throughout the first 4 weeks postpartum, all compounds were present in lesser concentrations in breast milk than in serum, including nortriptyline (milk:serum = 0.74) and the more plentiful *E*-10-OH-nortriptyline (milk:serum=0.70). No tricyclic or metabolites were measurable in the infant's serum by termination of the study on day 26, at which time his estimated 'dose' of TCA (including *E*-10-OH-nortriptyline) was 80-fold lower than his mother's.[85]

Against these benign findings, isolated cases of serious toxicity related to a TCA metabolite present in breast milk stand out. An 8-week-old nursing infant experienced sedation, hypotonia, and depressed respiration following 6 weeks of doxepin therapy (up to 75 mg/day) taken by her mother.[89] Although low concentrations of doxepin and its demethyl-metabolite were measured in the mother's milk, and the infant's serum contained only trace amounts of doxepin, demethyl-doxepin was present at similar serum concentrations in both mother and (at a mean concentration of 62 μg/L) baby. The authors of this case report explain that 'paths of metabolism for demethyl-doxepin include hydroxylation and conjugation with glucuronic acid, both being limited in the newborn'.[89] In this instance, cessation of breast-feeding led to a complete clinical recovery of the infant within 24 hours. A similar case published at about the same time[90] described a 10-week-old infant whose mother was being treated with doxepin 150 mg/day. After 43 days of nursing, the infant's serum concentration of doxepin was undetectable, but that of demethyl-doxepin was 15 μg/L; this infant, however, was clinically asymptomatic. Similarly, in a later British case,[91] no effect on development was observed in a child who had been exposed to appreciable amounts of dothiepin and northiaden in breast milk. A more recent case report from Germany, however, has again described an association between maternal doxepin use and toxicity in a breast-feeding newborn infant.[92] Hospitalised 9 days after birth due to hypotonia, poor feeding with vomiting and weight loss, and drowsiness, the infant was found to have a plasma concentration of doxepin and of *N*-demethyl-doxepin below the lower limit of detection (10 μg/L). His mother, who was taking 35 mg/day of doxepin, was providing in her breast milk only 2.5% of her weight-adjusted dose to her baby daily. Nonetheless, following cessation of nursing, all of the infant's symptoms cleared within 48 hours.[92]

On balance, the current consensus is that in most new mothers taking TCAs, the benefits of breast-feeding outweigh the potential risks.[10,93,94] The risk of toxicity from accumulated tricyclics and active metabolites appears to be greatest in very young infants (aged 10 weeks or less), possibly because of decreased metabolic activity of the immature liver or newborn hyperbilirubinaemia,[13,85,92] particularly when the antidepressant was used during pregnancy and not started postpartum.[94] The potential clinical role of infant serum concentration monitoring is under study.[13,94]

1.1.1b Exogenous Factors Affecting Metabolism

The metabolism of TCAs, and consequently the formation of tricyclic metabolites, can be influenced by a variety of exogenous factors that have direct or indirect effects on the liver oxidative enzyme system.

Ethanol: Gastrointestinal irritation and reduced plasma protein concentrations associated with chronic ethanol ingestion may interfere with usual TCA pharmacokinetics.[95] A triphasic pattern of ethanol effects on TCA hepatic metabolism has been described:[68] acutely, ethanol reduces first-pass metabolism, while chronically inducing liver metabolising enzymes.[2] Alcohol abuse to the point of cirrhosis and portocaval shunting again is associated with less first-pass metabolism of tricyclics.[68] Shoaf and Linnoila[95] pointed out that many studies of alcohol use in patients fail to control for the confounding variable of smoking.

Smoking: Decreased steady-state plasma concentrations of TCAs are commonly observed in association with cigarette smoking.[2,95] In the hepatic oxidase system, the P450 1A2 enzyme is specifically induced by the polyaromatic hydrocarbons present in cigarette smoke.[95,96] Studies focused on tricyclic-treated smokers have found enhanced *N*-demethylation[36,45,97] and glucuronidation,[36] while hydroxylation is not directly affected.[36,97,98]

Other medications: Drug-drug interactions can influence tricyclic pharmacokinetics at various steps in their metabolic pathways.[2,10] For example, drugs that reduce hepatic blood flow, e.g. β-blockers or cimetidine, will decrease first-pass metabolism of TCAs.[2,68] In terms of the production of tricyclic metabolites, most recent interest has centred on drugs that interfere with CYP2D6-mediated hydroxylation and related P450 isoenzyme functions.[8,13,68,99] Concomitant neuroleptics, for example, are associated with modestly elevated TCA concentrations, apparently by interfering with the hydroxylation pathway of tricyclic metabolism.[2,55] Of particular current clinical significance is the competitive inhibition of CYP2D6 by some of the newer SSRIs, most notably fluoxetine and paroxetine.[100,101] These TCA-SSRI interactions are associated with often-dramatic elevations of steady-state TCA plasma concentrations, ascribed to reduced clearance via hydroxylation but with demethylation unaffected.[8,68,100]

Demethylated metabolites, including the secondary amine metabolites of tertiary amine tricyclics, may rise disproportionately in such cases of SSRI inhibition of CYP2D6, as a result of impairment of the second, hydroxylation step of TCA metabolism.[101] Such interactions may assume particular importance in cases of TCA overdose, where parent drug and metabolite concentrations are already in the toxic range.[48]

Continued systematic observation of such drug-drug interactions is furthering the understanding of TCA metabolism and metabolite production. In one example, Jefferson[66] noted significant declines in steady-state plasma concentrations of the tricyclic, doxepin, as well as of its demethyl-metabolite, when the nonsteroidal anti-estrogen agent, tamoxifen, a substrate and probable inducer of the P450 3A4 isoenzyme, was added to ongoing TCA therapy.[67] Confirming the long term clinical observation that concomitant barbiturate administration lowers TCA concentrations, von Bahr and associates[102] experimentally demonstrated that the reduction in nortriptyline plasma concentrations observed after 2 days of added pentobarbital treatment was associated with a substantial increase in metabolic clearance of the tricyclic by 10-hydroxylation. Although most nortriptyline hydroxylation is under CYP2D6 control, stimulation of CYP3A4 by pentobarbital has been hypothesised as responsible for the increased hydroxylation of the TCA in this drug-drug interaction.[102,103] Similarly, CYP3A4 induction by carbamazepine has been linked to the reduction in plasma concentrations of both enantiomers of concomitant mianserin and of (*S*)-8-hydroxy-mianserin, with less effect on demethyl-mianserin concentrations.[24,56]

1.1.2 Developmental Factors

Even in the absence of support from controlled clinical trials, TCAs and other antidepressants are being prescribed increasingly to children and adolescents.[80,81,104,105] The hepatic metabolism and first-order elimination of most psychotropic medications are primarily under genetic control, as reviewed above, with similar efficacy in an individual across the life cycle.[2] As reviewed by Geller,[106] developmental considerations yielding more robust metabolism and elimination of psychotropic compounds in children and adolescents compared with adults include, in younger patients, relatively greater hepatic capacity, more efficient renal functioning, and relatively less adipose tissue.[81] Treatment of children with tertiary amine tricyclics, such as imipramine, is commonly associated with relatively higher steady-state concentrations of the secondary amine form, e.g. desipramine, than is commonly observed in adults.[4,5,107] Fixed-dose studies have demonstrated in children and adolescents the expected wide inter-individual range of steady-state plasma TCA concentrations and of hydroxy-metabolite clearance rates,[42,104,107,108] but a more narrow range of secondary amine tricyclic hydroxy-metabolite steady-state plasma concentrations compared with other drug forms.[107]

The most comprehensive comparison of TCA pharmacokinetics across age groups was reported by Wilens and associates,[42] who administered fixed weight-adjusted doses of desipramine to >100 children, adolescents, and adults. Both desipramine and, surprisingly, hydroxy-desipramine plasma concentrations per dose rose with age. The ratio of plasma concentrations of hydroxy-desipramine:desipramine failed to correlate with age in this[42] and in an earlier study of young patients with desipramine-treated attention deficit hyperactivity disorder.[108] It is likely that the more efficient hepatic oxidative metabolism of TCAs in children, which had been expected to produce relatively higher circulating concentrations of tricyclic hydroxy-metabolites,[42] was offset by the more active renal clearance present in younger patients (see below). These findings are consistent with the need for higher weight-corrected TCA doses in children and adolescents.[78,104] The pharmacodynamic implications of the failure to observe excessive hydroxy-desipramine concentrations in children in light of recent concern over possible cardiotoxicity of desipramine in this age group are discussed below.

1.1.3 Renal Clearance of Metabolites

Knowledge of the mechanisms of *production* of TCA metabolites has been growing over the past two decades. So too, has an appreciation of the important role of *renal excretion* in mediating the concentrations and thus the activity of these often-potent breakdown products.[2] The measured steady-state plasma concentrations of TCA metabolites represent the net balance of metabolite production (by hepatic biotransformation of the parent compound) and elimination (typically renal excretion of polar forms of the drug).[2,68]

Similar to lithium, for decades the only psychotropic drug eliminated without undergoing transformation (gabapentin, an anticonvulsant under study in mood and anxiety disorders,[109] is also not metabolised by the liver), the metabolites, especially those formed by hydroxylation, are dependent on renal mechanisms for their clearance from the body, following glucuronidation to increase their polarity.[2,110] Reviewing the pharmacokinetics of antidepressant clearance in detail, Lane[110] pointed out that without any change in metabolic clearance by the liver, reduced renal function would be expected to substantially increase the plasma concentrations of metabolites that account for at least 10% of the dose of the parent drug in the urine, a description clearly fitting the TCAs.[2,68] Even dothiepin, with its unusual *S*-oxidation metabolic pathway,[23] is susceptible to the influence of impaired renal function, as its predominant sulphoxide metabolite is excreted solely unchanged in the urine.[5]

Among the variables that can affect kidney function, the 2 that have the greatest influence on the renal clearance of TCA metabolites are *age* and *disease*. As previously noted, Wilens and associates'[42] data appear to indirectly address this issue at the low end of the age range, with the finding that hydroxy-desipramine plasma concentrations per weight-corrected desipramine dose were actually lower in children than in adults, despite the presumed greater production of the metabolite in the former.

Most of the established data, and clinical importance of this phenomenon, lie at the other end of the age spectrum. By the early 1980s an increased plasma concentration ratio of hydroxy-metabolite to parent drug in the elderly was established for the secondary amine TCAs nortriptyline[32] and desipramine.[111] In our laboratory Kitanaka and colleagues[111] demonstrated that the relative increase in unconjugated 2-OH-desipramine plasma concentrations in the elderly versus young adults was accounted for by diminishing renal clearance of the metabolite with age ($r = -0.73$). Nelson et al.[49,112] have noted that the reduced tricyclic plasma protein binding commonly observed in the elderly may lead to especially high *free* concentrations of TCA hydroxy-metabolites in older patients.

These findings were extended to nortriptyline by Young and associates,[113] who described relatively increased plasma concentrations of the predominant *E*-10-hydroxy-metabolite in elderly depressed patients as a function of age-associated decreased renal clearance. Similar results were reported by Schneider et al.,[114] although in that study an age effect on plasma *E*-10-OH-nortriptyline concentrations independent of creatinine clearance also appeared operative. The investigators hypothesised that an age effect in addition to that on renal function, involving protein binding (see above), hepatic drug oxidation, or lean body mass, might play a role in determining nortriptyline metabolite concentrations in the elderly.[114] In contrast, a subsequent multicentre trial of nortriptyline at doses titrated to achieve therapeutic plasma concentrations of the parent compound in 38 older depressed patients failed to confirm a relative increase in hydroxy-nortriptyline concentrations.[115]

This research in otherwise physically healthy psychiatric patients is complemented by comparative study of individuals with impaired renal function. Naturalistic investigations in the UK[116] and the US[117] documented similar, and expected, handling of any of several TCAs by depressed patients with chronic renal failure, including individuals undergoing haemodialysis. Plasma concentrations of parent tricyclics were unchanged. Relative plasma concentrations of *unconjugated* hydroxy-metabolites were comparable to those seen in control subjects with normal kidney function,[116] although there was evidence of their delayed elimination.[117] Most strikingly, steady-state plasma concentrations of *conjugated* hydroxy-tricyclic compounds were up to 20-fold higher in the chronic renal failure patients than in the control group,[116,117] which was presumed due to impaired elimination of the conjugates in the patients with kidney dysfunction.[118]

1.2 Pharmacodynamic Aspects

Having presented the evidence for substantial concentrations of tricyclic metabolites in blood and CSF during routine use of TCAs, we turn now to the demonstration of their biological activity. Depending on the drug, the individual taking the medication, and the particular circumstances of its use, the role of the metabolites may be additive to or conflicting with that of the parent drug, in terms of both therapeutic and adverse effects.

1.2.1 Biochemical Effects of TCA Metabolites

Preclinical Studies

More than 20 years passed between the introduction of TCAs and the demonstration that their hydroxy-metabolites possessed *in vitro* acute biochemical activity similar to that of the parent compounds: presynaptic reuptake inhibition of monoamine neurotransmitters.[32,119] Earlier it had been appreciated that the demethylated metabolites of the tertiary amine tricyclics, i.e. the secondary amines, such as nortriptyline and desipramine, were TCAs in their own right. The 2-hydroxy-metabolites of imipramine and desipramine inhibit noradrenaline uptake to a similar extent to their parent compounds,[119-121] but inhibit reuptake of serotonin with only half the potency. Amitriptyline and nortriptyline are twice as potent noradrenaline reuptake inhibitors as are their 10-OH-metabolites,[32] with no difference between the (+)- and (–)-enantiomers of *E*-10-OH-nortriptyline.[22] However, unlike amitriptyline and, to a lesser extent, nortriptyline, their hydroxy-metabolites do not inhibit the reuptake of serotonin.[32,121]

The example of a related TCA, clomipramine, illustrates an important interaction between the pharmacokinetics and pharmacodynamics of this family of drugs: while the parent compound is a potent inhibitor of *serotonin* reuptake, its demethyl-metabolite selectively blocks reuptake of *noradrenaline*.[18,20,27,119,121,122] *In vitro* data from Núñez and Perel[122] show similar serotonin and noradrenaline reuptake inhibition potency between 8-OH-clomipramine and the parent drug. The mixed action of TCA plus active metabolites is one of the ways in which the new generation of SSRIs differs from the older tricyclics (see below).

Other classical animal screening tests for antidepressant activity, including reversal of reserpine-induced ptosis and decreased motor activity, demonstrate the similarity between TCA hydroxy-metabolites and parent tricyclics.[119] While the putative prodrug, lofepramine, is inactive in the rat forced swim model of depression, its demethylated derivatives, including demethyl-lofepramine and demethyl-desipramine as well as desipramine, do show antidepressant activity.[12] Moreover, a rat model was utilised to document that tricyclic metabolites cross the blood-brain barrier and appear in brain and CSF after chronic TCA administration.[119,123]

Clinical Studies

Direct and indirect measures of noradrenergic transmission have been used to infer the acute and chronic pharmacodynamic profile of antidepressants and their metabolites.[124] For example, the significant elevations in supine and standing plasma noradrenaline concentrations – the latter associated with increased pulse rate – observed in healthy volunteers given single oral doses of *E*-10-OH-nortriptyline[37] have been interpreted as reflections of the metabolite-induced noradrenaline reuptake inhibition.

Reductions in concentrations of the major noradrenaline metabolite, 3-methoxy-4-hydroxyphenylglycol (MHPG) in accessible bodily fluids, particularly CSF and urine, are associated with repeated administration of noradrenaline reuptake inhibitors, including the TCAs and/or their metabolites.[22,120,124] The coexistence of tricyclic hydroxy-metabolites with their parent compounds in the usual treatment situation has made it difficult to dissect out the role of the metabolites per se, for instance in the 30 to 80% decrease in CSF MHPG concentrations observed during chronic treatment with nortriptyline or desipramine.[120,124,125] However, the more modest decline in CSF concentrations of the primary metabolite of serotonin, 5-hydroxy-indoleacetic acid (5-HIAA) during nortriptyline treatment was correlated with the CSF concentration of the parent tricyclic, and not of the hydroxy-metabolite.[125] Moreover, related platelet studies revealed serotonin reuptake inhibition induced by nortriptyline to be approximately 7-fold more potent than that associated with *E*-10-OH-nortriptyline.[126]

Again, direct administration of *E*-10-OH-nortriptyline proved helpful in elucidating its *in vivo* biochemical actions in several patients,[40] including a slight but significant reduction in CSF MHPG, without effect on concentrations of 5-HIAA in CSF. Hydroxy-metabolites of other TCAs also appear to lack effect on serotonergic measures.[120,124] The 'mixed' acute biochemical actions of clomipramine treatment are demonstrable with measurement of drug blood concentrations: plasma clomipramine concentrations correlate with the observed decrease in CSF 5-HIAA concentrations, whereas the noradrenaline-reuptake inhibiting metabolite, demethyl-clomipramine correlates with reduction in MHPG concentrations in CSF.[18]

1.2.2a Adverse Effects of TCA Metabolites

Preclinical Studies

A major limiting factor in the clinical use of TCAs has been a substantial adverse effect burden for many patients.[8,9] Understanding the role of the metabolites of these medications in producing or ameliorating the adverse effects that accompany routine use of these agents could offer new opportunities for prevention or treatment of these unwanted actions. Most interest and data, in both preclinical and human models, have focused on the anticholinergic and cardiovascular actions of tricyclics and their metabolites.

Anticholinergic activity: The potent binding of TCAs to central and peripheral muscarinic acetylcholine receptors permits a valid and reliable laboratory procedure to determine relative receptor affinities, which have been shown to correlate well with clinical anticholinergic effects.[127,128] The general ranking of cholinergic receptor binding for this class of antidepressants is: tertiary amines > secondary amines > demethylated metabolites > hydroxylated metabolites.[127-129]

Thus for the amitriptyline family, nortriptyline itself possesses 20% of the binding potency of amitriptyline,[127,128] while *Z*-10-OH-nortriptyline in turn is only 11% as potent as nortriptyline.[129] In turn, the *E*-10-OH-nortriptyline is half as potent as its *Z*-isomer, i.e. nortriptyline is nearly 18-times more anticholinergic than its *E*-10-hydroxy-metabolite in a whole brain model,[129] fuelling the interest in the use of this noradrenaline reuptake blocking metabolite as an antidepressant drug in its own right.[22] Directly comparing muscarinic receptor binding of nortriptyline and its *E*-10-OH-metabolite in cerebral cortex and various other organs of the guinea-pig, Nilvebrant and Nordin[130] found *E*-10-OH-nortriptyline consistently to show 10- to 12-times lower affinity than the parent compound. The hydroxy-metabolites of amitriptyline are more potent at binding to the muscarinic receptor than are those of nortriptyline, and are more in the order of desipramine.[127-129]

Similar findings for the substantially anticholinergic tertiary amine TCA, clomipramine and its metabolites have been reported,[121] with muscarinic receptor binding potency of clomipramine > demethyl-clomipramine >>> 8-OH-clomipramine > 8-OH-demethyl-clomipramine. As is true for other tested TCAs,[127,128] *N*-demethylation of tricyclic compounds was associated with a moderate reduction of *in vitro* anticholinergic potency, such that demethyl-clomipramine was about 2.5-times less potent than clomipramine, while 8-OH-demethyl-clomipramine was less potent than 8-OH-clomipramine by a similar percentage.[121] Hydroxylation has an even greater effect,[128,129] such that 8-OH-clomipramine is 10- to 12-times less potent at muscarinic receptor binding than clomipramine, and 8-OH-demethyl-clomipramine has 10-times less anticholinergic potency than demethyl-clomipramine.[121]

Thus, just as *E*-OH-nortriptyline is an equipotent noradrenaline reuptake inhibitor but with fewer anticholinergic properties than nortriptyline,[22] 8-OH-clomipramine is a serotonin reuptake blocker of similar magnitude to its parent TCA, while possessing a very small anticholinergic burden *in vitro*.[121] These favourable laboratory profiles suggest that future development of TCAs may focus on the therapeutic use of tricyclic hydroxy-metabolites.[22,121]

Although desipramine is 1.7-times less potent than nortriptyline in the muscarinic receptor binding assay,[127,128] its 2-OH-metabolite has 32-fold still less affinity for the receptor, rendering 2-OH-desipramine >3-fold less anticholinergic than *E*-10-OH-nortriptyline *in vitro*.[129] While imipramine is more than twice as anticholinergic as desipramine in this model,[131] 2-OH-imipramine shows 13-fold weaker cholinergic receptor binding than its parent compound. Still lower binding affinities to the muscarinic cholinergic receptor awaited the development of the SSRIs and the other new generation antidepressants, as will be reviewed below.

Cardiovascular effects: Two animal studies have provided evidence of differential cardiotoxicity of the hydroxy-metabolites of imipramine (increased toxicity) and nortriptyline (reduced cardiac adverse effects). In the former case,[132] markedly reduced left ventricular function with diminished cardiac output was produced in anaesthetised dogs administered intravenous 2-hydroxy-imipramine; in contrast, the parent tricyclic caused much less, and delayed, cardiac depression. Confounding variables included the highly invasive nature of the procedure and lack of plasma concentration monitoring of drug or metabolite.[123] Another study in dogs,[133] however, found 2-OH-imipramine to be twice as potent as imipramine in reversing cardiac arrhythmias induced by ouabain. More recently, a different animal model, the unanaesthetised pig, has served to demonstrate an apparent increase in cardiotoxicity for intravenous 2-OH-imipramine, with significantly more severe cardiac arrhythmias and depressed cardiac motility and output, with hypotension, compared with imipramine.[52] In contrast, *E*-10-OH-nortriptyline in this system was essentially free of the cardiotoxicity, including decreased cardiac output and arrhythmias, that marked both its parent TCA and its *Z*-isomer.[52,134]

Clinical Human Studies

As with all actions of TCAs, the role of active metabolites in producing the myriad of common adverse effects associated with use of this class of drugs is difficult to discern, given their coexistence with parent and other forms of the medications in the usual treatment situation.[8,22] Other than the limited option of administration of a purified metabolite itself,[38] understanding of the range of actions of tricyclic metabolites has come from correlations of plasma concentrations of metabolites with pharmacodynamic measures in individuals with a range of metabolic profiles for parent TCAs.[22] As with the preclinical data described above, the key examples of classical TCA adverse effects *in vivo* include anticholinergic and cardiovascular actions; newer tricyclic-like compounds exhibit unique toxicities related to their active metabolites.

Anticholinergic effect: Paralleling the *in vitro* muscarinic receptor binding data reviewed above,[128] the anticholinergic adverse effects of TCAs, while ubiquitous, are highly variable.[8,135] These commonly include dryness of the mucous membranes, constipation, blurred vision, and the often more serious urinary retention and a range of cognitive toxicities.[8] In general, the tertiary amine tricyclics are more anticholinergic than their demethyl-metabolites, i.e. secondary amine TCAs. Although correlations between TCA plasma concentrations and anticholinergic effects have been identified,[136] these adverse effects generally are maximal at subtherapeutic plasma concentrations. While desipramine has the lowest anticholinergic activity among the classical TCAs, its potency is still appreciable.[135,136] Lofepramine, which is extensively metabolised to desipramine, also affords a mild anticholinergic profile among the TCAs.[6,8,137]

The *in vitro* receptor binding data also suggest a lower anticholinergic potency for tricyclic hydroxy-metabolites compared with their parent drugs. This is supported by a case of an extremely rapid hydroxylator of debrisoquine and nortriptyline, who was treated with high doses of nortriptyline.[70] Despite the generation of an unusually high plasma 10-OH-nortriptyline: nortriptyline ratio of nearly 8:1, anticholinergic adverse effects were minimal, apparently eliminating the hydroxy-metabolite from consideration as a major contributor to these actions.[22,70]

Subsequently, this group introduced the paradigm of administration of hydroxy-nortriptyline itself to healthy volunteers and to depressed patients. Encouraged by the absence of spontaneous reports of dryness of the mouth among the first group of volunteers receiving single oral doses of *E*-10-OH-nortriptyline,[37] Nordin and associates[22,125] went on to directly compare a specific anticholinergic action (reduction of salivary flow) of single equimolar doses of nortriptyline and its hydroxy-metabolite in a placebo-controlled crossover trial of 8 healthy men. As expected, the 37% salivary flow decrease observed with nortriptyline was significantly greater than the 21% reduction associated with *E*-10-OH-nortriptyline; the latter was not significantly different from the 13% change after placebo.[22,125] Although similar *in vivo* results would be anticipated for the hydroxy-metabolites of other TCAs,[121] to date specific human studies are lacking.

Cardiovascular effects: Ranging from benign increases in heart rate to potentially lethal slowing of cardiac conduction, the class of TCAs exerts a host of effects on the cardiovascular system.[8,109,138] Again, most of the extant data failed to account for active tricyclic metabolites, leaving their role in producing these actions unknown. It can be generalised that the orthostatic hypotension commonly observed during treatment with the tertiary amine TCAs is less likely to occur when their demethyl-metabolite derivatives, i.e. secondary amines, such as nortriptyline, are prescribed;[8] this may relate to differences in affinity for the α_1-receptor.

The quinidine-like membrane stabilisation and resulting slowing of impulse conduction may suppress pre-existing premature atrial or ventricular contractions but precipitate bundle-branch or complete heart block, presenting a risk of arrhythmias or even sudden death in individuals with underlying heart disease.[8,138] In physically healthy individuals, TCA plasma concentrations correlate with the innocuous prolongation of electrocardiogram (ECG) parameters during routine administration.[139] However, in cases of serious TCA toxicity, including intentional overdose[48] and, possibly, slow tricyclic metabolisers with supratherapeutic blood concentrations,[140,141] widening of the QRS complex on the ECG is typical, and has been correlated with red blood cell concentrations of tricyclic demethyl-metabolites.[142] Even TCAs with longstanding reputations for cardiovascular safety, including doxepin and dothiepin, are capable of inducing the usual tricyclic adverse effects.[8] Claims for a benign cardiovascular profile for the most recently developed TCA, lofepramine[137] must be reconciled with the extensive metabolism of this drug to desipramine, as reviewed above.

Much of the ongoing work exploring the relationship of tricyclic metabolites to cardiovascular parameters focuses on the extremes of the life cycle: children and the elderly. In the case of the former, reports of sudden death in several children receiving desipramine prompted an intensive study of the cardiac effects of this drug in 71 paediatric patients by Biederman and associates.[143] Despite comprehensive 24-hour monitoring, no evidence of desipramine-associated cardiac abnormalities were found, and cardiac parameters failed to correlate with desipramine dose or plasma concentration; however, desipramine metabolites were not assayed.[143] It has been noted above that in the related study of developmental factors in desipramine pharmacokinetics[42] no excessive accumulation of the potentially cardiotoxic desipramine hydroxy-metabolite was found in children or adolescents. Analysis of standard ECGs in that patient sample[144] revealed little relationship between ECG parameters and desipramine or OH-desipramine plasma concentrations in children and adolescents; for all age groups, the observed association between ECG abnormalities and higher concentrations of the tricyclic and its hydroxy-metabolite was modest and felt to be clinically unimportant for either young or old depressed patients.[144]

The situation may be different in the elderly.[111] Initial clinical reports[145,146] documented surprisingly small effects on heart rate and blood pressure during desipramine treatment of older depressed patients, despite substantial plasma 2-OH-desipramine concentrations. Subsequently, Kutcher et al.[147] challenged the claimed lack of desipramine cardiotoxicity in this patient population, citing, in the context of therapeutic desipramine blood concentrations in elderly depressives, a 40% incidence of potentially serious ECG abnormalities, some of which correlated with hydroxy-desipramine plasma concentrations.

For nortriptyline as well the cardiovascular effects of hydroxy-metabolites may be more pronounced in the elderly than in young, physically healthy volunteers or depressed patients. On the one hand, the extensive metaboliser described by Bertilsson et al.[70] – a 40-year-old woman – suffered no cardiovascular ill effects during nortriptyline treatment despite the development of extreme supratherapeutic 10-OH-nortriptyline plasma concentrations. Similarly, no significant changes in heart rate, blood pressure, or serial ECGs were observed in healthy volunteers given a single dose of hydroxy-nortriptyline[22] or in 5 depressed patients treated with 10-OH-nortriptyline.[40]

On the other hand, hydroxy-nortriptyline – at least at the relatively high plasma concentrations described in the elderly[111] – may be cardiotoxic in this more vulnerable population. Young and associates[148] described a 68-year-old man who developed left bundle-branch block and congestive heart failure in association with very high (2- to 4-fold the usual equal-to-twice plasma parent drug concentrations) plasma concentrations of 10-OH-nortriptyline. In a series of 18 elderly depressives treated with nortriptyline, this group[149] reported in 8 individuals ECG abnormalities, primarily prolonged PR intervals, which were correlated with *E*-10-OH-nortriptyline plasma concentrations. The experience of Schneider and colleagues[150] in a series of 21 nortriptyline-treated ambulatory elderly depressed patients was similar: the 4 patients who developed cardiac conduction during the trial exhibited significantly greater *E*-10-OH-nortriptyline plasma concentrations (but similar parent drug concentrations) than the others. For the group as a whole, increases with PR interval on the ECG was associated with increasing nortriptyline concentration, while QRS duration and QTc interval prolongation were related to increasing *Z*-10-OH-nortriptyline concentration.[150]

Thus, to date the strongest evidence for the cardiotoxicity of TCA hydroxy-metabolites comes from studies of elderly patients, who generate higher concentrations of these metabolites than do younger individuals and who may be more sensitive to their effects.[22,148-151]

Toxicities of Metabolites of TCA-Related Antidepressants: Although their introduction in the 1970s and 1980s was accompanied by the hope of enhanced efficacy and/or reduced adverse effects compared with the standard TCAs, the initial group of 'new generation' antidepressants proved in some cases to possess new problems of their own.[6] Two TCA-like compounds, amoxapine (a tricyclic that is itself the *N*-demethylated metabolite of loxapine, an antipsychotic) and maprotiline (a tetracyclic), both noradrenaline reuptake inhibitors, illustrate the role of active metabolites in mediating new toxicities beyond those typical of the tricyclic class.[56]

Amoxapine is hydroxylated in the 7 and 8 positions to compounds which share the potent noradrenaline reuptake blocking action of the parent drug; the metabolites also slightly inhibit reuptake of serotonin. Of great significance to the toxicity, if not efficacy, of this drug is the dopamine receptor blocking activity of amoxapine and its 7-OH metabolite. Radioreceptor assay shoes that amoxapine and 7-OH-amoxapine possess dopamine receptor binding activity comparable to that of the neuroleptics thioridazine and haloperidol, respectively.[6,152,153] Another pharmacokinetic factor of note is that while the half-lives of amoxapine and its 7-OH metabolite are short (10 and 4 hours, respectively), that of 8-OH-amoxapine is 30 hours (table I).[2,152] Steady-state plasma concentrations of the 8-OH-metabolite may be as high as 3- to 10-times those of the parent drug, potentially dominating the clinical picture.[5]

On the positive side, the neuroleptic action of amoxapine and one of its metabolites offers clear benefit to the patient suffering from psychotic depression, who typically fails to respond to an antidepressant alone and requires addition of an antipsychotic drug.[9,109,154] However, the dopamine-blocking action of amoxapine and its 7-OH metabolite carries with it the risk of any of the host of neuroleptic adverse effects. These range from galactorrhoea and amenorrhoea with hyperprolactinaemia[155] to the various extrapyramidal and motor syndromes (e.g. dystonic reactions, akathisia, parkinsonism, akinesia, neuroleptic malignant syndrome, and withdrawal and tardive dyskinesias).[6,8,10,56,156-158] In overdose amoxapine presents with an unusual clinical profile, consisting of a disproportionate number of seizures and fatalities,[48,159] despite relatively mild cardiovascular toxicity;[6,56] however, the role of amoxapine metabolites in producing this pattern of overdose toxicities has not been elucidated.

Maprotiline had also been hailed two decades ago as ushering in a new generation of antidepressant medications,[56] only to see concerns about its adverse effects overshadow its therapeutic efficacy.[6,9,160] The primary toxicity associated with the routine use of maprotiline is a disproportionate incidence of seizures,[6,8] which have been described in patients both with and without underlying neurological pathology. This has resulted in a ceiling of 225mg on the recommended daily dose, to be reached only with a week-long slow upward titration, similar to the situation with the more recently developed amfebutamone (bupropion) [see below].

The pharmacokinetics of maprotiline are proving instructive. Its unusually long elimination half-life of about 2 days,[2] double that of most TCAs, promotes drug accumulation with daily dosing. Moreover, its primary desalkyl-metabolite, normaprotiline, with a half-life at least as long as its parent compound,[5] accumulates as well, with a steady-state ratio of metabolite:maprotiline plasma concentrations of 1:2. Neurotoxic activity by this metabolite is consistent with the clinical data. Thus, in the largest series (N = 98) of maprotiline-associated seizures, Dessain et al.[161] found most to have occurred at high dosages which may have been stable for many weeks, with no apparent relationship between seizure occurrence and either rapid rise of dose or high plasma drug concentrations. These investigators speculated that an active metabolite of maprotiline with a long half-life might accumulate in some patients at high doses and induce seizures; normaprotiline appears to fit this description.[5,8]

1.2.3 TCA Metabolites and Antidepressant Response

Having established that pharmacologically active metabolites coexist in the circulation and in brain with parent tricyclic compounds during TCA treatment, we next turn to the evidence that specifically addresses the relationship between tricyclic metabolites and clinical response to TCAs. Of course, in terms of the demethyl-metabolites of the tertiary amine tricyclics, i.e. the secondary amines such as nortriptyline and desipramine, their relatively greater potency as antidepressants compared with their parent drugs has been convincingly established for more than 3 decades.[9,68] In the case of the hydroxy-metabolites of the TCAs, although, as noted above, their biochemical activity generally mimics that of the parent tricyclic, the evidence for the metabolites' role in producing clinical response *in vivo* is less clear.[162]

Amitriptyline: Data from two studies[62,163] suggested that OH-nortriptyline and possibly also OH-amitriptyline[163] contribute, with amitriptyline and nortriptyline, to a maximal total TCA plasma concentration, above which clinical response is unlikely, during amitriptyline treatment. However, no conclusions could be reached about specific antidepressant potency of the hydroxy-metabolites in the presence of the parent tricyclic compounds. Furthermore, detailed analysis of complete blood concentration data in 29 outpatients taking a fixed (150mg) daily dose of amitriptyline failed to identify minimal therapeutic concentration or curvilinear concentration:response relationships for any combination of amitriptyline, nortriptyline, and their hydroxy-metabolites.[163]

Nortriptyline: By removing the confounding presence of amitriptyline and its 10-OH-metabolite, administration of nortriptyline has better enabled assessment of the antidepressant efficacy of its OH-metabolites. Nortriptyline itself has long been known to demonstrate a curvilinear relationship ('therapeutic window') between steady-state plasma concentrations and clinical effect.[22,164] Adding 10-OH-nortriptyline to the equation, Nordin and colleagues[35,125,165] reported the range of plasma concentrations of nortriptyline and of its OH-metabolite (the latter range being more restricted) in clinical responders to nortriptyline; only 19% of nonresponders to this tricyclic were found to have plasma drug concentrations within the window of these two measures. These Karolinska Institute investigators found a significant positive correlation ($r = 0.62$) between CSF 10-OH-nortriptyline concentrations and antidepressant clinical response in 26 patients;[35,125] this linear relationship was thought due to the dearth of very high nortriptyline or hydroxy-metabolite concentrations in this patient sample.

Such supratherapeutic concentrations of nortriptyline or 10-OH-nortriptyline, with putative postsynaptic-receptor blocking properties, have been invoked as responsible for the upper limit on the nortriptyline blood concentration 'therapeutic window'.[9,22,125,164] For example, the extremely rapid nortriptyline hydroxylator described by Bertilsson et al.[70] generated seemingly therapeutic nortriptyline concentrations on quite high daily doses of the drug; despite this, his failure to respond was ascribed to the concurrent greatly supratherapeutic plasma 10-OH-nortriptyline concentrations.[70]

Further evidence that high plasma *E*-10-OH-nortriptyline concentrations may impair the antidepressant efficacy of nortriptyline in geriatric patients was presented by Young and colleagues;[166] in their sample of 37 elderly depressives, nortriptyline nonresponders were found to have higher plasma *E*-10-OH-nortriptyline plasma concentrations and greater OH-nortriptyline:nortriptyline ratios than responders to treatment.[166] At the other end of the age continuum, in a pharmacokinetically controlled study targeting parent TCA plasma concentrations in nortriptyline-treated depressed children, Geller and colleagues[104] were unable to distinguish clinical responders from nonresponders on the basis of total, *cis*-, or *trans*-10-OH-nortriptyline concentrations; however, as with most of the child and adolescent antidepressant literature[80,81,105] the response rate to active drug was very low, possibly obscuring any blood concentration:outcome relationship.[104]

The Swedish group cited above also has pioneered the introduction of *E*-10-OH-nortriptyline as an antidepressant drug in its own right.[22] During a 3-week open trial of this metabolite, up to 225 mg/day, in 5 patients with major depression,[22,40] total plasma *E*-10-nortriptyline concentrations and reductions in CSF MHPG concentrations were appreciable but somewhat lower than these investigators had observed in an earlier treatment trial with nortriptyline;[125] the mean 56% drop in unblinded depression ratings in the metabolite-treated group was consistent with, although could not prove, clinical efficacy of 10-OH-nortriptyline, suggesting the need for controlled clinical trials of this potential 'new' treatment of depression.[9,40,125]

Imipramine/Clomipramine: Despite a wealth of data describing complete drug and metabolite blood concentrations during imipramine treatment of depression in children[107] and adults,[4,43-45] there is little evidence that the addition of hydroxy-metabolite data has assisted clinical care. Most studies of steady-state kinetics of imipramine[43,45,107] or clomipramine[19] have not reported clinical correlations with plasma TCA concentration measures. In part, this may reflect the commonly accepted finding that imipramine plasma concentrations are correlated with clinical antidepressant effect without evidence of an upper limit, enabling this tricyclic to be administered in rising doses until a therapeutic effect or toxicity intervenes.[9] Träskman and associates[18] did find plasma concentrations of demethyl-clomipramine to correlate with antidepressant response to clomipramine in a biochemically defined patient subgroup, i.e. those with high baseline CSF concentrations of the serotonin metabolite, 5-HIAA. However, much research over the ensuing decade failed to support such efforts at biochemically subtyping depression and matching specific antidepressant mechanisms of action in treatment, because of the loss of acute biochemical specificity of antidepressant action during chronic treatment.[9,120,124,167] A more recent multicentre Danish trial also found only weak negative correlations between serum concentrations of clomipramine and/or demethyl-clomipramine and depression ratings during double-blind treatment with clomipramine.[50]

Perhaps more telling are the observations of Brosen, Gram, and their colleagues:[44] with daily imipramine dose optimised to achieve a therapeutic imipramine + desipramine plasma concentration, 11 of 12 patients with 'endogenous' depression but none of 4 subjects with 'neurotic' depression showed at least partial response to the TCA. In this instance, the medication-responsivity of the subtype of depressive illness apparently was more important in achieving the desired clinical response than was knowledge of tricyclic hydroxy-metabolite concentrations, which were obtained only retrospectively.[44] Similarly, as has been noted, despite the frequent use of antidepressant medications in children and adolescents, there remains scant support from the controlled trial literature for this practice in the treatment of depression, at least for the older class of drugs.[80,81,105] Consequently, any effort at relating TCA hydroxy-metabolite concentrations to clinical outcome in a paediatric population would be premature.[107] However, in another indication for tricyclics in children, enuresis, hydroxy-metabolite data have proven informative.[4,82,120] The anti-enuretic effect of imipramine was positively correlated with imipramine + desipramine blood concentrations in 29 boys,[4] a relationship that was strengthened by the addition of both OH-imipramine and OH-desipramine concentrations to the formula.

Desipramine: Using fixed-dose designs, two of three clinical trials of desipramine[168,169] identified minimal therapeutic plasma concentrations of parent drug for clinical response, but none was able to relate 2-OH-desipramine concentrations to antidepressant efficacy of the drug.[168-170] Adopting the rationale that the antidepressant effects of OH-desipramine might be obscured by the higher concentrations of desipramine itself in a fixed-dose study,[171] Nelson and associates[162] modified their protocol to permit the adjustment of desipramine dose to reach a targeted fixed plasma concentration of the parent compound (the same strategy as was used by Geller et al.[104] in their trial of nortriptyline in depressed children). Use of this strategy in 34 depressed inpatients showed that, while clinical response remained correlated more closely with desipramine than with OH-desipramine plasma concentrations, the combined total of drug + metabolite concentrations produced the strongest correlation for each assessed outcome measure.[162] As with other studies of imipramine or desipramine,[4,44,169] even with the inclusion of 2-OH-metabolite data, there was no evidence for an upper limit on therapeutic plasma drug concentrations.[162]

Once again, findings regarding TCA metabolites in the treatment of depression do not always generalise to the use of these medications in other disorders. Although the efficacy of desipramine in boys with attention deficit hyperactivity disorder was demonstrated in a double-blind trial,[108] neither desipramine nor OH-desipramine plasma concentrations, nor their combination, correlated with behavioural improvement, in contrast to the earlier experience with imipramine for childhood enuresis.[4]

2. Selective Serotonin Reuptake Inhibitors

With the development and widespread use of a new generation of antidepressant medications,[6,56] the near monopoly of the TCAs in the treatment of moderate-to-severe depressive illness has come to a close over the past 2 decades.[9] In addition to the oldest class of antidepressants, the monoamine oxidase inhibitors (MAOIs), to which additional members have been added, the current armamentarium against depression features a host of new categories of medications, most notably the SSRIs and related serotonergic compounds, the noradrenaline-serotonin reuptake blockers, at least one selective noradrenergic reuptake inhibitor, and amfebutamone.[6,9,109,172] All are clinically effective antidepressants, offering in most cases a milder adverse effect profile than the older tricyclics.[8] In terms of pharmacokinetics, however, including the formation of active metabolites, there is considerable heterogeneity, even within a single drug class.[6,172] Moreover, especially when compared with that of the >40-year-old TCAs, the database on the pharmacology of the new generation antidepressants remains incomplete, leaving some pertinent questions difficult to answer at present.[6,68,109,172]

2.1 SSRIs

Our consideration of the newer compounds begins with the SSRIs, which, despite the toxicity-related early withdrawal from the market of the first prototype, zimeldine (zimelidine),[6] have gone on to become the most widely prescribed antidepressant medications in the world. The several representative members of this drug class in this discussion share as a primary action the acute pharmacological property of blocking the presynaptic reuptake of serotonin, with little interaction with other transmitter systems and receptors.[173]

In a variety of *in vivo* and *ex vivo* preparations, the most common rank order potency of serotonin reuptake inhibition of these drugs is: paroxetine > citalopram > sertraline > fluvoxamine > fluoxetine.[172-176] Citalopram is most selective for serotonin reuptake inhibition,[174] particularly its *S*-enantiomer[177] and fluoxetine, the least.[11] At the other extreme, the TCA clomipramine, while a potent serotonin reuptake inhibitor in its own right (see above), in actual clinical use becomes a mixed transmitter reuptake blocker because of the selective noradrenergic action of its demethyl-metabolite.[27] In contrast, the metabolites of the SSRIs, where they exert any pharmacological effect at all, tend to reinforce the serotonergic activity of their parent compounds.[11,172,173,176]

Below, we first review the pharmacokinetics, including metabolism and metabolite formation and elimination, of the key members of this class, and weigh the evidence supporting – in only some cases – the pharmacological and clinical activity of SSRI metabolites. The role of metabolites in contributing to the therapeutic or adverse effects of SSRIs in clinical practice is discussed. Finally, returning to a topic introduced above, the pharmacogenetic implications of SSRI interactions with other drugs are addressed.

2.2 Pharmacokinetic Aspects of Metabolite Formation

Much as with the tricyclics, the SSRIs vary considerably with respect to several pharmacokinetic parameters, including elimination half-life, formation of active metabolites, induction of hepatic oxidative enzymes, volume of distribution, and plasma protein binding. They also share a number of common pharmacological properties, such as slow rate of absorption, metabolism by the liver, and minimal or absent binding to muscarinic, histaminic, or other receptors commonly associated with TCA adverse effects.[8,11,68,109] Pharmacokinetic and related pharmacodynamic factors applicable to the individual agents are highlighted in the following sections and compared in table II.

2.2.1 Fluoxetine

Despite a number of pharmacokinetic and pharmacodynamic disadvantages, fluoxetine, the first successfully mass-marketed SSRI, remains an extremely popular and effective treatment not only for depression, but for obsessive-compulsive disorder, bulimia, and a variety of mild-to-moderate mood and anxiety disorders.[6,9,109,178,179] Its pharmacokinetic hallmark is an unusually long elimination half-life of 1 to 3 days.[6,173,176] Moreover, it is arguably the only SSRI with a therapeutically important active metabolite, norfluoxetine, formed by *N*-demethylation, that is approximately equipotent to fluoxetine in serotonin reuptake inhibition and the plasma concentration of which may exceed that of its parent compound on chronic administration.[5,6,11,173,176,178]

The metabolite's uniquely lengthy half-life (7 to 15 days) contributes to difficulty with dose titration, as the effects of fluoxetine and norfluoxetine may gradually build up to the point of toxicity over a period of weeks.[8,68,176] Moreover, washout of fluoxetine and its major metabolite is quite prolonged after drug discontinuation.[180] This not only extends unwanted medication effects, but poses a risk of interaction with subsequently introduced medications for up to 8 weeks.[180,181] Such interactions can include those with MAOIs (implicated in serotonin syndrome induction in combination with fluoxetine)[8,182] and TCAs, phenothiazines, and the atypical antipsychotic, risperidone (the metabolism of which may be impaired by fluoxetine-associated CYP2D6 inhibition, as noted above).[68,178,183,184] While, as with all SSRIs, fluoxetine is relatively safe in overdose,[8,178,185] residual fluoxetine and norfluoxetine after discontinuation of therapeutic doses may heighten the toxicity of subsequent TCA overdose as a result of drug-drug interaction.[48] On the other hand, the long half-lives of fluoxetine and norfluoxetine mitigate against withdrawal symptoms in the event of treatment interruption or discontinuation.[109]

Norfluoxetine competitively inhibits CYP2D6 oxidative metabolism to an extent approximately equal to that of fluoxetine,[183] and the metabolite is a more potent inhibitor of CYP3A3/4 than the parent SSRI.[181] Current evidence suggests that fluoxetine's inhibition of the enzymes responsible for its own metabolism may be responsible for its nonlinear pharmacokinetics on repeated dosing.[68,173,186]

Both fluoxetine and norfluoxetine occur as different enantiomers with somewhat distinct profiles of activity, e.g. *R*-norfluoxetine is a considerably weaker serotonin reuptake inhibitor than the parent drug or its own *S*-enantiomer.[187,188] During steady-state fluoxetine administration, plasma concentrations of the *S*-enantiomers of both fluoxetine and norfluoxetine are more than twice those of the respective *R*-enantiomers of the parent SSRI or its metabolite.[189] While both enantiomers of racemic fluoxetine contribute to the drug's inhibition of serotonin transport, and presumably to its antidepressant effect, the shorter half-life and 6-fold lower potency of CYP2D6 inhibition of *R*-fluoxetine and *R*-norfluoxetine compared with their *S*-counterparts have prompted suggestions that a single *R*-fluoxetine isomer could exert a greater benefit:risk ratio than the racemic compound.[176,177] Therapeutically, norfluoxetine augments the enhanced natural killer cell activity that accompanies successful fluoxetine or other serotonergic antidepressant treatment.[190] As is true of all of the SSRIs, plasma concentrations of fluoxetine and norfluoxetine do not appear related to antidepressant response in either acute or maintenance treatment.[176,191-193]

Both fluoxetine and norfluoxetine are highly (>90%) protein-bound.[186] Limited data on the impact of various endogenous and external factors on the pharmacokinetics of fluoxetine and norfluoxetine include a growing consensus that their plasma concentrations are no higher in elderly compared with younger patients.[68,178,186,194] Preliminary experience suggests similar pharmacokinetics of fluoxetine and norfluoxetine in children and adults.[195] One study of the effect of alcohol-induced liver disease revealed tripling and doubling of the half-lives of fluoxetine and norfluoxetine, respectively.[196] Renal dysfunction does not affect the elimination of fluoxetine or norfluoxetine,[197] with typical plasma concentrations of both reported during treatment of depressed patients on haemodialysis.[198]

A growing but still incomplete and uncontrolled database supports the safety and effectiveness of fluoxetine and other SSRIs when indicated during pregnancy or in the postpartum period.[93,109] Approximately 10% of a nursing mother's daily dose of fluoxetine appears in breast milk.[199] However, fluoxetine and norfluoxetine concentrations in the plasma of nursing infants have been below the limits of detection,[200] and no adverse effects on infant development have been observed in these children.[199,200]

The fluorinated structure of fluoxetine and norfluoxetine has permitted the application of a new assay technique, nuclear magnetic resonance spectroscopy, to quantitate brain concentrations of these compounds during fluoxetine treatment.[201,202] Limited data demonstrate accumulation of fluoxetine and its metabolite to concentrations in brain several-fold corresponding plasma concentrations,[201] but current methodology does not yet permit separate measurement of norfluoxetine brain concentrations.

2.2.2 Sertraline

As with fluoxetine, sertraline is primarily *N*-demethylated in the liver. Although most work has focused on the polymorphic P450 isoenzyme CYP2C19, with a contribution by CYP2C9,[203] evidence points to a role for several cytochromes in sertraline *N*-demethylation.[204] Thus, in contrast to TCAs, alteration in activity of any single CYP isoenzyme, whether due to genetic or exogenous factors, is unlikely to significantly affect sertraline pharmacokinetics.[203,204] The resulting metabolite, demethyl-sertraline, exhibits a relatively prolonged elimination half-life (62 to 104 hours), in this case triple that of the parent SSRI's 24 hours.[11,68,172,173,176,187] At steady-state, plasma concentrations of demethyl-sertraline average >60% higher than those of the parent drug.[176] Another major difference from fluoxetine is the sertraline demethyl-metabolite's much weaker (approximately 5 to 10% of sertraline's potency) serotonin reuptake inhibition activity compared with the parent drug.[5,11,176,205] Perhaps related to sertraline's (and demethyl-sertraline's) relatively limited inhibition of hepatic P450 microsomal enzymes,[68,183,187] it follows linear kinetics at usual therapeutic doses and elicits few drug-drug interactions.[173,184,206] It is highly bound to plasma proteins. Sertraline's

Table II. Active metabolites of representative newer antidepressants. For references to the information in this table, see section 2 of the main text

Parent drug	Active metabolites	Mean elimination half-life (h)	Special characteristics
Selective serotonin reuptake inhibitors			
Fluoxetine		2 days	Norfluoxetine is equipotent to the parent drug in inhibition of serotonin (5-hydroxytryptamine; 5-HT) reuptake and CYP2D6 activity. The extremely long half-life of the metabolite delays achievement of steady-state and of drug washout. Elimination half-lives are further lengthened during repeated administration
	Norfluoxetine	11 days	
Sertraline		24	Despite a long elimination half-life, the clinical contribution of the metabolite is probably limited, due to its weak inhibition of serotonin reuptake
	Demethyl-sertraline	66	
Citalopram		33	The weak potency, low blood concentrations and limited blood-brain barrier penetration of the metabolites suggest little contribution to the clinical efficacy of the parent compound
	Demethyl-citalopram	NA	
	Didemethyl-citalopram	NA	
Paroxetine	None	20	The parent drug is metabolised to inactive byproducts. The half-life of paroxetine lengthens during repeated administration, due to interference with its own metabolism
Fluvoxamine	None	16	A longer elimination half-life is seen with repeated administration. None of 11 metabolites is pharmacologically active
Other newer antidepressants			
Venlafaxine		5	The predominant *O*-demethyl-metabolite is equivalent to venlafaxine in blocking serotonin reuptake, although the parent drug is twice as potent a noradrenaline reuptake inhibitor. The other metabolites contribute little to the actions of venlafaxine. As with other newer antidepressants, e.g. nefazodone and amfebutamone, the presence of an active metabolite with a relatively long half-life suggests that multiple daily administration may be unnecessary
	O-demethyl-venlafaxine	11	
	N,O-didemethyl-venlafaxine	NA	
	N-demethyl-venlafaxine	NA	
Nefazodone		3	At steady-state, concentrations of the long half-life triazoledione metabolite, a potent serotonin receptor blocker, predominate. The hydroxy-metabolite has a similar neuropharmacological profile to the parent drug. In contrast to trazodone, *m*-chlorophenylpiperazine contributes little to the actions of nefazodone
	Hydroxy-nefazodone	3	
	Triazoledione	18	
	m-Chlorophenyl-piperazine	6	
Amfebutamone (bupropion)		10	Concentrations of the parent drug are low compared with those of the 3 lone half-life metabolites in both plasma (where the hydroxy-metabolite predominates) and CSF (where threohydro-amfebutamone concentrations are highest). The metabolites, especially hydroxy-amfebutamone, appear to contribute to the therapeutic and adverse effects of the parent drug
	Hydroxy-amfebutamone	22	
	Threohydro-amfebutamone	20	
	Erythrohydro-amfebutamone	27	
Mirtazapine		20-40	Racemic mixture; *S*(+)-enantiomer (mean half-life = 10h) but not *R*(–)-enantiomer (mean half-life = 18h) is sensitive to effects of poor CYP2D6 metaboliser status
	Demethyl-mirtazapine	25	
Reboxetine		12-16	Metabolism of both enantiomers impaired by concurrent CYP3A4 inhibitors
	O-demethyl-reboxetine	NA	

CYP = cytochrome P450; **NA** = data not available.

pharmacokinetics are unaffected by age,[176,187,194] but as with other drugs of this class, its half-life is prolonged in the face of liver disease.[176]

As with fluoxetine, sertraline and its *N*-demethyl-metabolite can be measured in breast milk of nursing mothers in a dose-dependent fashion.[207] In several small case series, very low concentrations (often below the limits of detection of commercial labs) of sertraline and/or demethyl-sertraline were detected in the plasma of breast-feeding infants whose mothers were undergoing sertraline treatment.[207-209] An increasing gradient of drug concentration in each breast milk sample has been identified, with the highest sertraline and metabolite concentrations appearing in the 'hind' milk obtained 7 to 10 hours after a maternal dose.[207] Stowe and associates[207] noted the importance of *N*-demethyl-sertraline monitoring to ascertain infant drug exposure in those cases where the parent drug cannot be measured in the child. To date no adverse effects have been reported in infants ingesting the low doses of sertraline or other SSRIs and metabolites found in breast milk.[207-209]

In summary, sertraline occupies an 'intermediate' position among the SSRIs[181] in possessing a pharmacologically weakly active metabolite that may contribute – but probably modestly – to the serotonin reuptake inhibition and clinical effects of the parent compound;[11,68,173,187] whether this metabolite contributes to adverse effects is unknown.

2.2.3 Citalopram

Temporarily suspended from clinical use and investigation in the mid-1980s because of reported toxicity during animal testing,[6] citalopram has since been proven safe and effective in the treatment of depression. Used throughout much of the world, it is the most recent SSRI to be approved for marketing in the US. Along a continuum of metabolite activity, citalopram represents the point of demarcation, between the *active* metabolites of fluoxetine and, possibly, sertraline, on the one hand, and the clearly *inactive* byproducts of paroxetine and fluvoxamine, on the other.[5]

In the case of citalopram, its principal *N*-demethyl-metabolite is both less potent in blocking serotonin reuptake *in vitro* (by a factor of 4 to 10) as well as less selective, with the metabolite inhibiting noradrenaline uptake some 11-times more potently than does citalopram.[5,11,174] Moreover, didemethyl-citalopram, although weaker in inhibiting reuptake of both of these transmitters, does possess serotonin uptake blocking properties comparable to TCAs such as imipramine.[174] In addition to the lower potency of the metabolites compared with the parent compound, the lower plasma concentrations and reduced penetration of the blood-brain barrier by the metabolites have led to the conclusion that, in the actual clinical situation, any antidepressant contribution by citalopram metabolites is likely to be minimal.[174,181,210]

Like sertraline, citalopram shows linear pharmacokinetics.[173] And, similar to fluoxetine, citalopram is a racemic compound.[181] However, while both enantiomers of fluoxetine show serotonin reuptake inhibiting activity, most of the biological activity of citalopram, the most selective of the current SSRIs, resides in the *S*-isomer.[176,177] Clinical trials of the possible antidepressant role of *S*-citalopram are currently in progress.

The demethylation of citalopram is mediated primarily by hepatic P450 cytochromes 3A4 and 2C19, with a secondary role for CYP2D6.[211] Citalopram's modest effect on P450 isoenzymes, consisting of slight inhibition of CYP1A2, 2C19, and 2D6, is consistent with the dearth of reported drug-drug interactions with this SSRI.[109,176,211]

The relatively long (33-hour) elimination half-life of citalopram (up to 2 days for the demethyl-metabolite) is further prolonged in the elderly.[176,187] Because of diminished clearance and increased steady-state concentrations in older patients, reduced dosage of citalopram in the elderly has been recommended.[74,194] Quantification of *S*-citalopram plasma concentrations may be especially important in the elderly.[74] The extent of plasma protein binding, only 50%, is the lowest among all SSRIs.[174,187] As with most antidepressants, elimination of citalopram consists mainly of renal excretion of some parent drug but mostly metabolites, in free and glucuronidated form.[212] While moderate renal function impairment is associated with reduced renal elimination of citalopram, demethyl-citalopram, and didemethyl-citalopram, no dosage adjustment is generally necessary.[213] On the other hand, the significant decrease in citalopram clearance associated with impaired hepatic function, such as that accompanying cirrhosis, results in a doubling of the drug's half-life and generally requires a reduction in the usual daily dosage.[213]

Experience to date with infants' ingestion of citalopram and its metabolites in breast milk is similar to that with the other SSRIs. On the basis of a limited number of uncontrolled case reports from Scandinavia, nursing infants are estimated to receive 3 to 6% of their mothers' weight-adjusted daily dose.[214,215] In most cases, serum drug concentrations in the infants have been very low, and no adverse effects observed.[214,215] The one exception was a recent case of impaired sleep described in one breast-feeding infant, associated with the baby's serum citalopram concentration of 12.7 μg/L;[216] with a 50% reduction in the mother's 40 mg/day dose of citalopram and partial substitution of formula for breast milk, symptoms resolved.

Minor metabolites of citalopram formed by deamination mediated in part by monoamine oxidases type A and B appear to be pharmacologically inactive.[217]

2.2.4 Paroxetine

The straightforward extensive metabolism of paroxetine, primarily but apparently not exclusively mediated by hepatic CYP2D6,[218,219] yields no clinically active metabolites.[173,176,220] Although superficially the pharmacokinetics of this drug resemble those of the TCAs, with a 24-hour half-life (permitting once-daily dosing) and 95% plasma protein binding,[176,187] the considerable inhibition of P450 2D6 activity by paroxetine, like fluoxetine, renders this SSRI susceptible to interference with its own metabolism and consequent nonlinear kinetics.[172,173] Thus, in response to dose increases, paroxetine blood concentrations and half-life rise disproportionately.[187,219]

The significant CYP2D6 inhibition properties of paroxetine, like those of fluoxetine, also raise the possibility of drug-drug interactions, e.g. with concurrent TCAs.[183,206] Compared with pretreatment baseline, the addition of single dose metoprolol to healthy volunteers following 6 days of daily paroxetine 20mg administration resulted in a doubling of maximum plasma concentrations and elimination half-life of metoprolol;[221] corresponding cardiovascular effects demonstrated prolonged β-blockade resulting from this interaction. The M2 metabolite of paroxetine, which has not been identified in human plasma to date,[176] although lacking serotonin reuptake inhibiting activity, possesses CYP2D6 inhibiting potential similar to the parent SSRI.[181]

As with most SSRIs, during clinical use of paroxetine in the elderly, higher plasma drug concentrations and longer half-lives are common.[194,222] It is recommended that paroxetine treatment of older individuals begin with a lower than usual daily dose, e.g. 10mg, with gradual upward titration, given the greater effect of nonlinear kinetics in disproportionate rises in plasma concentrations with dose increases in the elderly.[194] Lower doses are also required in the presence of severe, but possibly not modest hepatic or renal dysfunction.[176]

As suggested for TCAs and other SSRIs, paroxetine appears safe for postpartum use by women who are breast-feeding.[223] Doses received by nursing infants are in the order of 1 to 3% of the maternal weight-corrected dose.[223,224] As with other studied antidepressants, highest paroxetine concentrations are found in the later (hind) portions of breast milk samples. However, in contrast to sertraline, no diurnal pattern of milk excretion of once-daily paroxetine has been identified.[225] Nonetheless, the failure of paroxetine serum concentrations in nursing infants to reach quantifiable concentrations in most cases, coupled with the absence of active metabolites and the lack of reported toxicity, have provided reassurance about the low risk of breast-feeding by women taking paroxetine.[223,224] Stowe and colleagues,[225] however, note that given the reliability of the appearance of paroxetine in breast milk samples, nursing infants must be considered to be exposed to the drug while breast-feeding.

2.2.5 Fluvoxamine

Approved in the US solely for the treatment of obsessive-compulsive disorder, fluvoxamine has been used extensively for more than 15 years in many countries in the treatment of depression.[175,179] Although extensively metabolised by oxidative enzymes in the liver, none of fluvoxamine's 11 metabolites (9 of which have been definitively identified) has proven to be pharmacologically active.[173,175,176,226] The half-life of fluvoxamine, 16 hours after a single dose, appears to be prolonged by several hours during repeated administration;[226] as with fluoxetine and paroxetine, nonlinear pharmacokinetics have been described for fluvoxamine.[173,176] Its plasma protein binding of 77% is intermediate among the SSRIs.[176,226]

Smoking is associated with reduced peak serum concentrations and lower areas under the serum concentration *vs* time curve following single dose fluvoxamine.[227] A longer half-life of fluvoxamine has been reported in patients with liver, but not renal disease.[175,226] Young and elderly individuals, both healthy volunteers and depressed patients, show similar kinetics of this SSRI.[194]

In contrast to fluoxetine and paroxetine, fluvoxamine does not produce CYP2D6 inhibition.[183] Rather, fluvoxamine is associated with drug-drug interactions due to its inhibition of CYP1A2 and 2C19.[173,184,228] Fluvoxamine 's unique profile of P450 enzyme subtype inhibition is discussed further below.

2.3 Pharmacodynamic Actions of SSRI Metabolites

Because of the absence of a purified metabolite suitable for direct human administration, such as in the case of *E*-10-OH-nortriptyline,[22] for the newer antidepressants, including SSRIs, the relative roles of parent drugs and their metabolites must be inferred. Most commonly this takes the form of correlating blood concentrations of individual medications and each of their metabolites with various therapeutic and adverse effects. A minor contribution by a given metabolite to the total drug concentration may, however, generate an inadequate 'signal-to-noise' ratio to tease out small metabolite actions.

2.3.1 SSRI Metabolites and Antidepressant Response

Norfluoxetine is the only SSRI metabolite felt to possess clinically important antidepressant activity (see above). With a flat dose-response curve,[68,187] it is not surprising that to date no meaningful relationship has been identified between SSRI parent drug or metabolite plasma concentrations and antidepressant efficacy of these medications.[174,191,222,229,230] However, most assays thus far have failed to differentiate the more (*S*-) from the less potent (*R*-) serotonin reuptake inhibiting enantiomers of norfluoxetine.[230] Moreover, in the case of norfluoxetine, the very long half-life of this metabolite (see above) confounds the issue further because of the possible failure to reach steady-state during an acute trial of fluoxetine.[176,229] However, this pharmacokinetic feature is being applied therapeutically in an effort to utilise intermittent (weekly) dosing of fluoxetine for antidepressant maintenance.[109,191]

2.3.2 Adverse Effects of SSRI Metabolites

As in the case of the therapeutic effects of SSRIs, most of the adverse actions associated with this class of medications are unrelated to plasma concentration of either parent SSRI or major metabolites.[222] Again, the main exception to date has been norfluoxetine, which in one study[231] was identified in disproportionately high plasma concentrations among the substantial minority of fluoxetine-treated depressed patients who developed new-onset sedation.

A single case report associated fluoxetine, and not norfluoxetine, with the primarily central nervous system toxicity of a neonate born to a fluoxetine-treated mother.[232] At birth, cord blood concentration of fluoxetine was 26 μg/L and of norfluoxetine, 54 μg/L, while by 96 hours later the infant was asymptomatic, despite the persistence of higher metabolite concentrations.[232] As reviewed above, as in the case of TCAs, small but quantifiable concentrations of SSRIs and their metabolites are present in the breast milk and infants' serum of nursing mothers being treated with these antidepressants. Consistent with those data, apparent withdrawal symptoms have been reported in a nursing infant whose mother abruptly discontinued sertraline, which she had been taking for a year, 3 weeks postpartum.[233] The apparent relative safety of SSRIs during pregnancy and lactation has been noted,[109] although more definitive research utilising maternal and infant drug and metabolite plasma concentrations is required.

2.3.3 Pharmacogenetics of SSRI Metabolites

With some variability across compounds, all of the SSRIs have been implicated in the inhibition of one or more of the hepatic P450 enzyme systems responsible for the metabolism of antidepressants and other psychotropic drugs.[8,68,176,183,187] As blockade of serotonin reuptake and P450 subtype inhibition are independent properties of the SSRIs and their metabolites, even therapeutically 'inactive' metabolites may contribute to enzyme inhibition and drug-drug interactions of the parent SSRI. Examples include *norfluoxetine*, which is equipotent with fluoxetine in both serotonin reuptake blockade and inhibition of CYP2D6,[187] with consequent interaction between fluoxetine and TCAs.[8,68,100,187] Moreover, norfluoxetine exerts greater inhibitory effect than its parent compound on another P450 isoenzyme, 3A4, which contributes to the hydroxylation of alprazolam[234] and the demethylation of tertiary amine TCAs.[67,176,187,234,235]

Demethyl-sertraline, although not equivalent to its parent drug in blocking serotonin reuptake, possesses similar 2D6 inhibitory properties to sertraline[187,234] and presumably contributes to drug-drug interactions *in vivo*.[68,176,183,187] As sertraline itself is metabolised in part by CYP3A4, it is subject to interaction with drugs affecting that isoenzyme.[66] On the other hand, the primary (M2) metabolite of paroxetine, which does not possess serotonin reuptake inhibiting activity, demonstrates one-third the potency of the parent SSRI on 2D6 inhibition.[176,187,234,236] In contrast to the other SSRIs studied to date, the P450 inhibitory actions of fluvoxamine *in vitro* do not involve 2D6, but rather 3A3/4 and 1A2.[176,183,234,235,237] To date, no metabolites of fluvoxamine have been studied in association with this SSRI's effects on the P450 system. For further discussion of the pharmacogenetics of SSRIs, the reader is referred to the comprehensive reviews by Bertilsson and Dahl[73] and by Coutts and Urichuk.[60]

3. Venlafaxine

A phenylephrine derivative, venlafaxine, represents a new class of serotonin and (less potently) noradrenaline reuptake inhibitor antidepressants that bear many resemblances to the SSRIs.[109,238] With a dual mechanism of action, at least at higher doses, venlafaxine is reminiscent of the older tertiary amine TCAs, but without the multitude of receptor interaction and cardiac conduction effects responsible for the various adverse actions long associated with the tricyclics.[8] As is the case with fluoxetine, the major metabolite of venlafaxine is pharmacologically active, with a profile of activity similar to the parent compound.

3.1 Pharmacokinetic Aspects of Metabolite Formation

As a substrate for metabolism by CYP2D6 and 3A3/4, venlafaxine in humans produces multiple demethylated and conjugated metabolites[239,240] and may interact with inducers and inhibitors of these hepatic isoenzymes.[66,67] Venlafaxine inhibition of 2D6 is weak compared with fluoxetine and paroxetine.[183,238,241] Studies with healthy volunteers have demonstrated that venlafaxine also does not influence metabolism mediated by CYP3A4[242] or 1A2.[243] As with most antidepressants, venlafaxine has a large volume of distribution, but its plasma protein binding (<30%) is unusually low.[238] With a short elimination half-life of only 5 hours, venlafaxine requires 2- or 3-times daily dosing, at least early in treatment, and demonstrates an ascending dose-response curve, in contrast to the flat dose-response relationship seen with the SSRIs.[187,238] Less frequent dosing can be achieved by use of a long-acting 'extended-release' preparation.[109]

Formed by CYP2D6 activity in the liver, the major, *O*-demethyl-metabolite of venlafaxine possesses a longer (11-hour) half-life than the parent drug and accounts for the majority of the renal elimination of a single dose of venlafaxine.[11,238,244] Saturability of the *O*-demethylation pathway results in slightly nonlinear pharmacokinetics with repeated venlafaxine administration.[181,194] The brain-to-blood distribution of venlafaxine and its major metabolite has not yet been defined.[181] Minor metabolites *N,O*-didemethyl- and *N*-demethyl-venlafaxine together make up about one-sixth of elimination of a venlafaxine dose.

As reviewed by Holliday and Benfield,[238] clearance of both venlafaxine and its *O*-demethyl-metabolite are substantially reduced in the presence of renal[245] or hepatic dysfunction. The modest decline in venlafaxine clearance, with a corresponding slight rise in steady-state concentration, seen with advanced age is felt to be clinically insignificant and does not warrant dose adjustment in older patients.[109,194,238] At the other end of the life cycle, venlafaxine and its active demethyl-metabolite easily pass from maternal circulation into breast milk, with preliminary case reports describing measurable concentrations of *O*-demethyl-venlafaxine in the plasma of nursing infants so exposed.[246] While to date no adverse effects have been reported from ingestion of venlafaxine and its metabolite in breast milk, more definitive study is required.

3.2 Pharmacodynamic Actions of Venlafaxine Metabolites

In preclinical models, both venlafaxine and its major, *O*-demethyl-metabolite display potent and equivalent serotonin reuptake inhibition, with less effect on noradrenaline reuptake blockade (venlafaxine twice as potent in the latter effect as the metabolite).[239] The two minor metabolites are orders of magnitude weaker in these actions than *O*-demethyl-venlafaxine.[239] Animal models for screening of antidepressant activity also have shown the *O*-demethyl-metabolite to be pharmacologically active.[239] Coupled with the pharmacokinetic data,[244] including appreciable plasma concentrations in human studies, these results provide evidence that the *O*-demethyl-metabolite of venlafaxine contributes to the antidepressant efficacy of this compound in humans,[11,238,239] and may permit less frequent dosing under steady-state conditions, even with the standard-release preparation (table II).

To date, no published studies have evaluated the relationship of blood concentrations of venlafaxine and its metabolites to antidepressant efficacy. The role, if any, of *O*-demethyl-venlafaxine or the other metabolites in producing the common adverse effects reported during venlafaxine administration, such as nausea, insomnia, and increased diastolic blood pressure[109,238] is unknown.

4. Trazodone

Developed in Italy as a somewhat serotonergic 'second generation' antidepressant,[56,247] trazodone has evolved into a specialised role as a supplemental hypnotic drug often used in combination with nonsedating new generation antidepressants, such as SSRIs, or even older agents, e.g. MAOIs.[8] Although its efficacy as a straightforward antidepressant has been questioned,[6,8] trazodone has generated considerable interest because of a major metabolite with serotonin agonist properties.

4.1 Pharmacokinetic Aspects of Metabolite Formation

Well-absorbed and highly protein bound, trazodone undergoes extensive hepatic metabolism. For antidepressant use it is administered in multiple daily doses because of its short biphasic elimination half-lives, consisting of an initial alpha phase (3 to 6 hours) followed by a slower (5 to 9 hours) beta phase.[2,247] Its major metabolite, *m*-chlorophenylpiperazine (mCPP), with a longer (4 to 14 hours) half-life than trazodone, reaches higher concentrations in brain than in plasma.[5,247,248] At steady-state, mCPP plasma concentrations are about 20% those of the parent compound.[5,249] Other known metabolites of trazodone include the *p*-hydroxy and *N*-oxide compounds, as well as the propionic acid derivative resulting from *N*-dealkylation and removal of the mCPP moiety; however, to date no pharmacological or clinical activity has been ascribed to these minor trazodone metabolites.[2,247]

4.2 Pharmacodynamic Actions of mCPP

The complex actions of trazodone itself on serotonergic systems, including weak serotonin reuptake inhibition and serotonin receptor antagonism, may account for the anti-serotonin effects reported at low doses of this drug.[56] However, at higher doses, trazodone appears to have serotonergic activity, which may be accounted for by the direct serotonin ($5\text{-}HT_{2c}$) receptor agonist properties of mCPP.[247,250,251] It is thus tempting to assign mCPP a major role in the therapeutic action of trazodone. However, this remains premature. Studies attempting to relate trazodone plasma concentrations to clinical response are few and contradictory,[247] and none has analysed the relationship between mCPP concentrations and antidepressant outcome. Indeed, overshadowing any such research are the questions raised about the equivalence of the clinical efficacy of trazodone compared with other antidepressants.[56,247] In one study, the efficacy of fluoxetine added to ongoing trazodone treatment in depressed inpatients was associated with increased trazodone and mCPP plasma concentrations, presumably due to fluoxetine-induced CYP2D6 inhibition;[252] however, interpretation is limited by the short duration and low dosage of the trazodone-only phase prior to the addition of fluoxetine.

At present, most of the interest in mCPP relates to its value as a pharmacological probe in several mental disorders. This metabolite has been described as 'the most extensively used probe of serotonin function in psychiatry'.[253] Orally or intravenously administered mCPP has behavioural, primarily stimulatory effects which are potentially anxiogenic in either healthy volunteers and, to a possibly greater extent, in patients with anxiety disorders.[253-257] Exacerbation of positive symptoms in neuroleptic-free patients with schizophrenia[258] and blunted cortisol response in newly detoxified alcoholic men following intravenous mCPP have also been reported.[259] In depression, however, this use of mCPP has not proven fruitful to date; other than less drowsiness and blunted growth hormone release in depressed patients compared with healthy volunteers, the behavioural and neuroendocrine responses of these two groups to intravenous infusion of mCPP were similar.[260]

Other disorders of putative serotonergic pathophysiology, such as obsessive-compulsive disorder (OCD) continue to attract more interest in the information provided by mCPP. Temporary worsening of OCD symptoms in some patients following mCPP challenge[261-264] may be blocked by serotonin receptor antagonists[263] or by successful clinical treatment with clomipramine[261] or fluoxetine.[262] It remains unclear to what extent such data reflect the underlying pathology of OCD and/or the mechanisms of anti-OCD action of such serotonergic antidepressants.[109,264]

Returning to the more common circumstance accounting for mCPP in the blood and brains of depressed patients, i.e. as the major active metabolite of trazodone, the above data suggest that this metabolite could be responsible for anxiogenic or otherwise stimulatory adverse effects of the parent compound. However, such reactions to trazodone are not common.[8,56,247] Speculation and further investigation continue to focus on the putative role of mCPP in producing whatever antidepressant effect can be seen in trazodone-treated patients.

5. Nefazodone

Even as the use of trazodone in the treatment of depression was declining[9] came the more recent development of the structurally similar antidepressant compound, nefazodone. This newer agent also possesses a dual mechanism of serotonergic action, blocking serotonin (5-HT_{2a}) receptors and, at higher doses, inhibiting serotonin reuptake.[247] Lacking the α-adrenoceptor antagonist properties of trazodone, nefazodone has less propensity to cause orthostatic hypotension, sedation, and, probably, priapism.[8,109] Administered twice daily, nefazodone appears to be an effective antidepressant with antianxiety effects as well, a mild adverse effect profile, and a generally linear dose-response curve, with a possible fall-off at high doses, at which point nonlinear kinetics are noted.[265] Nefazodone is extensively bound to plasma proteins.

Drug-drug interactions are possible as a result of the P450 3A3/4 inhibiting properties of nefazodone.[67,266-269] Both nefazodone and its hydroxy-metabolite, but not mCPP, are more potent inhibitors of CYP3A4 than norfluoxetine or fluvoxamine.[270] Thus, reduced clearance and increased plasma concentrations and clinical effects of alprazolam are observed in the presence of concomitant nefazodone.[268,271] Coadministration of nefazodone and carbamazepine results in the inhibition of carbamazepine metabolism by nefazodone and the induction of nefazodone metabolism – with reduced concentrations of the parent drug and all three main metabolites – by carbamazepine.[272] Nefazodone may be safely coadministered with lithium.[273]

5.1 Pharmacokinetic Aspects of Metabolite Formation

Multiple metabolites result from the extensive *N*-dealkylation and aliphatic and aromatic hydroxylation undergone by nefazodone after oral dosing,[274,275] primarily mediated by CYP3A4.[270] The triazole ring structure of nefazodone leads to a relatively lower metabolism to mCPP compared with trazodone. At steady-state, mCPP plasma concentrations are only 1 to 10% those of nefazodone.[274,275] Two other, more prominent metabolites of nefazodone have been identified. Alpha-hydroxynefazodone, with steady-state plasma concentrations 30 to 45% those of the parent compound, shares nefazodone's short (3 to 4 hour) half-life.[265,268,269,274,275] With a considerably longer 12- to 18-hour half-life, the triazoledione metabolite achieves plasma concentrations up to 10-fold higher than those of nefazodone during chronic dosing and more stable over the dosing interval than concentrations of either the parent drug or other metabolites (table II).[265] Several additional metabolites of nefazodone remain poorly characterised.[274,275] The brain:blood distribution of nefazodone and its metabolites is not well defined.[181] In rodent models little hydroxy-nefazodone enters the brain after nefazodone administration;[276] although the parent compound enters the brain, its concentration there is many times smaller than that of mCPP.

While the pharmacokinetics of nefazodone and its hydroxy-metabolite are nonlinear, those of mCPP formed after administration of nefazodone are linear.[181,265,277] Reduced clearance of parent drug and hydroxy-nefazodone is observed in patients with hepatic cirrhosis, after both single and, to a lesser extent, repeated doses of nefazodone compared with healthy volunteers;[265] the increase in systemic exposure to mCPP was even greater in the patients with cirrhosis, while exposure to the triazoledione metabolite of nefazodone was unaffected by the liver disease. Although exposure to mCPP at steady-state nefazodone doses is unaffected by age, elderly women develop significantly higher and more sustained nefazodone and hydroxy-nefazodone plasma concentrations at steady-state compared with younger individuals and older men,[278] suggesting that nefazodone be introduced at lower doses in older patients.[194]

5.2 Pharmacodynamic Actions of Nefazodone Metabolites

The kinetic data demonstrate that mCPP plays even less of a role in the action of nefazodone than in the case of trazodone (see above). In further contrast to trazodone, there is good evidence for the pharmacological activity of the other two major metabolites of nefazodone, which are not produced by the metabolism of trazodone. Specifically, hydroxy-nefazodone shares the same neuropharmacological profile, qualitatively and quantitatively, as its parent drug,[11] rendering it analogous to norfluoxetine, reviewed above. On the other hand, the triazoledione metabolite shares only one of the biochemical actions of nefazodone – blockade of 5-HT_{2a} receptors – and does so in a more selective manner than the parent compound;[11] this metabolite does not inhibit serotonin reuptake, as does nefazodone. Thus, the triazoledione metabolite, sharing the major pharmacological action of nefazodone, may contribute significantly to the therapeutic efficacy of the latter.[265] Moreover, the longer half-life of this metabolite suggests that less frequent dosing of nefazodone, e.g. once, rather than twice daily, may be sufficient to maintain the antidepressant effect.[109]

6. Amfebutamone (Bupropion)

The introduction of amfebutamone (bupropion) as a new generation antidepressant in North America in the mid-1980s offered apparently novel mechanisms of antidepressant action but also new toxicities.[6,8] In addition to a fundamentally noradrenergic mode of action, amfebutamone may have effects on dopamine function.[11,279-281] This has implications for this medication's spectrum of therapeutic activity, e.g. amfebutamone is under study for the treatment of attention deficit hyperactivity disorder and is now marketed for smoking cessation, as well as risks, such as the precipitation of psychosis, as will be discussed below.[6,8,109,282]

Increased risk of seizures at high doses, first evident in patients with eating disorders, delayed the introduction of the drug into clinical use and led to the US Food and Drug Administration recommended labelling of a daily dosage ceiling of 450mg, administered three times/day, with each dose no greater than 150mg.[8] On the other hand, the lack of amfebutamone effects on serotonergic systems avoids some adverse effects commonly encountered with use of SSRIs and other newer antidepressants, such as sexual dysfunction.[6,8,109] Extensive research into the metabolites of amfebutamone suggests some contribution to the therapeutic effect of the drug and an even greater role in some of the toxicity associated with this compound.[5,7,283]

6.1 Pharmacokinetic Aspects of Metabolite Formation

The unique unicyclic aminoketone structure of amfebutamone undergoes hepatic side-chain oxidative cleavage and hydroxylation at the terminal methyl group, as well as reduction of the intact aminoketone to an aminoalcohol. In healthy volunteers this metabolism, after a single dose, results in three major metabolites, which possess elimination half-lives 2- to 3-times longer than the approximately 10 hours of the parent compound.[82,284] While amfebutamone and its metabolites threohydro-amfebutamone (TB) and erythrohydro-amfebutamone (EB) are neither metabolised by nor inhibit CYP2D6, plasma concentrations of the active metabolite, hydroxy-amfebutamone (HB) are increased in poor 2D6 metabolisers.[285]

Under actual therapeutic conditions, Golden and colleagues at the US National Institute of Mental Health[286] intensively studied the pharmacokinetics of amfebutamone, using both blood and CSF sampling, during a 3- to 6-week clinical trial in 10 depressed patients, representing 12 separate courses of treatment. In both compartments studied, all three metabolites predominated over amfebutamone in every patient. In CSF, TB concentrations were 40-times higher than those of the parent compound, while those of each of the other two metabolites,

EB and HB, were 6-times greater than amfebutamone CSF concentrations. Plasma metabolite concentrations (which also exceeded those of amfebutamone) were strongly correlated with the respective CSF measures.[286] Although HB predominated in plasma, the much lower (50 *vs* 96%) degree of protein binding of TB suggested higher pharmacologically active concentrations of the latter amfebutamone metabolite in brain. Abrupt discontinuation of amfebutamone in one patient led to confirmation of earlier findings of very long (up to 50 hours in the case of TB) elimination half-lives of amfebutamone metabolites,[286] which could ultimately prove to be a rationale for less frequent dosing of immediate-release amfebutamone in some patients (table II); a slow-release formulation of amfebutamone permits twice-daily dosing.[287] Steady-state plasma concentrations of TB and EB are strongly correlated, suggesting similar mechanisms of formation or clearance of these amfebutamone metabolites.[288]

The effects of alcohol-related liver disease on single-dose amfebutamone kinetics were studied by DeVane and associates;[289] their only significant finding was of a 50% longer elimination half-life of HB in the hepatic disease group. Amfebutamone is safely used routinely in the elderly and patients with cardiac disease.[8] However, limited data suggest the potential for reduced clearance of amfebutamone and its metabolites at standard doses in older individuals,[194] especially in the case of HB and TB.[288] Given reports that amfebutamone may have particular value in the treatment of bipolar depression,[8,290] Ketter et al.[291] investigated the effects of concurrent mood stabilisers on amfebutamone kinetics. They found marked reduction in single dose amfebutamone plasma concentrations, with concomitant rise in HB concentrations, in the presence of carbamazepine. Valproate also increased concentrations of HB, without change in concentrations of amfebutamone.[291]

6.2 Pharmacodynamic Actions of Amfebutamone Metabolites

Therapeutic effects: In animal behavioural tests used for screening antidepressants, amfebutamone metabolites HB and TB demonstrate approximately half the potency of the parent compound.[280,283,292] Acute amfebutamone administration in a rat model was associated with a rapid and significant reduction in firing of noradrenergic neurons in the locus ceruleus,[280] a property shared equipotently by HB. Firing rates of dopaminergic, but not serotonergic neurons, are also reduced by high doses of amfebutamone.[281] In clinical studies amfebutamone is associated with enhanced efficiency of noradrenergic transmission, as reflected by an increased excretion of the hydroxy-metabolite of melatonin, increased plasma MHPG concentrations, and reduced whole-body noradrenaline turnover.[279,281,287,293] At least the hydroxy-metabolite of amfebutamone is felt to share or predominate in these actions.[281,283] Plasma concentrations of amfebutamone and its metabolites in depressed patients undergoing treatment have not proven consistently helpful in guiding treatment,[68,286,292] but excessive concentrations have been related to poor outcome and toxicity in some patients, as reviewed below. In one open fixed-dose study, TB plasma concentrations correlated modestly but significantly with post-treatment depression rating scores.[287]

Adverse effects: The most detailed account of the relationship of amfebutamone metabolites to poor outcome and toxicity of the drug comes from the study of Golden et al.,[286] employing amfebutamone doses up to 900 mg/day, in which significantly higher plasma concentrations of each of the 3 metabolites were observed in nonresponders compared with clinical responders to amfebutamone. This was most clearly illustrated in the case of HB, which demonstrated plasma concentrations >1250 μg/L in all 5 nonresponders, while each of the 7 amfebutamone responders had HB plasma concentrations below 1200 μg/L. These high HB concentrations correlated significantly post-treatment with plasma concentrations of homovanillic acid (HVA), the major metabolite of dopamine, which rose only in the amfebutamone non-responders,[279,286] most of whom developed psychotic symptoms.[282] Modest elevations in plasma HVA concentrations during treatment with slow-release amfebutamone have not been associated with psychosis.[287] Although the major feared adverse effect of amfebutamone, seizures, appears to be dose related,[6,8] no specific association of this toxicity with patterns of metabolite production or distribution has been described.

An unusual laboratory problem associated with amfebutamone metabolites has been reported: cross-reactivity and, hence, false positive results, of amfebutamone and its three major metabolites, especially EB, with a screening urinary immunoassay for amphetamines.[294] This is to be distinguished from those MAOIs which are actually metabolised to amphetamine derivatives, as will be reviewed in a later section.

7. Other Newer Antidepressants

A seemingly continuous stream of new antidepressants has been marketed over the past two decades. Among those compounds which have appeared on the worldwide market since we last examined antidepressant metabolites[295] are mirtazapine and reboxetine.[109] Although knowledge of metabolites of these drugs is at an early stage, the foregoing emphasise the importance of recognising the potential role of metabolites as contributing to the therapeutic and/or adverse effects of any antidepressant.

7.1 Mirtazapine

The unique mechanism of action of mirtazapine, a tetracyclic compound related to mianserin, yields enhanced noradrenergic and serotonergic neurotransmission via presynaptic α_2-adrenergic receptor blockade.[247] Although antihistamine effects result in sedation at low doses, as well as weight gain, the blockade of 5-HT_2 and 5-HT_3 receptors by mirtazapine appears responsible for the low incidence of SSRI-like gastrointestinal and sexual dysfunction adverse effects associated with the newer agent.[8,109,247,296]

Metabolised by several P450 subfamilies, including CYP1A2, 2D6, and 3A4, mirtazapine follows the common path of demethylation and oxidation, followed by metabolite conjugation. With linear kinetics and approximately 85% plasma protein binding, mirtazapine demonstrates an elimination half-life of 20 to 40 hours, averaging 21.5 hours.[297] Mirtazapine is marketed as a racemic mixture, with pharmacokinetic differences between its enantiomers. Half-life and steady-state plasma concentrations are greater for the *R*(–)-enantiomer, while only the *S*(–)-enantiomer is metabolised more slowly by CYP2D6 poor metabolisers.[181,298] Limited data suggest that young men may demonstrate shorter half-lives and lower steady-state plasma concentrations of mirtazapine than young women or older persons of either gender.[194] With little effect on P450 isoenzymes, mirtazapine is involved in few drug-drug interactions.[299]

Among the 4 primary metabolites of mirtazapine, the unconjugated demethyl-metabolite appears most pharmacologically active, although less so than the parent compound.[296,297] Its pharmacological profile is similar to that of mirtazapine, but with 5- to 10-times less potency and half the area under the plasma concentration *vs* time curve of the parent drug; the metabolite's contribution to the therapeutic and adverse activity of this novel antidepressant is estimated at only 5 to 10% of the total.[296,298] Liver and moderate renal impairment are associated with a 30% reduction in oral mirtazapine clearance.[299]

7.2 Reboxetine

The newest antidepressant to be marketed in the US, this selective noradrenaline reuptake inhibitor has been available throughout the world for several years.[109] While its mechanism of action is reminiscent of the tricyclics, reboxetine's dearth of receptor affinity and cardiovascular effects other than tachycardia results in an adverse effect profile more consistent with a new-generation antidepressant.[8]

Pharmacologically, reboxetine exists as a mixture of *R,R* (-) and a more potent but pharmacodynamically similar *S,S* (+) enantiomer. Its elimination half-life of 12 to 16 hours permits twice-daily administration.[109] The extensive metabolism of reboxetine appears mediated mainly by CYP3A4, without involvement of CYP2D6.[300,301] By means of CYP3A-mediated 2-*O*-dealkylation of the ethoxyphenoxy ring, each enantiomer of reboxetine is metabolised to one primary product, *O*-desethyl-reboxetine, as well as three minor metabolites, two of which are formed by oxidation of the ethoxy aromatic ring. Steady-state concentrations of reboxetine metabolites are low, and to date their entry into the brain and their pharmacological activity have not been shown.[181,300]

Reduced clearance of both enantiomers of reboxetine, by a quarter to a third, can be demonstrated with the concurrent administration of the antifungal agent, ketoconazole, an inhibitor of CYP3A4 activity.[302] In human liver microsomes, ketoconazole, but not inhibitors of other CYP isoenzymes, significantly reduces the formation of *O*-desethyl-reboxetine.[301] In the presence of this CYP3A4 inhibitor, the elimination half-life of *S*-reboxetine increased by 31%, while that of the *R*-enantiomer rose by 45%.[302]

Inducers of CYP3A4 activity, such as carbamazepine, would be expected to speed reboxetine metabolism, but the pharmacological and clinical effects of such an interaction await study. While both reboxetine enantiomers are weak competitive inhibitors of CYP2D6 and 3A4 *in vitro*,[301] this does not appear to be clinically relevant. For example, reboxetine does not affect the pharmacokinetic or pharmacodynamic profile of the benzodiazepine, alprazolam, a 3A4 substrate, in contrast to nefazodone.[268,271]

8. Monoamine Oxidase Inhibitors

The original class of antidepressants – accidentally discovered[1] – MAOIs – have generally been overlooked in consideration of pharmacokinetics and metabolites.[2,303,304] This relates to these drugs' unusual 'hit-and-run' pharmacodynamics on the degradative enzyme MAO in brain and gut, whereby the actions of these antidepressants – long outlasting the MAOIs' physical presence – have appeared unrelated to acute kinetics and blood concentrations of the drug or of any metabolites.[8,9,303] Thus, most research on the biochemical and clinical effects of MAOIs has focused on the long term consequences of MAO inhibition, not the direct effects of the medications. Even the short term, e.g. one week, washout of classical MAO inhibitors does not reverse their biochemical actions, which are dependent on the weeks-long process of regeneration of the enzyme. In contrast, the newer reversible MAOIs are not associated with such long-lasting effects in the absence of medication in the blood.[303,304]

Recent attention to the metabolites of both older and newer, reversible MAOIs has focused on their structural and pharmacological resemblance to amphetamines, with possible implications for the acute short term stimulant effect experienced by some patients in the first several hours after MAOI dosing.[68]

8.1 Classical Nonselective MAOIs

Since the serendipitous observation in the early 1950s that iproniazid therapy for tuberculosis was associated with unexplained euphoria in some patients,[1,303] MAOIs entered the therapeutic armamentarium as nonselective irreversible inhibitors of both subtypes of monoamine oxidase. Through the 1970s such nonselective drugs as phenelzine, tranylcypromine, and isocarboxazid waxed and waned in popularity. Their use was influenced on the one hand by concerns over potential hypertensive reactions and the development of seemingly safer and more effective antidepressant compounds, and on the other by research demonstrating the efficacy of MAOIs – in some cases surpassing that of the tricyclics – in various subtypes of depression, e.g. bipolar or atypical, as well as in panic and other anxiety disorders.[9,303,304] While much ongoing research attends the development of new, safer reversible and selective MAOIs, the classical drugs, particularly phenelzine and tranylcypromine, remain the standard MAOIs in current use throughout the world.[303,304]

8.1.1 Phenelzine

Even decades after the introduction of this standard MAOI, considerable disagreement about the metabolism of phenelzine was rife in the field.[303] It is known that phenelzine is a well absorbed, short (1.5 to 4 hour) half-life drug.[304] The slow increase in steady-state plasma concentrations of phenelzine over the first 6 to 8 weeks of treatment has been interpreted as reflecting nonlinear kinetics due to inhibition of phenelzine metabolism by the drug itself, or by its metabolites.[303-305] The assumption that phenelzine, like the structurally similar isoniazid, is metabolised by acetylation, led to a string of studies in the 1960s and 1970s yielding inconsistent findings regarding the relationship between acetylator status and either clinical response to or adverse effects of phenelzine treatment (reviewed by Mallinger and Smith[305]). The premise that phenelzine is primarily acetylated now appears to have been flawed,[303-305] with acetylation more likely a minor metabolic pathway of this MAOI.[306] Instead, the majority of an administered dose of phenelzine appears in urine in the form of phenylacetic acid (PAA) or 4-OH-PAA, which are considered pharmacologically inactive.[305,306] In part, PAA may be formed directly by the action of MAO on phenelzine.[305,306] Of greater interest is the alternative metabolic pathway for phenelzine that produces β-phenylethylamine (PEA),[305,306] an endogenous amphetamine-like compound that easily crosses the blood-brain barrier.[307] PEA is the most likely candidate for an active metabolite of phenelzine (and may play a minor role in the action of the newer selective drugs, such as deprenyl [selegiline]),[307] but to date no research has documented its contribution to either the therapeutic or adverse effects of this MAOI. In turn, PEA is metabolised by MAO-type B to PAA,[305,306] which as noted is subject to 4-hydroxylation.

Additionally, phenelzine itself is ring-hydroxylated, and 4-OH-phenelzine may be converted to 4-OH-PAA.[306] There is no evidence that either of these metabolites is pharmacologically active. The elevation of brain GABA concentrations associated with phenelzine treatment has been ascribed to still unidentified metabolites of this MAOI.[306]

8.1.2 Tranylcypromine

For this other standard MAOI there is a more complete database on pharmacokinetics,[305] but the question of amphetamine-like active metabolites has not been fully resolved.[306] Tranylcypromine is rapidly absorbed and eliminated, with a half-life of <3 hours.[308,309] There may be differences in the kinetics of the (+) and (–) isomers of tranylcypromine – the medication as prescribed is the racemic mixture – but the few studies of this have been contradictory.[305] The two stereoisomers also differ in their primary acute biochemical action: irreversible MAO inhibition (+) versus catecholamine reuptake inhibition (–), but the clinical significance of this distinction is unknown.[310]

Some cardiovascular effects have been related to tranylcypromine dose[311] or blood concentrations during chronic administration.[305] Orthostatic drop in systolic blood pressure and corresponding orthostatic rise in pulse rate at the time of peak tranylcypromine concentrations after dosing correlated positively with that plasma tranylcypromine concentration in one investigation.[308] In a related study, tranylcypromine concentrations at a later (5-hour post-dose) time point was inversely correlated with clinical antidepressant response.[309] In those important pharmacokinetic investigations by Mallinger and associates[308,309] no tranylcypromine metabolites were accounted for.[305] A subsequent report by Keck et al.[311] described a positive correlation between the acute elevation in supine blood pressure after tranylcypromine and the MAOI dose. That investigation was particularly noteworthy for its prospective documentation of the absence of amphetamine or methamphetamine in any plasma samples obtained from patients during tranylcypromine treatment.[311]

Indeed, the best evidence for the existence of active byproducts of tranylcypromine comes from the literature on overdose. A report of amphetamine in the plasma of a patient who took an overdose of racemic tranylcypromine[312] led to a fruitless search for amphetamine in the blood and urine of 8 patients in a crossover study who took either isomer of tranylcypromine for a single dose (N = 5) or, in the case of 3 neurological patients, for 3 days.[310] Although no amphetamine was identified in any subject, PEA was increased in blood after (+) tranylcypromine. As noted, later prospective efforts at assaying amphetamine-like metabolites of tranylcypromine also were unsuccessful.[306,311,313]

However, occasional reports of tranylcypromine abuse[314] and dependence[315,316] continue to suggest stimulant-like properties of the drug – presumably the parent compound – particularly at high doses. This might also relate to reports of apparently spontaneous hypertensive reactions during tranylcypromine treatment[317] and the belatedly appreciated danger of hypertensive crises from a rapid switch from a hydrazine MAOI, e.g. phenelzine or isocarboxazid, to tranylcypromine.[8] The well-described, and feared, potentially dangerous interactions between classical MAOIs and catecholaminergic or serotonergic drugs or other exogenous substances[8,109,303,304] also do not appear to involve mediation by any active antidepressant metabolites.

8.1.3 Isocarboxazid

This nonselective, irreversible MAOI is being prescribed with decreasing frequency as its manufacture has become inconsistent in parts of the world.[109] Although isocarboxazid may act through the production of benzylhydrazine as an active metabolite,[5] no peer-reviewed studies of this MAOI's pharmacokinetics have been published.[305,306]

8.2 Selective MAOIs

The recent development of MAOIs selective for either of the two functionally distinct forms of the enzyme has sought to capitalise on potential advances in therapeutic efficacy and/or reduced toxicity.[8,318] While clorgiline, an irreversible inhibitor of MAO-type A[6] has proven to be a potent antidepressant in bipolar and unipolar patients, for many individuals it offers no particular pharmacokinetic or pharmacodynamic advantage or distinction.[318] However, on an investigational basis clorgiline occupied a special niche as an effective treatment for rapid-cycling bipolar disorder in low doses, with few adverse effects.[319] Representatives of two relatively new categories of MAOIs – one directed at each subtype of MAO – are particularly relevant to the consideration of active metabolites.

8.2.2 Selective MAO-B Inhibition: Deprenyl (Selegiline)

Selegiline (*l*-deprenyl) is a selective MAO-B inhibitor (the *d*-isomer lacks MAO inhibition). Low doses are well established as an adjunct to standard treatments for Parkinson's disease. In contrast, the role of the drug in the treatment of depression is less well defined.[6,303] This relates to the loss of the MAO-B selectivity of selegiline's enzyme inhibitory action as the daily dose is raised to the 30mg antidepressant range.[6,8] Even at the 10 mg/day standard antiparkinsonian dose concentration, however, selegiline has proven extremely interesting in terms of potentially active metabolites in the stimulant class.

Oral selegiline is rapidly absorbed and quickly reduces MAO activity in platelets (type B enzyme).[6,303,320] Modern imaging techniques can document the entry of selegiline into the brain – to a greater extent than the MAO-A inhibitor, clorgiline – within seconds after intravenous administration.[321] The half-life of the parent compound is extremely short (<2 hours). A transdermal formulation of selegiline, which produces higher and more sustained plasma concentrations of the parent drug than orally administered selegiline, is showing promise in early clinical antidepressant trials.[322] Extensive stereoselective (with no racemic transformation) hepatic (and, to a far lesser degree, lung and kidney) microsomal metabolism results in production of norselegiline (*l*-demethyl-selegiline), which is further metabolised to *l*-amphetamine (and which, in turn, is subsequently *p*-hydroxylated).[306] Selegiline is also directly metabolised to *l*-methamphetamine,[306,321] which, like amphetamine, is subjected to further *p*-hydroxylation.

Early studies demonstrated the presence of *l*-amphetamine in human brain after the therapeutic use of low dose selegiline in Parkinson's disease.[323] Subsequent advances in assay methodology have permitted the similar measurement of demethyl-selegiline and *l*-methamphetamine as well as *l*-amphetamine in blood, urine, and CSF of patients and healthy volunteers after single or repeated doses of selegiline.[305,307,321,324] Following multiple doses of the drug, *l*-methamphetamine predominates in CSF and urine, with mean CSF concentrations of 15 μg/L, versus 7 μg/L for *l*-amphetamine and 1 μg/L for demethyl-selegiline, which has the shortest half-life of the metabolites.[321] The accumulation of selegiline metabolites reported in the past[323] has not been observed using more sensitive techniques.[321] Following discontinuation of selegiline, metabolites continue to be excreted for an additional one to 5 days.[305]

The pharmacodynamic role of the metabolites of selegiline, which may possess MAO-A reversible inhibitory properties of their own,[305] is unclear. In support of a possible therapeutic role of the conversion of selegiline to methamphetamine and amphetamine, Karoum and associates[307] noted that the observed biochemical effects of selegiline were better explained as actions of the metabolites than of parent drug.

8.2.3 Moclobemide

The reversibility of the selective MAO-A inhibitors, such as moclobemide, confers an additional margin of safety compared with the older drugs of this class.[8,109,303,318] Additionally, with a new emphasis on short-term drug action, the role of pharmacokinetics with reversible inhibitors of MAO-A (RIMAs) is considerably more important than was the case with the classical irreversible MAOIs.[305] For example, the time course of moclobemide's action incorporates a brief elimination half-life of <2 hours, with MAO-A inhibition of 8 to 10 hours' duration after a dose, returning to baseline within one day.[305] An even shorter-acting RIMA, toloxatone, produces MAO-A inhibition that wanes between doses.[8,305] While drug-drug interactions involving the irreversible MAOIs focus on pharmacodynamic responses,[8] those related to the RIMAs, as with the other antidepressants under discussion, also deal with kinetic alterations, e.g. the reduced clearance of moclobemide associated with concurrent cimetidine.[325] On the other hand, abrupt discontinuation of tertiary amine TCAs does not affect the kinetics of subsequently introduced moclobemide or of its two major metabolites.[326]

As with most antidepressants, moclobemide undergoes extensive hepatic oxidative metabolism. There is evidence that one or more of the involved metabolic pathways may saturate on repeated dosing, with subsequent reduced clearance and increased bioavailability and half-life of drug.[305,325,327] Two major metabolites of moclobemide are formed. The primary one (Ro 12-8095), produced by hydroxylation of the morpholine ring, with subsequent lactam formation, is pharmacologically inactive.[305,306,328] *N*-oxidation of the morpholine ring of moclobemide produces an *active* metabolite (Ro 12-5637), with steady-state blood concentrations somewhat lower than those of the parent compound; plasma concentrations of metabolite Ro 12-8095 are similar to those of moclobemide.[306,328,329] Pharmacogenetic data point to a role of CYP2C19 in the hydroxylation of moclobemide, such that plasma concentrations of metabolite Ro 12-8095 are lower in poor than in extensive metabolisers of *S*-mephenytoin.[329] Aromatic hydroxylation is an additional minor metabolic pathway of this RIMA. The active *N*-oxide metabolite Ro 12-5637 accounts for 20 to 30% of a moclobemide dose in urine, while the unchanged parent drug and the inactive lactam metabolite Ro 12-8095 cannot be identified because of extensive subsequent metabolism.[328] Ultimately as many as 20 metabolites of moclobemide can be identified in human body fluids.[181] In contrast to moclobemide itself, some of the drug's minor open-ring metabolites in a rat model demonstrate MAO-B inhibitory activity.[181]

As with older antidepressants, studies with moclobemide have examined its kinetics in various physiological states. For instance, Pons et al.[330] investigated a sample of lactating women under treatment with moclobemide. Based on the low concentrations of parent drug and Ro 12-8095 metabolite assayed in breast milk, it was estimated that a nursing infant would ingest in a feeding a dose of moclobemide approximating 1% of the mother's dose, controlling for weight,[330] an amount of medication presumed safe. Of note was the absence of the active moclobemide metabolite Ro 12-5637 in breast milk.[330] On the other hand, renal impairment has been found associated with lengthened disposition half-life and greater peak concentrations of Ro 12-5637 after single-dose moclobemide.[331] The relative distribution of this active metabolite into the brain, compared with parent moclobemide, remains under investigation.[181]

With the growing understanding of the pharmacokinetics of moclobemide metabolites, research attention is now turning to an appreciation of their potential contribution to the antidepressant actions of this relatively new compound. The role of an *O*-demethylated active metabolite of brofaromine, and of an additional poorly characterised but possibly active metabolite in the mechanisms of action of that RIMA also await further study.[306]

9. Conclusions

Serendipity has marked the history of psychopharmacology. One result of this phenomenon has been the introduction and even widespread use of many antidepressant compounds prior to a complete understanding of their mechanisms of action. A frequently hidden source of variance mediating the actions of a wide group of older and newer antidepressant medications is the presence of pharmacologically active metabolites. These may play a role, either significant or minor, in producing the therapeutic and/or toxic effects of antidepressant drugs. Indeed, the presence of active metabolites may amplify or nullify effects of the more visible parent compound.

Careful attention to active metabolites, at both the medication development and postmarketing stages, including the assurance of bioequivalence of generic formulations,[153] is necessary to maximise the benefit:risk ratio of antidepressants. Accounting for the pharmacokinetic and pharmacodynamic actions of putative active metabolites may explain some unexpected drug-drug interactions and cases of apparent nonresponse or intolerance to antidepressant medications.

References

1. Rudorfer MV, Linnoila M, Potter WZ. Accidental antidepressants: search for specific action. In: Dahl SG, Gram LF, Paul SM, et al, editors. Clinical pharmacology in psychiatry. IV. Selectivity in psychotropic drug action: promises or problems? Heidelberg: Springer-Verlag, 1987: 157-66
2. Rudorfer MV, Potter WZ. Pharmacokinetics of antidepressants. In: Meltzer HY, editor. Psychopharmacology: the third generation of progress. New York: Raven Press, 1987: 1353-63
3. Hammer W, Sjöqvist F. Plasma levels of monomethylated tricyclic antidepressants during treatment with imipramine-like compounds. Life Sci 1967; 6: 1895-903

4. Potter WZ, Calil HM, Sutfin T, et al. Active metabolites of imipramine and desipramine in man. Clin Pharmacol Ther 1982; 31: 393-401
5. Caccia S, Garattini S. Pharmacokinetic and pharmacodynamic significance of antidepressant drug metabolites. Pharmacol Res 1992; 26: 317-29
6. Rudorfer MV, Potter WZ. Antidepressants: a comparative review of the clinical pharmacology and therapeutic use of the 'newer' versus the 'older' drugs. Drugs 1989; 37: 713-38
7. Potter WZ, Manji HK. Antidepressants, metabolites, and apparent drug resistance. Clin Neuropharmacol 1990; 13 Suppl. 1: S45-53
8. Rudorfer MV, Manji HK, Potter WZ. Comparative tolerability profiles of the newer versus older antidepressants. Drug Saf 1994; 10: 18-46
9. Potter WZ, Rudorfer MV, Manji HK. The pharmacologic treatment of depression. N Engl J Med 1991; 325: 633-42
10. Potter WZ, Manji HK, Rudorfer MV. Tricyclics and tetracyclics. In: Schatzberg AF, Nemeroff CB, editors. The American Psychiatric Press Textbook of Psychopharmacology. 2nd ed. Washington, DC: American Psychiatric Press, 1998: 199-218
11. Sanchez C, Hyttel J. Comparison of the effects of antidepressants and their metabolites on reuptake of biogenic amines and on receptor binding. Cell Mol Neurobiol 1999; 19: 467-89
12. Kelly JP, Leonard BE. An investigation of the antidepressant properties of lofepramine and its desmethylated metabolites in the forced swim and olfactory bulbectomized rat models of depression. Eur Neuropsychopharmacol 1999; 9: 101-5
13. Rudorfer MV, Potter WZ. Metabolism of tricyclic antidepressants. Cell Mol Neurobiol 1999; 19: 373-409
14. Watkins PB. Role of cytochromes P450 in drug metabolism and hepatotoxicity. Semin Liver Dis 1990; 10: 235-50
15. Shen WW, Lin K-M. Cytochrome P450 monooxygenases and interactions of psychotropic drugs. Int J Psychiatry Med 1991; 21: 47-56
16. Shen WW. Cytochrome P450 monooxygenases and interactions of psychotropic drugs: a five-year update. Int J Psychiatry Med 1995; 25: 271-84
17. Rudorfer MV, Lane EA, Chang W-H, et al. Desipramine pharmacokinetics in Chinese and Caucasian volunteers. Br J Clin Pharmacol 1984; 17: 433-40
18. Träskman L, Åsberg M, Bertilsson L, et al. Plasma levels of chlorimipramine and its demethyl metabolite during treatment of depression. Clin Pharmacol Ther 1979; 26: 600-10
19. Linnoila M, Insel T, Kilts C, et al. Plasma steady-state concentrations of hydroxylated metabolites of clomipramine. Clin Pharmacol Ther 1982; 32: 208-11
20. Balant-Gorgia AE, Gex-Fabry M, Balant LP. Clinical pharmacokinetics of clomipramine. Clin Pharmacokinet 1991; 20: 447-62
21. Young RC, Dhar AK, Kutt H, et al. Isomers of 10-hydroxynortriptyline in geriatric depression. Ther Drug Monit 1988; 10: 164-7
22. Nordin C, Bertilsson L. Active hydroxymetabolites of antidepressants: emphasis on E-10-hydroxy-nortriptyline. Clin Pharmacokinet 1995; 28: 26-40
23. Lancaster SG, Gonzalez JR. Dothiepin: a review of its pharmacodynamic and pharmacokinetic properties, and therapeutic efficacy in depressive illness. Drugs 1989; 38: 123-47
24. Eap CB, Yasui N, Kaneko S, et al. Effects of carbamazepine coadministration on plasma concentrations of the enantiomers of mianserin and of its metabolites. Ther Drug Monit 1999; 21: 166-70
25. Alvan G, Borga O, Lind M, et al. Concentrations of parent drug and major metabolites in plasma. Eur J Clin Pharmacol 1977; 11: 219-24
26. Mellström B, Alvan G, Bertilsson L, et al. Nortriptyline formation after single oral and intramuscular doses of amitriptyline. Clin Pharmacol Ther 1982; 32: 664-7
27. Golden RN, Gilmore JH, Carson SW. Antidepressant challenge tests: the interface of pharmacokinetics and pharmacodynamics. Psychopharmacol Bull 1991; 27: 611-7
28. Liedholm H, Liden A. Food intake and the presystemic metabolism of single doses of amitriptyline and nortriptyline. Fundam Clin Pharmacol 1998; 12: 636-42
29. Hawes EM. N+-glucuronidation, a common pathway in human metabolism of drugs with a tertiary amine group. Drug Metab Dispos 1998; 26: 830-7
30. Dahl-Puustinen M-L, Åberg-Wistedt A, Bertilsson L. Glucuronidation of amitriptyline in man in vivo. Toxicology 1989; 65: 37-9
31. Ziegler VE, Fuller TA, Biggs JT. Nortriptyline and 10-hydroxynortriptyline plasma concentrations. J Pharm Pharmacol 1976; 28: 849-50
32. Bertilsson L, Mellström B, Sjöqvist F. Pronounced inhibition of noradrenaline uptake by 10-hydroxy-metabolites of nortriptyline. Life Sci 1979; 25: 1285-92
33. Bock J, Giller E, Gray S, et al. Steady-state plasma concentrations of cis- and trans- 10-OH amitriptyline metabolites. Clin Pharmacol Ther 1982; 31: 609-16
34. Young RC, Alexopoulos GS, Shamoian CA, et al. Plasma 10-hydroxynortriptyline in elderly depressed patients. Clin Pharmacol Ther 1984; 35: 540-4
35. Nordin C, Bertilsson L, Siwers B. CSF and plasma levels of nortriptyline and its 10-hydroxy metabolite. Br J Pharmacol 1985; 20: 411-3
36. Edelbroek PM, Zitman FG, Knoppert-van der Klein EAM, et al. Therapeutic drug monitoring of amitriptyline: impact of age, smoking and contraceptives on drug and metabolite levels in bulimic women. Clin Chim Acta 1987; 165: 177-87
37. Bertilsson L, Nordin C, Otani K, et al. Disposition of single oral doses of E-10-hydroxynortriptyline in healthy subjects, with some observations on pharmacodynamic effects. Clin Pharmacol Ther 1986; 40: 261-7
38. Bertilsson L, Dahl-Puustinen M-L, Nordin C. E-10-hydroxynortriptyline: effects and disposition of a potential novel antidepressant. In: Dahl SG, Gram LF, editors. Clinical pharmacology in psychiatry. Berlin: Springer-Verlag, 1989: 52-9
39. Dahl-Puustinen M-L, Perry TL, Dumont E, et al. Stereoselective disposition of racemic E-10-hydroxynortriptyline in human beings. Clin Pharmacol Ther 1989; 45: 650-6
40. Nordin C, Bertilsson L, Dahl-Puustinen M-L, et al. Treatment of depression with E-10-hydroxynortriptyline: a pilot study on biochemical effects and pharmacokinetics. Psychopharmacology 1991; 103: 287-90
41. Potter WZ, Calil HM, Zavadil AP III, et al. Steady-state concentrations of hydroxylated metabolites of tricyclic antidepressants in patients: relationship to clinical effect. Psychopharmacol Bull 1980; 16: 32-4
42. Wilens TE, Biederman J, Baldessarini RJ, et al. Developmental changes in serum concentrations of desipramine and 2-hydroxydesipramine during treatment with desipramine. J Am Acad Child Adolesc Psychiatry 1992; 31: 691-8
43. Gram LF, Bjerre M, Kragh-Sørensen P, et al. Imipramine metabolites in blood of patients during therapy and after overdose. Clin Pharmacol Ther 1983; 33: 335-42
44. Brosen K, Gram LF, Klysner R, et al. Steady-state levels of imipramine and its metabolites: significance of dose-dependent kinetics. Eur J Pharmacol 1986; 30: 43-9

45. Sutfin T, Perini G, Molnar G, et al. Multiple-dose pharmacokinetics of imipramine and its major active and conjugated metabolites in depressed patients. J Clin Psychopharmacol 1988; 8: 48-53
46. Cooke RG, Warsh JJ, Stancer HC, et al. The nonlinear kinetics of desipramine and 2-hydroxydesipramine in plasma. Clin Pharmacol Ther 1984; 36: 343-9
47. Preskorn S, Irwin H. Toxicity of tricyclic antidepressants: kinetics, mechanism, intervention. A review. J Clin Psychiatry 1982; 43: 151-6
48. Jarvis MR. Clinical pharmacokinetics of tricyclic antidepressant overdose. Psychopharmacol Bull 1991; 27: 541-50
49. Nelson JC, Mazure C, Jatlow PI. Clinical implications of the pharmacokinetics of tricyclic antidepressants. In: Dahl SG, Gram LF, editors. Clinical pharmacology in psychiatry. Berlin: Springer-Verlag, 1989: 219-27
50. Danish University Antidepressant Group (DUAG). Clomipramine dose-effect study in patients with depression: clinical end points and pharmacokinetics. Clin Pharmacol Ther 1999; 66: 152-65
51. DeVane CL, Jusko W. Plasma concentration monitoring of hydroxylated metabolites of imipramine and desipramine. Drug Intell Clin Pharm 1981; 15: 263 -6
52. Pollock BG, Perel JM. Hydroxy metabolites of tricyclic antidepressants: evaluation of relative cardiotoxicity. In: Dahl SG, Gram LF, editors. Clinical pharmacology in psychiatry. Berlin: Springer-Verlag, 1989: 232-6
53. Pollock BG, Perel JM, Altieri L, et al. Debrisoquine hydroxylation phenotyping in geriatric psychopharmacology. Psychopharmacol Bull 1992; 28: 163-8
54. Neilsen KK, Gram LF. Steady-state plasma levels of clomipramine and its metabolites: impact of sparteine/debrisoquine oxidation polymorphism. Eur J Pharmacol 1992; 43: 405-11
55. Balant-Gorgia AE, Balant LP, Genet C, et al. Importance of oxidative polymorphism and levomepromazine treatment on the steady-state blood concentrations of clomipramine and its major metabolites. Eur J Clin Pharmacol 1986; 31: 449-55
56. Rudorfer MV, Golden RN, Potter WZ. Second-generation antidepressants. Psychiatr Clin North Am 1984; 7: 519-34
57. Rudorfer MV. Pharmacokinetics of psychotropic drugs in special populations. J Clin Psychiatry 1993; 54 Suppl. 9: 50-4
58. Lin K-M, Smith MW. Psychopharmacotherapy in the context of culture and ethnicity. In: Ruiz P, editor. Ethnicity and psychopharmacology. Vol. 19. Washington, DC: American Psychiatric Press, Inc., 2000. In press
59. DeVane CL. Pharmacogenetics and drug metabolism of newer antidepressant agents. J Clin Psychiatry 1994; 55 Suppl. 12: 38-45
60. Coutts RT, Urichuk LJ. Polymorphic cytochromes P450 and drugs used in psychiatry. Cell Mol Neurobiol 1999; 19: 325-54
61. Skjelbo, E, Brosen K, Hallas J, et al. The mephenytoin oxidation polymorphism is partially responsible for the N-demethylation of imipramine. Clin Pharmacol Ther 1991; 49: 18-23
62. Breyer-Pfaff U, Pfandl B, Nill K, et al. Enantioselective amitriptyline metabolism in patients phenotyped for two cytochrome P450 isozymes. Clin Pharmacol Ther 1992; 52: 350-8
63. Pollock BG. Recent developments in drug metabolism of relevance to psychiatrists. Harv Rev Psychiatry 1994; 2: 204-13
64. Venkatakrishnan K, Greenblatt DJ, von Moltke LL, et al. Five distinct human cytochromes mediate amitriptyline N-demethylation in vitro: dominance of CYP 2C19 and 3A4. J Clin Pharmacol 1998; 38: 112-21
65. Mellström B, Bertilsson L, Säwe J, et al. E- and Z-10-hydroxylation of nortriptyline: relationship to polymorphic debrisoquine hydroxylation. Clin Pharmacol Ther 1981; 30: 189-93
66. Jefferson JW. Tamoxifen-associated reduction in tricyclic antidepressant levels in blood. J Clin Psychopharmacol 1995; 15: 223-4
67. Ketter TA, Flockhart DA, Post RM, et al. The emerging role of cytochrome P450 3A in psychopharmacology. J Clin Psychopharmacol 1995; 15: 387-98
68. Preskorn SH. Pharmacokinetics of antidepressants: why and how they are relevant to treatment. J Clin Psychiatry 1993; 54 Suppl. 9: 14-34
69. Sjöqvist F. Pharmacogenetics of antidepressants. In: Dahl SG, Gram LF, editors. Clinical pharmacology in psychiatry. Berlin: Springer-Verlag, 1989: 181-91
70. Bertilsson L, Åberg-Wistedt A, Gustafsson LL, et al. Extremely rapid hydroxylation of debrisoquine: a case report with implication for treatment with nortriptyline and other tricyclic antidepressants. Ther Drug Monit 1985; 7: 478-80
71. Bertilsson L, Dahl M-L, Sjöqvist F, et al. Molecular basis for rational megaprescribing in ultrarapid hydroxylators of debrisoquine [letter]. Lancet 1993; 341: 63
72. Johansson I, Lundqvist E, Bertilsson L, et al. Inherited amplification of an active gene in the cytochrome P450 CYP2D locus as a cause of ultrarapid metabolism of debrisoquine. Proc Natl Acad Sci USA 1993; 90: 11825-9
73. Bertilsson L, Dahl M-L. Polymorphic drug oxidation: relevance to the treatment of psychiatric disorders. CNS Drugs 1996; 5: 200-23
74. Foglia JP, Pollock BG, Kirshner M, et al. Plasma levels of citalopram enantiomers and metabolites in elderly patients. Psychopharmacol Bull 1997; 33: 109-12
75. Dawkins K, Potter WZ. Gender differences in pharmacokinetics and pharmacodynamics of psychotropics: focus on women. Psychopharmacol Bull 1991; 27: 417-26
76. Gex-Fabry M, Balant-Gorgia AE, Balant LP, et al. Clomipramine metabolism: model-based analysis of variability factors from drug monitoring data. Clin Pharmacokinet 1990; 19: 241-55
77. Nordin C. CSF/plasma ratio of 10-hydroxynortriptyline is influenced by sex and body height. Psychopharmacology 1993; 113: 222-4
78. Ben Musa A, Smith CS. Neonatal effects of maternal clomipramine therapy [abstract]. Arch Dis Child 1979; 54: 405
79. Schimmell MS, Katz EZ, Shaag Y, et al. Toxic neonatal effects following maternal clomipramine therapy. Clin Toxicol 1991; 29: 479-84
80. Rudorfer MV. Challenges in medication clinical trials. Psychopharmacol Bull 1993; 29: 35-44
81. Vitiello B, Jensen PS. Developmental perspectives in pediatric psychopharmacology. Psychopharmacol Bull 1995; 31: 75-81
82. Young RC. Hydroxylated metabolites of antidepressants. Psychopharmacol Bull 1991; 27: 521-32
83. Wisner KL, Perel JM, Foglia JP. Serum clomipramine and metabolite levels in four nursing mother-infant pairs. J Clin Psychiatry 1995; 56: 17-20
84. Wisner KL, Perel JM. Serum nortriptyline levels in nursing mothers and their infants. Am J Psychiatry 1991; 148: 1234-6
85. Wisner KL, Perel JM, Findling RL, Hinnes RL. Nortriptyline and its hydroxymetabolites in breastfeeding mothers and newborns. Psychopharmacol Bull 1997; 33: 249-51
86. Bader TF, Newman K. Amitriptyline in human breast milk and the nursing infant's serum. Am J Psychiatry 1980; 137: 855-6
87. Brixen-Rasmussen L, Halgrener J, Jorgensen A. Amitriptyline and nortriptyline excretion in human breast milk. Psychopharmacology 1982; 76: 94-5
88. Breyer-Pfaff U, Nill K, Entenmann A, et al. Secretion of amitriptyline and metabolites into breast milk [letter]. Am J Psychiatry 1995; 152: 812-3
89. Matheson J, Pande H, Alersten AR. Respiratory depression caused by N-desmethyldoxepin in breast milk [letter]. Lancet 1985; 2: 1124

90. Kemp J, Ilett KF, Booth J. Excretion of doxepin and N-desmethyldoxepin in human milk. Br J Clin Pharmacol 1985; 20: 479-84
91. Buist A, Janson H. Effect of exposure to dothiepin and northiaden in breast milk on child development. Br J Psychiatry 1995; 167: 370-3
92. Frey OR, Scheidt P, von Brenndorff AI. Adverse effects in a newborn infant breast-fed by a mother treated with doxepin. Ann Pharmacother 1999; 33: 690-3
93. Yoshida K, Smith B, Kumar R. Psychotropic drugs in mothers' milk: a comprehensive review of assay methods, pharmacokinetics and of safety of breast-feeding. J Psychopharmacol 1999; 13: 64-80
94. Birnbaum CS, Cohen LS, Bailey JW, et al. Serum concentrations of antidepressants and benzodiazepines in nursing infants: a case series. Pediatrics 1999; 104: e11
95. Shoaf SE, Linnoila M. Interaction of ethanol and smoking on the pharmacokinetics and pharmacodynamics of psychotropic medications. Psychopharmacol Bull 1991; 27: 577-94
96. Fleischmann R, Remmer H, Starz U. Induction of cytochrome P-448 iso-enzymes and related glucuronyltransferases in the human liver by cigarette smoking. Eur J Clin Pharmacol 1986; 30: 475-80
97. Mellström B, Säwe J, Bertilsson L, et al. Amitriptyline metabolism: association with debrisoquine hydroxylation in nonsmokers. Clin Pharmacol Ther 1986; 39: 369-71
98. Perry PJ, Browne JL, Prince RA, et al. Effects of smoking on nortriptyline plasma concentrations in depressed patients. Ther Drug Monit 1986; 8: 279-84
99. Spina E, Perucca E. Newer and older antidepressants: a comparative review of drug interactions. CNS Drugs 1994; 2: 479-97
100. Bergstrom RF, Peyton AL, Lemberger L. Quantification and mechanism of the fluoxetine and tricyclic antidepressant interaction. Clin Pharmacol Ther 1992; 51: 239-48
101. Leucht S, Hackl HJ, Steimer W, et al. Effect of adjunctive paroxetine on serum levels and side-effects of tricyclic antidepressants in depressive inpatients. Psychopharmacology 2000; 147: 378-83
102. von Bahr C, Steiner E, Koike Y, et al. Time course of enzyme induction in humans: effect of pentobarbital on nortriptyline metabolism. Clin Pharmacol Ther 1998; 64: 18-26
103. Venkatakrishnan K, von Moltke LL, Greenblatt DJ. Nortriptyline E-10-hydroxylation in vitro is mediated by human CYP2D6 (high affinity) and CYP3A4 (low affinity): implications for interactions with enzyme-inducing drugs. J Clin Pharmacol 1999; 39: 567-77
104. Geller B, Cooper TB, Graham DL, et al. Pharmacokinetically designed, double-blind, placebo-controlled study of nortriptyline in 6-to-12-year olds with major depressive disorder. J Am Acad Child Adolesc Psychiatry 1992; 31: 34-44
105. Hazell P, O'Connell D, Heathcote D. Efficacy of tricyclic drugs in treating child and adolescent depression: a meta-analysis. BMJ 1995; 310: 897-901
106. Geller B. Psychopharmacology of children and adolescents: pharmacokinetics and relationships of plasma/serum levels to response. Psychopharmacol Bull 1991; 27: 401-9
107. Preskorn SH, Bupp SJ, Weller EB, et al. Plasma levels of imipramine and metabolites in 68 hospitalized children. J Am Acad Child Adolesc Psychiatry 1989; 28: 373-5
108. Donnelly M, Zametkin AJ, Rapoport JL, et al. Treatment of childhood hyperactivity with desipramine: plasma drug concentration, cardiovascular effects, plasma and urinary catecholamine levels, and clinical response. Clin Pharmacol Ther 1986; 39: 72-81
109. Hyman SE, Rudorfer MV. Mood and anxiety disorders. In: Scientific American Medicine. New York: Scientific American, 2000. In press
110. Lane EA. Renal function and the disposition of antidepressants and their metabolites. Psychopharmacol Bull 1991; 27: 533-40
111. Kitanaka I, Ross RJ, Cutler NR, et al. Altered hydroxydesipramine concentrations in elderly depressed patients. Clin Pharmacol Ther 1982; 31: 51-5
112. Nelson JC, Atillasoy E, Mazure C, et al. Hydroxydesipramine in the elderly. J Clin Psychopharmacol 1988; 8: 428-33
113. Young RC, Alexopoulos GS, Dhar AK, et al. 10-hydroxynortriptyline and renal function in elderly depressives. Biol Psychiatry 1987; 22: 1283-7
114. Schneider LS, Cooper TB, Suckow RE, et al. Relationship of hydroxynortriptyline to nortriptyline concentration and creatinine clearance in depressed elderly outpatients. J Clin Psychopharmacol 1990; 10: 333-7
115. Ng Ying Kin NMK, Klitgaard N, Nair NPV, et al. Clinical relevance of serum nortriptyline and 10-hydroxy-nortriptyline measurements in the depressed elderly: a multicenter pharmacokinetic and pharmacodynamic study. Neuropsychopharmacology 1996; 15: 1-6
116. Dawling S, Lynn K, Rosser R, et al. Nortriptyline metabolism in chronic renal failure: metabolite elimination. Clin Pharmacol Ther 1982; 32: 322-9
117. Lieberman JA, Cooper TB, Suckow RF, et al. Tricyclic antidepressant and metabolite levels in chronic renal failure. Clin Pharmacol Ther 1985; 37: 301-7
118. Potter WZ, Lane EA, Rudorfer MV. Hydroxy metabolite concentrations: role of renal clearance. In: Gram LF, Usdin E, Dahl SG, et al., editors. Clinical pharmacology in psychiatry: bridging the experimental-therapeutic gap. London: Macmillan Press, 1983: 203-16
119. Potter WZ, Calil HM, Manian A, et al. Hydroxylated metabolites of tricyclic antidepressants. Biol Psychiatry 1979; 14: 601-13
120. Javaid JI, Perel JM, Davis JM. Inhibition of biogenic amine uptake by imipramine, desipramine, 2 OH-imipramine and 2 OH-desipramine in rat brain. Life Sci 1979; 24: 21-8
121. Potter WZ, Rudorfer MV, Lane EA. Active metabolites of antidepressants: pharmacodynamics and relevant pharmacokinetics. In: Usdin E, Bertilsson L, Sjöqvist F, editors. Frontiers in biochemical and pharmacological research in depression. New York: Raven Press, 1984: 373-90
122. Núñez R, Perel JM. Comparative neurotransmitter reuptake and anticholinergic potencies of the 8-hydroxy metabolites of clomipramine. Psychopharmacol Bull 1995; 31: 217-21
123. Potter WZ, Calil HM. Metabolites of tricyclic antidepressants: biological activity and clinical implications. In: Usdin E, editor. Clinical pharmacology in psychiatry. New York: Elsevier North Holland Inc., 1981: 311-24
124. Potter WZ, Rudorfer MV, Linnoila M. New clinical studies support a role of norepinephrine in antidepressant action. In: Barchas JD, Bunney Jr WE, editors. Perspectives in psychopharmacology: a collection of papers in honor of Earl Usdin. New York: Alan R. Liss Inc., 1988: 495-513
125. Nordin C, Bertilsson L, Siwers B. Clinical and biochemical effects during treatment with nortriptyline: the role of 10-hydroxynortriptyline. Clin Pharmacol Ther 1987; 42: 10-9
126. Malmgren R, Åberg-Wistedt A, Bertilsson L. Serotonin uptake inhibition during treatment of depression with nortriptyline caused by parent drug and not by 10-hydroxymetabolites. Psychopharmacology 1987; 92: 169-72
127. Snyder SH, Yamamura HI. Antidepressants and the muscarinic acetylcholine receptor. Arch Gen Psychiatry 1977; 34: 236-9
128. Richelson E, Nelson AL. Antagonism by antidepressants of neurotransmitter receptors of normal human brain in vitro. J Pharmacol Toxicol Methods 1984; 230: 94-102
129. Wagner A, Ekqvist B, Bertilsson L, et al. Weak binding of 10-hydroxymetabolites of nortriptyline to rat brain muscarinic acetylcholine receptors. Life Sci 1984; 35: 1379-83
130. Nilvebrant L, Nordin C. Affinity of nortriptyline and its E-10-hydroxy metabolite for muscarinic receptors. Pharmacol Toxicol 1991; 68: 64-7

131. El-Fakahany E, Richelson E. Antagonism by antidepressants of muscarinic acetylcholine receptors of human brain. Br J Pharmacol 1983; 78: 97-102
132. Jandhyala BS, Steenberg ML, Perel JM, et al. Effects of several tricyclic antidepressants on the hemodynamics and myocardial contractility of anesthetized dogs. Eur J Pharmacol 1977; 42: 403-10
133. Wilkerson RD. Antiarrhythmic effects of tricyclic antidepressant drugs in ouabain-induced arrhythmias in the dog. J Pharmacol Exp Ther 1978; 206: 666-74
134. Pollock BG, Everett G, Perel JM. Comparative cardiotoxicity of nortriptyline and its isomeric 10-hydroxymetabolites. Neuropsychopharmacology 1992; 6: 1-10
135. Nierenberg AA, Cole JO. Antidepressant adverse drug reactions. J Clin Psychiatry 1991; 52 Suppl. 6: 40-7
136. Rudorfer MV, Young RC. Anticholinergic effects and plasma desipramine levels. Clin Pharmacol Ther 1980; 28: 703-6
137. Lancaster SG, Gonzalez JR. Lofepramine: a review of its pharmacodynamic and pharmacokinetic properties, and therapeutic efficacy in depressive illness. Drugs 1989; 37: 123-40
138. Glassman AH, Roose SP, Bigger Jr JT. The safety of tricyclic antidepressants in cardiac patients: risk-benefit reconsidered. JAMA 1993; 269: 2673-5
139. Rudorfer MV, Young RC. Desipramine: cardiovascular effects and plasma levels. Am J Psychiatry 1980; 137: 984-6
140. Preskorn SH, Fast GA. Therapeutic drug monitoring for antidepressants: efficacy, safety, and cost effectiveness. J Clin Psychiatry 1991; 52 Suppl. 6: 23-33
141. Bluhm RE, Wilkinson GR, Shelton R, et al. Genetically determined drug-metabolizing activity and desipramine-associated cardiotoxicity: a case report. Clin Pharmacol Ther 1993; 53: 89-95
142. Amitai Y, Erickson T, Kennedy EJ, et al. Tricyclic antidepressants in red cells and plasma: correlation with impaired intraventricular conduction in acute overdose. Clin Pharmacol Ther 1993; 54: 219-27
143. Biederman J, Baldessarini RJ, Goldblatt A, et al. A naturalistic study of 24-hour electrocardiographic recording and echocardiographic findings in children and adolescents treated with desipramine. J Am Acad Child Adolesc Psychiatry 1993; 32: 805-13
144. Wilens TE, Biederman J, Baldessarini RJ, et al. Electrocardiographic effects of desipramine and 2-hydroxydesipramine in children, adolescents, and adults treated with desipramine. J Am Acad Child Adolesc Psychiatry 1993; 32: 798-804
145. Nelson JC, Jatlow PI, Bock J. Major adverse reactions during desipramine treatment: relationship to drug plasma concentrations, concomitant antipsychotic treatment and patient characteristics. Arch Gen Psychiatry 1982; 39: 1055-61
146. Cutler NR, Zavadil A, Linnoila M, et al. Effects of chronic desipramine on plasma norepinephrine concentrations and cardiovascular parameters in elderly depressed women: a preliminary report. Biol Psychiatry 1984; 19: 549-56
147. Kutcher SP, Reid K, Dubbin JD, et al. Electrocardiogram changes and therapeutic desipramine and 2-hydroxy-desipramine concentrations in elderly depressives. Br J Psychiatry 1986; 148: 676-9
148. Young RC, Alexopoulos GS, Shamoian CA, et al. Heart failure associated with high plasma 10-hydroxynortriptyline levels. Am J Psychiatry 1984; 141: 432-3
149. Young RC, Alexopoulos GS, Kent E, et al. Plasma 10-hydroxynortriptyline and ECG changes in elderly depressed patients. Am J Psychiatry 1985; 142: 866-8
150. Schneider LS, Cooper TB, Severson JA, et al. Electrocardiographic changes with nortriptyline and 10-hydroxynortriptyline in elderly depressed outpatients. J Clin Psychopharmacol 1988; 8: 402-8
151. McCue RE, Georgotas A, Nagachandran N, et al. Plasma levels of nortriptyline and 10-hydroxynortriptyline and treatment-related electrocardiographic changes in the elderly depressed. J Psychiatr Res 1989; 23: 73-9
152. Calvo B, Garcia MJ, Pedraz JL, et al. Pharmacokinetics of amoxapine and its active metabolites. Int J Clin Pharmacol Ther Toxicol 1985; 23: 180-5
153. Midha KK, Hubbard JW, McKay G, et al. The role of metabolites in a bioequivalence study II: amoxapine, 7-hydroxyamoxapine, and 8-hydroxyamoxapine. Int J Clin Pharmacol Ther 1999; 37: 28-38
154. Anton Jr RF, Burch Jr EA. Amoxapine versus amitriptyline combined with perphenazine in the treatment of psychotic depression. Am J Psychiatry 1990; 147: 1203-8
155. Gelenberg AJ, Cooper DS, Doller JC, et al. Galactorrhea and hyperprolactinemia associated with amoxapine therapy: report of a case. JAMA 1979; 242: 1900-1
156. Lydiard RB, Gelenberg AJ. Amoxapine: an antidepressant with some neuroleptic properties? Pharmacotherapy 1981; 1: 163-78
157. Huang CC. Persistent tardive dyskinesia associated with amoxapine therapy. Am J Psychiatry 1986; 143: 1069-70
158. Taylor NE, Schwartz HI. Neuroleptic malignant syndrome following amoxapine overdose. J Nerv Ment Dis 1988; 176: 249-51
159. Litovitz TL, Troutman WG. Amoxapine overdose. JAMA 1983; 250: 1069-71
160. Cassidy SL, Henry JA. Fatal toxicity of antidepressant drugs in overdose. BMJ 1987; 295: 1021-4
161. Dessain EC, Schatzberg AF, Woods BT, et al. Maprotiline treatment in depression: a perspective on seizures. Arch Gen Psychiatry 1986; 43: 86-90
162. Nelson JC, Mazure C, Jatlow PI. Antidepressant activity of 2-hydroxydesipramine. Clin Pharmacol Ther 1988; 88: 283-8
163. Robinson DS, Cooper TB, Howard D, et al. Amitriptyline and hydroxylated metabolite plasma levels in depressed outpatients. J Clin Psychopharmacol 1985; 5: 83-8
164. Åsberg M, Cronholm B, Sjöqvist F, et al. Relationship between plasma levels and therapeutic effect of nortriptyline. BMJ 1971; 3: 331-4
165. Nordin C, Siwers B, Benitez J, et al. Plasma concentrations of nortriptyline and its 10-hydroxy metabolite in depressed patients: relationship to the debrisoquine hydroxylation metabolic ratio. Br J Clin Pharmacol 1985; 19: 832-5
166. Young RC, Alexopoulos GS, Shindledecker R, et al. Plasma 10-hydroxynortriptyline and therapeutic response in geriatric depression. Neuropsychopharmacology 1988; 1: 213-5
167. Potter WZ, Scheinin M, Golden RN, et al. Selective antidepressants and cerebrospinal fluid: lack of specificity on norepinephrine and serotonin metabolites. Arch Gen Psychiatry 1985; 42: 1171-7
168. Nelson JC, Bock JL, Jatlow P. Clinical implications of 2-hydroxydesipramine plasma concentrations. Clin Pharmacol Ther 1983; 33: 183-9
169. Kutcher SP, Shulman KI, Reed K. Desipramine plasma concentration and therapeutic response in elderly depressives: a naturalistic pilot study. Can J Psychiatry 1986; 31: 752-4
170. Amsterdam JD, Brunswick DJ, Potter WZ, et al. Desipramine and 2-hydroxydesipramine plasma levels in endogenous depressed patients: lack of correlation with therapeutic response. Arch Gen Psychiatry 1985; 42: 361-4
171. Bock JL, Nelson JC, Gray S, et al. Desipramine hydroxylation: variability and effect of antipsychotic drugs. Clin Pharmacol Ther 1983; 33: 322-8
172. Leonard BE. The comparative pharmacology of new antidepressants. J Clin Psychiatry 1993; 54: 3-15
173. Hiemke C, Hartter S. Pharmacokinetics of selective serotonin reuptake inhibitors. Pharmacol Ther 2000; 85: 11-28

174. Milne RJ, Goa KL. Citalopram: a review of its pharmacodynamic and pharmacokinetic properties, and therapeutic potential in depressive illness. Drugs 1991; 41: 450-77
175. Palmer KJ, Benfield P. Fluvoxamine: an overview of its pharmacological properties and review of its therapeutic potential in non-depressive disorders. CNS Drugs 1994; 1: 57-87
176. DeVane CL. Metabolism and pharmacokinetics of selective serotonin reuptake inhibitors. Cell Mol Neurobiol 1999; 19: 443-66
177. Owens MJ, Knight DL. The next generation SSRIs: a comparison of the transporter binding profile of R-fluoxetine and S-citalopram (LU 26-054) [abstract]. Presented at the 40th Annual New Clinical Drug Evaluation Unit (NCDEU) meeting; abstract no. 14; 2000 May 30-Jun 2; Boca Raton, FL, USA
178. Goodnick PJ. Pharmacokinetics of second generation antidepressants: fluoxetine. Psychopharmacol Bull 1991; 27: 503-12
179. Blier P, Bergeron R, Pineyro G, et al. Understanding the mechanism of action of serotonin reuptake inhibitors in obsessive-compulsive disorder: a step toward more effective treatments? In: Goodman WK, Rudorfer MV, Maser JD, editors. Obsessive-compulsive disorder: contemporary issues in treatment. Mahwah, New Jersey, USA: Lawrence Erlbaum Associates, 2000: 551-71
180. Pato MT, Murphy DL, DeVane CL. Sustained plasma concentrations of fluoxetine and/or norfluoxetine four and eight weeks after fluoxetine discontinuation. J Clin Psychopharmacol 1991; 11: 224-5
181. Caccia S. Metabolism of the newer antidepressants. An overview of the pharmacological and pharmacokinetic implications. Clin Pharmacokinet 1998; 34: 281-302
182. Coplan JD, Gorman JM. Detectable levels of fluoxetine metabolites after discontinuation: an unexpected serotonin syndrome [letter]. Am J Psychiatry 1993; 150: 837
183. Alfaro CL, Lam YWF, Simpson J, et al. CYP2D6 status of extensive metabolizers after multiple-dose fluoxetine, fluvoxamine, paroxetine, or sertraline. J Clin Psychopharmacol 1999; 19: 155-63
184. Daniel WA, Syrek M, Haduch A, et al. The influence of selective serotonin reuptake inhibitors (SSRIs) on the pharmacokinetics of thioridazine and its metabolites: in vivo and in vitro studies. Exp Toxicol Pathol 1999; 51: 309-14
185. Feireraband R. Benign course in a child with a massive fluoxetine overdose. J Fam Pract 1995; 41: 289-91
186. Bergstrom RF, Lemberger L, Faird NA, et al. Clinical pharmacology and pharmacokinetics of fluoxetine: a review. Br J Psychiatry 1988; 153 Suppl. 3: 47-50
187. Preskorn SH. Clinical pharmacology of selective serotonin reuptake inhibitors. Caddo, OK, USA: Professional Communications, Inc., 1996
188. Wong DT, Bymaster FP, Reid LR, et al. Norfluoxetine enantiomers as inhibitors of serotonin uptake in rat brain. Neuropsychopharmacology 1993; 8: 337-44
189. Torok-Both GA, Baker GB, Coutts RT, et al. Simultaneous determination of fluoxetine and norfluoxetine enantiomers in biological samples by gas chromatography with electron-capture detection. J Chromatography 1992; 579: 99-106
190. Frank MG, Hendricks SE, Johnson DR, et al. Antidepressants augment natural killer cell activity: in vivo and in vitro. Neuropsychobiology 1999; 39: 18-24
191. Burke WJ, Hendricks SE, McArthur-Campbell D, et al. Fluoxetine and norfluoxetine serum concentrations and clinical response in weekly versus daily dosing. Psychopharmacol Bull 1996; 32: 27-32
192. Amsterdam JD, Fawcett J, Quitkin FM, et al. Fluoxetine and norfluoxetine plasma concentrations in major depression: a multicenter study. Am J Psychiatry 1997; 154: 963-9
193. Brunswick DJ, Amsterdam JD, Fawcett J, et al. Fluoxetine and norfluoxetine plasma concentrations during relapse-prevention treatment [abstract]. Presented at the 40th Annual New Clinical Drug Evaluation Unit (NCDEU) meeting; abstract no. 24; 2000 May 30-Jun 2; Boca Raton, FL, USA
194. DeVane CL, Pollock BG. Pharmacokinetic considerations of antidepressant use in the elderly. J Clin Psychiatry 1999; 60 Suppl. 20: 38-44
195. Cohen L, Wilens T, Biederman J, et al. Pharmacokinetics of fluoxetine in pediatric patients [abstract]. Clin Pharmacol Ther 2000; 67: 129
196. Schenker S, Bergstrom RE, Wolen RL, et al. Fluoxetine disposition and elimination in cirrhosis. Clin Pharmacol Ther 1988; 44: 353-9
197. Aronoff GR, Bergstrom RF, Pottratz ST, et al. Fluoxetine kinetics and protein binding in normal and impaired renal function. Clin Pharmacol Ther 1984; 36: 138-44
198. Blumenfield M, Levy NB, Spinowitz B, et al. Fluoxetine in depressed patients on dialysis. Int J Psychiatry Med 1997; 27: 71-80
199. Taddio A, Ito S, Koren G. Excretion of fluoxetine and its metabolite, norfluoxetine, in human breast milk. J Clin Pharmacol 1996; 36: 42-7
200. Yoshida K, Smith B, Craggs M, et al. Fluoxetine in breast-milk and developmental outcome of breast-fed infants. Br J Psychiatry 1998; 172: 175-8
201. Renshaw PF, Guimaraes AR, Fava M, et al. Accumulation of fluoxetine and norfluoxetine in human brain during therapeutic administration. Am J Psychiatry 1992; 149: 1592-4
202. Miner CM, Davidson JRT, Potts NLS, et al. Brain fluoxetine measurements using fluorine magnetic resonance spectroscopy in patients with social phobia. Biol Psychiatry 1995; 38: 696-8
203. Xu ZH, Wang W, Zhao XJ, et al. Evidence for involvement of polymorphic CYP2C19 and 2C9 in the N-demethylation of sertraline in human liver microsomes. Br J Clin Pharmacol 1999; 48: 416-23
204. Greenblatt DJ, von Moltke LL, Harmatz JS, et al. Human cytochromes mediating sertraline biotransformation: seeking attribution. J Clin Psychopharmacol 1999; 19: 489-92
205. Sprouse J, Clarke T, Reynolds L, et al. Comparison of the effects of sertraline and its metabolite desmethylsertraline on blockade of central 5-HT reuptake in vivo. Neuropsychopharmacology 1996; 14: 225-31
206. Alderman J, Preskorn SH, Greenblatt DJ, et al. Desipramine pharmacokinetics when coadministered with paroxetine or sertraline in extensive metabolizers. J Clin Psychopharmacol 1997; 17: 284-91
207. Stowe ZN, Owens MJ, Landry JC, et al. Sertraline and desmethylsertraline in human breast milk and nursing infants. Am J Psychiatry 1997; 154: 1255-60
208. Mammen OK, Perel JM, Rudolph G, et al. Sertraline and norsertraline levels in three breastfed infants. J Clin Psychiatry 1997; 58: 100-3
209. Wisner KL, Perel JM, Blumer J. Serum sertraline and N-desmethylsertraline levels in breast-feeding mother-infant pairs. Am J Psychiatry 1998; 155: 690-2
210. Wikell C, Apelqvist G, Carlsson B, et al. Pharmacokinetic and pharmacodynamic responses to chronic administration of the selective serotonin reuptake inhibitor citalopram in rats. Clin Neuropharmacol 1999; 22: 327-36
211. Von Moltke LL, Greenblatt DJ, Grassi JM, et al. Citalopram and desmethylcitalopram in vitro: human cytochromes mediating transformation, and cytochrome inhibitory effects. Biol Psychiatry 1999; 46: 839-49
212. Dalgaard L, Larsen C. Metabolism and excretion of citalopram in man: identification of O-acyl- and N-glucuronides. Xenobiotica 1999; 29: 1033-41

213. Joffe P, Larsen FL, Pedersen V, et al. Single-dose pharmacokinetics of citalopram in patients with moderate renal insufficiency or hepatic cirrhosis compared with healthy subjects. Eur J Clin Pharmacol 1998; 54: 237-42
214. Jensen PN, Olesen OV, Bertelsen A, et al. Citalopram and desmethylcitalopram concentrations in breast milk and in serum of mother and infant. Ther Drug Monit 1997; 91: 236-9
215. Spigset O, Carieborg L, Ohman R, et al. Excretion of citalopram in breast milk. Br J Clin Pharmacol 1997; 44: 295-8
216. Schmidt K, Olesen OV, Jensen PN. Citalopram and breast feeding: serum concentration and side effects in the infant. Biol Psychiatry 2000; 47: 164-5
217. Rochat B, Kosel M, Boss G, et al. Stereoselective biotransformation of the selective serotonin reuptake inhibitor citalopram and its demethylated metabolites by monoamine oxidases in human liver. Biochem Pharmacol 1998; 56: 15-23
218. Bloomer JC, Woods FR, Haddock RE, et al. The role of cytochrome P4502D6 in the metabolism of paroxetine by human liver microsomes. Br J Clin Pharmacol 1992; 33: 521-3
219. Sindrup SH, Brosen K, Gram LF. Pharmacokinetics of the selective serotonin reuptake inhibitor paroxetine: nonlinearity and relation to the sparteine oxidation polymorphism. Clin Pharmacol Ther 1992; 51: 288-95
220. Gunasekara NS, Noble S, Benfield P. Paroxetine: an update of its pharmacology and therapeutic use in depression and a review of its use in other disorders. Drugs 1998; 55: 85-120
221. Hemeryck A, Lefebvre, RA, Eng CD, et al. Paroxetine affects metoprolol pharmacokinetics and pharmacodynamics in healthy volunteers. Pharmacol Ther 2000; 67: 283-91
222. Dechant KL, Clissold SP. Paroxetine: a review of its pharmacodynamic and pharmacokinetic properties, and therapeutic potential in depressive illness. Drugs 1991; 41: 225-53
223. Begg EJ, Duffull SB, Saunders DA, et al. Paroxetine in human milk. Br J Clin Pharmacol 1999; 48: 142-7
224. Ohman R, Hagg S, Carleborg L, et al. Excretion of paroxetine into breast milk. J Clin Psychiatry 1999; 60: 519-23
225. Stowe ZN, Cohen LS, Hostetter A, et al. Paroxetine in human breast milk and nursing infants. Am J Psychiatry 2000; 157: 185-9
226. Perucca E, Gatti G, Spina E. Clinical pharmacokinetics of fluvoxamine. Clin Pharmacokinet 1994; 27: 175-90
227. Spigset O, Carleborg L, Hedenmalm K, et al. Effect of cigarette smoking on fluvoxamine pharmacokinetics in humans. Clin Pharmacol Ther 1995; 58: 399-403
228. Carrillo JA, Ramos SI, Herraiz AG, et al. Pharmacokinetic interaction of fluvoxamine and thioridazine in schizophrenic patients. J Clin Psychopharmacol 1999; 19: 494-9
229. Kelly MW, Perry PJ, Holstad SG, et al. Serum fluoxetine and norfluoxetine concentrations and antidepressant response. Ther Drug Monit 1989; 11: 165-70
230. Kelsey JE, Nemeroff CB. Fluoxetine. In: Sadock BJ, Sadock VA, editors. Comprehensive textbook of psychiatry. 7th ed. Philadelphia: Lippincott Williams & Wilkins, 2000: 2438-44
231. Keck Jr PE, McElroy SL. Ratio of plasma fluoxetine to norfluoxetine concentrations and associated sedation. J Clin Psychiatry 1992; 53: 127-9
232. Spencer MJ. Fluoxetine (FLX) neonatal toxicity. Pediatrics 1993; 92: 721-2
233. Kent LSW, Laidlaw JDD. Suspected congenital sertraline dependence. Br J Psychiatry 1995; 167: 412-3
234. Von Moltke LL, Greenblatt DJ, Court MH, et al. Inhibition of alprazolam and desipramine hydroxylation in vitro by paroxetine and fluvoxamine: comparison with other selective serotonin reuptake inhibitor antidepressants. J Clin Psychopharmacol 1995; 15: 125-31
235. Hartter S, Wetzel H, Hammes E, et al. Inhibition of antidepressant demethylation and hydroxylation by fluvoxamine in depressed patients. Psychopharmacology 1993; 110: 301-8
236. Sindrup SH, Brosen K, Gram LF, et al. The relationship between paroxetine and the sparteine oxidation polymorphism. Clin Pharmacol Ther 1992; 51: 278-87
237. Fleishaker JC, Hulst LK. A pharmacokinetic and pharmacodynamic evaluation of the combined administration of alprazolam and fluvoxamine. Eur J Clin Pharmacol 1994; 46: 35-9
238. Holliday SM, Benfield P. Venlafaxine: a review of its pharmacology and therapeutic potential in depression. Drugs 1995; 49: 280-94
239. Muth EA, Moyer JA, Haskins JT, et al. Biochemical, neurophysiological, and behavioral effects of WY-45,233 and other identified metabolites of the antidepressant venlafaxine. Drug Dev Res 1991; 23: 191-9
240. Howell SR, Husbands GEM, Scatina JA, et al. Metabolic disposition of 14C-venlafaxine in mouse, rat, dog, rhesus monkey and man. Xenobiotica 1993; 23: 349-59
241. Amchin J, Zarycranski W, Taylor KP, et al. Effect of venlafaxine on the pharmacokinetics of risperidone. J Clin Pharmacol 1999; 39: 297-309
242. Amchin J, Zarycranski W, Taylor KP, et al. Effect of venlafaxine on the pharmacokinetics of alprazolam. Psychopharmacol Bull 1998; 34: 211-9
243. Amchin J, Zarycranski W, Taylor KP, et al. Effect of venlafaxine on CYP1A2-dependent pharmacokinetics and metabolism of caffeine. J Clin Pharmacol 1999; 39: k252-9
244. Klamerus KJ, Maloney K, Rudolph R, et al. Introduction of a composite parameter to the pharmacokinetics of venlafaxine and its active O-desmethyl metabolite. J Clin Pharmacol 1992; 32: 716-24
245. Troy SM, Schultz RW, Parker VD, et al. The effect of renal disease on the disposition of venlafaxine. Clin Pharmacol Ther 1994; 56: 14-21
246. Ilett KF, Hackett LP, Dusci LJ, et al. Distribution and excretion of venlafaxine and O-desmethylvenlafaxine in human milk. Br J Clin Pharmacol 1998; 45: 459-62
247. Golden RN, Dawkins K, Nicholas L, et al. Trazodone, nefazodone, bupropion, and mirtazapine. In: Schatzberg AF, Nemeroff CB, editors. The American Psychiatric Press textbook of psychopharmacology. 2nd ed. Washington, DC: American Psychiatric Press, 1998: 251-69
248. Caccia S, Ballabio M, Samanin R, et al. (-)-m-Chlorophenyl-piperazine, a central 5-hydroxytryptamine agonist, is a metabolite of trazodone. J Pharm Pharmacol 1981; 33: 477-8
249. Otani K, Mihara K, Yasui N, et al. Plasma concentrations of trazodone and m-chlorophenylpiperazine at steady state can be predicted from those after an initial dose of trazodone. Prog Neuropsychopharmacol Biol Psychiatry 1997; 21: 239-44
250. Mueller EA, Murphy DL, Sunderland T. Further studies of the putative serotonin agonist, m-chlorophenylpiperazine: evidence for a serotonin receptor mediated mechanism of action in humans. Psychopharmacology 1986; 89: 388-91
251. Seibyl JP, Krystal JH, Price LH, et al. Effects of ritanserin on the behavioral, neuroendocrine, and cardiovascular responses to meta chlorophenylpiperazine in healthy human subjects. Psychiatry Res 1991; 38: 227-36
252. Maes M, Estenberg H, Vandoolaeghe E, et al. Effects of trazodone and fluoxetine in the treatment of major depression: therapeutic pharmacokinetic and pharmacodynamic interactions through formation of meta-chlorophenylpiperazine. J Clin Psychopharmacol 1997; 17: 358-64

253. Kahn RS, Wetzler S. m-Chlorophenylpiperazine as a probe of serotonin function. Biol Psychiatry 1991; 30: 1139-66
254. Charney DS, Woods SW, Goodman WK, et al. Serotonin function in anxiety. Psychopharmacology 1987; 92: 14-24
255. Murphy DL, Mueller EA, Hill JL, et al. Comparative anxiogenic, neuroendocrine, and other physiologic effects of m-chlorophenylpiperazine given intravenously or orally to healthy volunteers. Psychopharmacology 1989; 98: 275-82
256. Kalus O, Wetzler S, Kahn RS, et al. A dose-response study of intravenous m-chlorophenylpiperazine in normal subjects. Psychopharmacology 1992; 106: 388-90
257. Stein DJ, Hollander E, Cohen L, et al. Serotonergic responsivity in trichotillomania: neuroendrocrine effects of m-chlorophenylpiperazine. Biol Psychiatry 1995; 37: 414-6
258. Krystal JH, Seibyl JP, Price LH, et al. m-Chlorophenylpiperazine effects in neuroleptic-free schizophrenic patients: evidence implicating serotonergic systems in the positive symptoms of schizophrenia. Arch Gen Psychiatry 1993; 50: 624-35
259. Krystal JH, Webb E, Cooney NL, et al. Serotonergic and noradrenergic dysregulation in alcoholism: m-chlorophenylpiperazine and yohimbine effects in recently detoxified alcoholics and healthy comparison subjects. Am J Psychiatry 1996; 153: 83-92
260. Anand A, Charney DS, Delgado PL, et al. Neuroendocrine and behavioral responses to intravenous m-chlorophenylpiperazine (mCPP) in depressed patients and healthy comparison subjects. Am J Psychiatry 1994; 151: 1626-30
261. Zohar J, Insel TR, Zohar-Kadouch RC, et al. Serotonergic responsivity in obsessive-compulsive disorder: effects of chronic clomipramine treatment. Arch Gen Psychiatry 1988; 45: 167-72
262. Hollander E, DeCaria C, Gully R, et al. Effects of chronic fluoxetine treatment on behavioral and neuroendocrine responses to meta-chloro-phenylpiperazine in obsessive-compulsive disorder. Psychiatry Res 1991; 36: 1-17
263. Pigott TA, Hill JL, Grady TA, et al. A comparison of the behavioral effects of oral versus intravenous mCPP administration in OCD patients and the effects of metergoline prior to IV mCPP. Biol Psychiatry 1993; 33: 3-14
264. Hollander E, Wong CM. Spectrum, boundary, and subtyping issues: implications for treatment-refractory obsessive-compulsive disorder. In: Goodman WK, Rudorfer MV, Maser JD, editors. Obsessive-compulsive disorder: contemporary issues in treatment. Mahwah, New Jersey, USA: Lawrence Erlbaum Associates, 2000: 3-22
265. Barbhaiya RH, Shukla UA, Natarajan CS, et al. Single- and multiple-dose pharmacokinetics of nefazodone in patients with hepatic cirrhosis. Clin Pharmacol Ther 1995; 58: 390-8
266. Kroboth PD, Folan MM, Lush RM, et al. Coadministration of nefazodone and benzodiazepines. I. Pharmacodynamic assessment. J Clin Psychopharmacol 1995; 15: 306-19
267. Barbhaiya RH, Shukla UA, Kroboth PD, et al. Coadministration of nefazodone and benzodiazepines. II. A pharmacokinetic interaction study with triazolam. J Clin Psychopharmacol 1995; 15: 320-6
268. Greene DS, Salazar DE, Dockens RC, et al. Coadministration of nefazodone and benzodiazepines. III. A pharmacokinetic interaction study of alprazolam. J Clin Psychopharmacol 1995; 15: 399-408
269. Greene DS, Salazar DE, Dockens RC, et al. Coadministration of nefazodone and benzodiazepines. IV. A pharmacokinetic interaction study with lorazepam. J Clin Psychopharmacol 1995; 15: 409-16
270. Von Moltke LL, Greenblatt DJ, Granda BW, et al. Nefazodone, meta-chlorophenylpiperazine, and their metabolities in vitro: cytochromes mediating transformation, and P450-3A4 inhibitory actions. Psychopharmacology 1999; 145: 113-22
271. Toney GB, Ereshefsky L, Lam YWF, et al. Effects of reboxetine and nefazodone on the pharmacokinetics and pharmacodynamics of alprazolam [abstract]. Presented at the 40th Annual New Clinical Drug Evaluation Unit (NCDEU) meeting; abstract no. 154; 2000 May 30-Jun 2; Boca Raton, FL, USA
272. Laroudie C, Salazar DE, Cosson JP, et al. Carbamazepine-nefazodone interaction in healthy subjects. J Clin Psychopharmacol 2000; 20: 46-53
273. Laroudie C, Salazar DE, Cosson JP, et al. Pharmacokinetic evaluation of co-administration of nefazodone and lithium in healthy subjects. Eur J Clin Pharmacol 1999; 54: 923-8
274. Franc JE, Duncan GF, Farmen RH, et al. High-performance liquid chromatographic method for the determination of nefazodone and its metabolites in human plasma using laboratory robotics. J Chromatogr B Biomed Appl 1991; 570: 129-38
275. Mayol RF, Cole CA, Luke GM, et al. Characterization of the metabolites of the antidepressant drug nefazodone in human urine and plasma. Drug Metab Dispos 1994; 22: 304-11
276. Nacca A, Guiso G, Fracasso C, et al. Brain-to-blood partition and in vivo inhibition of 5-hydroxytryptamine reuptake and quipazine-medicated behaviour of nefazodone and its main active metabolites in rodents. Br J Pharmacol 1998; 125: 1617-23
277. Barbhaiya RH, Shukla UA, Chaikin P, et al. Nefazodone pharmacokinetics: assessment of nonlinearity, intra-subject variability and time to attain steady-state plasma concentrations after dose escalation and de-escalation. Eur J Clin Pharmacol 1996; 50: 101-7
278. Barbhaiya RH, Buch AB, Greene DS. A study of the effect of age and gender on the pharmacokinetics of nefazodone after single and multiple doses. J Clin Psychopharmacol 1996; 16: 19-25
279. Golden RN, Rudorfer MV, Sherer MA, et al. Bupropion in depression. I. Biochemical effects and clinical response. Arch Gen Psychiatry 1988; 45: 139-43
280. Cooper BR, Wang CM, Cox RE, et al. Evidence that the acute behavioral and electrophysiological effects of bupropion (Wellbutrin) are mediated by a noradrenergic mechanism. Neuropsychopharmacology 1994; 11: 133-41
281. Ascher JA, Cole JO, Colin JN, et al. Bupropion: a review of its mechanism of antidepressant activity. J Clin Psychiatry 1995; 56: 395-401
282. Golden RN, James SP, Sherer MA, et al. Psychoses associated with bupropion treatment. Am J Psychiatry 1985; 142: 1459-62
283. Golden RN. Antidepressant profiles of bupropion and three metabolites: clinical and pre-clinical studies [letter]. Pharmacopsychiatry 1991; 24: 68
284. Laizure SC, DeVane CL, Stewart JT, et al. Pharmacokinetics of bupropion and its major basic metabolites in normal subjects after a single dose. Clin Pharmacol Ther 1985; 38: 586-9
285. Pollock BG, Sweet RA, Kirshner M, et al. Bupropion plasma levels and CYP2D6 phenotype. Ther Drug Monit 1996; 18: 581-5
286. Golden RN, DeVane CL, Laizure SC, et al. Bupropion in depression. II. The role of metabolites in clinical outcome. Arch Gen Psychiatry 1988; 45: 145-9
287. Goodnick PJ, Dominguez RA, DeVane CL, et al. Bupropion slow-release response in depression: diagnosis and biochemistry. Biol Psychiatry 1998; 44: 629-32
288. Silkey B, Preskorn SH, Golbeck A. Interindividual variability in steady-state plasma levels of bupropion and its major metabolites [abstract]. Presented at the 40th Annual New Clinical Drug Evaluation Unit (NCDEU) meeting; abstract no. 172; 2000 May 30-Jun 2; Boca Raton, FL, USA
289. DeVane CL, Laizure SC, Stewart JT, et al. Disposition of bupropion in healthy volunteers and subjects with alcoholic liver disease. J Clin Psychopharmacol 1990; 10: 328-32
290. Sachs GS, Lafer B, Stoll AL, et al. A double-blind trial of bupropion versus desipramine for bipolar depression. J Clin Psychiatry 1994; 55: 391-3
291. Ketter TA, Jenkins JB, Schroeder DH, et al. Carbamazepine but not valproate induces bupropion metabolism. J Clin Psychopharmacol 1995; 15: 327-33

292. Goodnick PJ. Pharmacokinetics of second generation antidepressants: bupropion. Psychopharmacol Bull 1991; 27: 513-9
293. Golden RN, Markey SP, Risby ED, et al. Antidepressants reduce whole-body norepinephrine turnover while enhancing 6-hydroxymelatonin output. Arch Gen Psychiatry 1988; 45: 150-4
294. Nixon AL, Long WH, Puopolo PR, et al. Bupropion metabolites produce false-positive urine amphetamine results. Clin Chem 1995; 41: 955-6
295. Rudorfer MV, Potter WZ. The role of metabolites of antidepressants in the treatment of depression. CNS Drugs 1997; 7: 273-312
296. Fawcett J, Barkin RL. Review of the results from clinical studies on the efficacy, safety and tolerability of mirtazapine for the treatment of patients with major depression. J Affect Disord 1998; 51: 267-85
297. Davis R, Wilde MI. Mirtazapine: a review of its pharmacology and therapeutic potential in the management of major depression. CNS Drugs 1996; 5: 389-402
298. Dahl ML, Voortman G, Alm C, et al. In vitro and in vivo studies on the disposition of mirtazapine in humans. Clin Drug Invest 1997; 13: 37-46
299. Holm KJ, Markham A. Mirtazapine: a review of its use in major depression. Drugs 1999; 57: 607-31
300. Holm KJ, Spencer CM. Reboxetine: a review of its use in depression. CNS Drugs 1999; 12: 65-83
301. Wienkers LC, Allievi C, Hauer MJ, et al. Cytochrome P-450-mediated metabolism of the individual enantiomers of the antidepressant agent reboxetine in human liver microsomes. Drug Metab Dispos 1999; 27: 1334-40
302. Herman BD, Fleishaker JC, Brown MT. Ketoconazole inhibits the clearance of the enantiomers of the antidepressant reboxetine in humans. Clin Pharmacol Ther 1999; 66: 374-9
303. Rudorfer MV. Monoamine oxidase inhibitors: reversible and irreversible. Psychopharmacol Bull 1992; 28: 45-57
304. Thase ME, Trivedi MH, Rush AJ. MAOIs in the contemporary treatment of depression. Neuropsychopharmacology 1995; 12: 185-219
305. Mallinger AG, Smith E. Pharmacokinetics of monoamine oxidase inhibitors. Psychopharmacol Bull 1991; 27: 493-502
306. Baker GB, Urichuk LJ, McKenna KF, et al. Metabolism of monoamine oxidase inhibitors. Cell Mol Neurobiol 1999; 19: 411-26
307. Karoum F, Chuang L-W, Eisler T, et al. Metabolism of (-) deprenyl to amphetamine and methamphetamine may be responsible for deprenyl's therapeutic benefit: a biochemical assessment. Neurology 1982; 32: 503-9
308. Mallinger AG, Edwards DJ, Himmelhoch JM, et al. Pharmacokinetics of tranylcypromine in patients who are depressed: relationship to cardiovascular effects. Clin Pharmacol Ther 1986; 40: 444-50
309. Mallinger AG, Himmelhoch JM, Thase ME, et al. Plasma tranylcypromine: relationship to pharmacokinetic variables and clinical antidepressant actions. J Clin Psychopharmacol 1990; 10: 176-83
310. Reynolds GP, Rausch WD, Riederer P. Effects of tranylcypromine stereoisomers on monoamine oxidation in man. Br J Clin Pharmacol 1980; 9: 521-3
311. Keck Jr PE, Carter WP, Nierenberg AA, et al. Acute cardiovascular effects of tranylcypromine: correlation with plasma drug, metabolite, norepinephrine, and MHPG levels. J Clin Psychiatry 1991; 52: 250-4
312. Youdim MBH, Aronson JK, Blau K, et al. Tranylcypromine (Parnate) overdose: measurement of tranylcypromine concentrations and MAO inhibitory activity and identification. Psychol Med 1979; 9: 377-82
313. Jefferson JW. Is tranylcypromine really metabolized to amphetamine? J Clin Psychiatry 1992; 53: 450-1
314. Brady KT, Lydiard RB, Kellner C. Tranylcypromine abuse. Am J Psychiatry 1991; 148: 1268-9
315. Briggs NC, Jefferson JW, Koenecke FH. Tranylcypromine addiction: a case report and review. J Clin Psychiatry 1990; 51: 426-9
316. Vartzopoulos D, Krull F. Dependence on monoamine oxidase inhibitors in high dose. Br J Psychiatry 1991; 158: 856-7
317. Keck PE, Pope HG, Nierenberg AA. Autoinduction of hypertensive reactions by tranylcypromine? J Clin Psychopharmacol 1989; 9: 48-51
318. Finberg JPM. Pharmacology of reversible and selective inhibitors of monoamine oxidase type A. Acta Psychiatr Scand 1995; 91 Suppl. 386: 8-13
319. Potter WZ, Murphy DL, Wehr TA, et al. Clorgyline: a new treatment for refractory rapid cycling disorder. Arch Gen Psychiatry 1982; 39: 505-10
320. Sunderland T, Cohen RM, Molchan S, et al. High-dose selegiline in treatment-resistant older depressive patients. Arch Gen Psychiatry 1994; 51: 607-15
321. Heinonen EH, Anttila MI, Lammintausta RAS. Pharmacokinetic aspects of l-deprenyl (selegiline) and its metabolites. Clin Pharmacol Ther 1994; 56: 742-9
322. Amsterdam JK, Bodkin JA. Transdermal selegiline in the treatment of patients with major depression: a double-blind, placebo-controlled trial [abstract]. Presented at the 40th Annual New Clinical Drug Evaluation Unit (NCDEU) meeting; abstract no. 15; 2000 May 30-Jun 2; Boca Raton, FL, USA
323. Reynolds GP, Riederer P, Sandler M, et al. Amphetamine and 2-phenylethylamine in post-mortem Parkinsonian brain after (-)deprenyl administration. J Neural Transm Park Dis Dement Sect 1978; 43: 271-7
324. Reynolds GP, Blau EK, Sandler M, et al. Deprenyl is metabolized to methamphetamine and amphetamine in man. Br J Clin Pharmacol 1978; 6: 542-4
325. Schoerlin MP, Mayersohn M, Hoevls B, et al. Cimetidine alters the disposition kinetics of the monoamine oxidase-A inhibitor moclobemide. Clin Pharmacol Ther 1991; 49: 32-8
326. Dingemanse J, Kneer J, Fotteler B, et al. Switch in treatment from tricyclic antidepressants to moclobemide: a new generation monoamine oxidase inhibitor. J Clin Psychopharmacol 1995; 15: 41-8
327. Schoerlin MP, Mayersohn M, Korn A, et al. Disposition kinetics of moclobemide, a monoamine oxidase-A enzyme inhibitor: single and multiple dosing in normal subjects. Clin Pharmacol Ther 1987; 42: 395-404
328. Fitton A, Faulds D, Goa KL. Moclobemide: a review of its pharmacological properties and therapeutic use in depressive illness. Drugs 1992; 43: 561-96
329. Gram LF, Guentert TW, Grange S, et al. Moclobemide, a substrate of CYP2C19 and an inhibitor of CYP2C19, CYP2D6, and CYP1A2: a panel study. Clin Pharmacol Ther 1995; 57: 670-7
330. Pons G, Schoerlin MP, Tam YK, et al. Moclobemide excretion in human breast milk. Br J Clin Pharmacol 1990; 29: 27-31
331. Schoerlin MP, Horber FF, Frey FJ, et al. Disposition kinetics of moclobemide, a new MAO-A inhibitor, in subjects with impaired renal function. J Clin Pharmacol 1990; 30: 272-84

Correspondence: *Matthew V. Rudorfer*, Division of Services and Intervention Research, National Institute of Mental Health, 6001 Executive Blvd, Rm 7163, MSC 9635, Bethesda, MD 20892-9635, USA
E-mail: mrudorfe@nih.gov

Sleep EEG Profile of Antidepressant Drugs
Pharmacological and Treatment Issues

Luc Staner, Rémy Luthringer and *Jean-Paul Macher*

FORENAP, Institute for Research in Neurosciences, Neuropharmacology and Psychiatry, Centre Hospitalier de Rouffach, Rouffach, France

A large empirical database supports the proposition that sleep dysregulation is closely linked to the underlying pathophysiology of depressive illness. Depressed patients almost invariably complain about their quality of sleep. Indeed, as many as 90% of patients with major depression will display some electroencephalographic (EEG)-verifiable sleep disruption.[1] Evidence for a common pathophysiology in sleep and depression comes from epidemiological longitudinal studies showing that patients with persistent insomnia complaints are 3 times more likely to develop depression within a 1-year follow-up period than patients without insomnia.[2] Moreover, sleep deprivation alters mood in 50% of patients[3] and can trigger mania in patients with bipolar disorders.[4,5] Finally, disturbances of the sleep-wake cycle can affect other biological rhythms that may be involved in depression, such as hypothalamic-pituitary adrenocortical system-related rhythms.[6]

Since the regulation of sleep appears to be related to the regulation of mood, understanding the effects of antidepressant medication on sleep may help to elucidate the interrelationship of sleep and mood in affective disorders. The purpose of this paper is to present the effects of antidepressants on sleep EEG and to discuss the possible pharmacological mechanisms involved. Relevant effects of antidepressant drugs on the sleep EEG of animals and of nondepressed patients, including healthy volunteers, will be discussed but not systematically reviewed.

1. Sleep Polygraphic Disturbances in Depression

Most sleep researchers have recognised 3 distinct states of existence: wakefulness, rapid eye movement (REM) sleep and non-REM sleep. REM sleep is also called 'paradoxical sleep' because of the close resemblance with the EEG of active wakefulness combined with a 'paradoxical' active inhibition of major muscle groups that seems to reflect a heavy sleep. Non-REM sleep is subdivided into four stages, with stage 1 being the lightest and stage 4 being the deepest sleep. Since slow 'delta' waves distinguish stages 3 and 4, these stages are often defined as delta sleep or slow-wave sleep (SWS). Normal sleep is characterised electrographically as recurrent cycles of non-REM and REM sleep of about 90 minutes in duration. In the successive cycles of the night, the durations of stages 3 and 4 decrease; furthermore, the proportion of the cycle occupied by REM sleep tends to increase – REM episodes occurring late in the night have more eye movement bursts than REM episodes occurring early in the night.[7]

When compared with healthy patients, depressed patients have been shown to have disturbances in sleep continuity and architecture as well as REM sleep disorganisation.[8] Lengthening of sleep latency, frequent nocturnal awakenings and early morning awakenings resulting in a decrease of total sleep time are the hallmarks of sleep continuity disturbances in major depression. Regarding sleep architecture, a deficit of SWS, especially during the first sleep cycle, has been consistently described. Disturbances in REM sleep organisation consist of an earlier onset of this sleep stage, a greater amount of REM sleep in the beginning of the night and an increase in actual REM activity and REM density during this sleep stage.[1,9] There is some evidence that these sleep abnormalities increase with the severity of the depression[10,11] and that they are more pronounced in older patients.[12,13] Furthermore, some studies, which controlled for the effects of these variables, have indicated a comparable sleep EEG in different subtypes of depression, including the bipolar/unipolar distinction,[14] but have suggested a role for endogenous and psychotic symptoms in the appearance of shortening of REM latency.[15,16]

It must be underlined that most of the reported sleep polysomnography changes are believed to be characteristic, although not specific, of major depressive disorders. For instance, sleep continuity disturbances and SWS reductions have also been observed in patients with anxiety disorders,[17-19] eating disorders,[20-22] alcohol (ethanol) dependence[23-25] or schizophrenia.[26-28] Shortening of REM latency could be demonstrated in antidepressant-responsive conditions, such as obsessive-compulsive disorder,[17] panic disorder,[18] comorbid depression and anorexia nervosa[29] or alcoholism[30] and, by some authors, in nondepressed patients with schizophrenia.[31]

Characteristic sleep EEG changes have been consistently identified in depressive illness. Some of these abnormalities seem to relate to the severity and/or the symptomatological profile of the acute depressive state. Although the specificity of this sleep EEG profile to depression is not fully established, it has to be noted that, according to Benca et al.,[8] the most widespread and most severe disturbances are found in patients with depressive disorders. Whether this abnormal sleep profile represents a state versus a trait marker for depressive illness is still a matter of debate. To some extent, the therapeutic effects of most antidepressant therapies may be related to their influences on sleep parameters. Therefore, the study of antidepressant drug-induced changes in the sleep EEG of healthy individuals and depressed patients could represent a valuable tool for investigating both normal sleep physiological processes and pathophysiological mechanisms involved in depressive illness.[32]

2. Effects of Antidepressant Drugs on Rapid Eye Movement (REM) Sleep

Changes in REM sleep variables are the best documented effects of most antidepressants on sleep polygraphic variables. Vogel et al.[33] reviewed 251 studies (from 1962 to 1989) of the influence of a variety of drugs (including antidepressants, antipsychotics, barbiturates, benzodiazepines, lithium, opioids, amine precursors and ethanol) on REM sleep in animals, healthy individuals and depressed patients. They concluded that all drugs producing large and sustained decreases of REM sleep time, followed on withdrawal by an REM rebound, have significant clinical efficacy in treating endogenous depression (table I). Conversely, reserpine, an old antihypertensive agent that induces high rates of depression, causes dramatic

Table I. Overview of the effects of antidepressant drugs on sleep EEG in patients with major depression

Drugs	EEG sleep effects		
	REM sleep	SWS	Sleep continuity
Nonspecific monoamine reuptake inhibitors			
Amitriptyline	↓↓↓	↑	↑↑↑
Clomipramine	↓↓↓	↑	↔↑
Desipramine	↓↓	↑	↑
Doxepin	↓↓	↑↑	↑↑↑
Imipramine	↓↓↓	↔	↔
Nortriptyline	↓↓↓	↑	↔
Trimipramine	↔	↔	↑↑↑
Noradrenergic and specific serotonergic antidepressants			
Mirtazapine	↓	↑	↑↑
Venlafaxine	↓↓↓	↔	↓
Monoamine oxidase inhibitors			
Moclobemide	↓	↔	↔
Phenelzine	↓↓↓	↔	↓
Selective serotonin reuptake inhibitors			
Citalopram	↓↓	↔	↓
Fluvoxamine	↓↓	↔	↓
Fluoxetine	↓↓	↔	↓
Paroxetine	↓↓	↔	↓
Sertraline	↓↓	↔	↔
Selective noradrenaline reuptake inhibitors			
Maprotiline	↓↓	↔	↑
Oxaprotiline	↓↓	↔	↔
Viloxazine	↓↓	↓	↓
Other antidepressant drugs			
Amfebutamone (bupropion)	↑	↓	↔
Amineptine	↔	↓	↔
Mianserin	↓	↔↑	↑↑
Nefazodone	↔↑	↔	↔
Tianeptine	↔	↔	↔
Trazodone	↔↓	↔↑	↑↑

↑ = increased; ↓ = decreased; ↔ = no change.
EEG = electroencephalogram; **REM** = rapid eye movement; **SWS** = slow-wave sleep.

increases in REM sleep and reduces REM latency.[34] In the same way, recent studies demonstrate that serotonin depletion after administration of a tryptophan-free amino acid drink significantly increased REM sleep and decreased REM latency in healthy individuals[35] and caused remission of depression in patients maintained on antidepressant medication.[36]

2.1 Nonspecific Monoamine Reuptake Inhibitors

In healthy individuals, tricyclic antidepressants (TCAs) almost invariably suppress REM sleep and increase REM latency. This effect occurs from the first night, appears to persist during continued administration, though some tolerance phenomenon may occur, and is followed by REM rebound upon withdrawal.[37-39]

The effects of TCAs on REM sleep are somewhat less pronounced in depressed patients. Some drugs such as clomipramine, amitriptyline, imipramine and nortriptyline have clear REM suppressant effects[40-42] which have even been shown to persist after withdrawal (clomipramine),[43-45] or, long term administration (up to 2 years; imipramine and nortriptyline).[46,47] However, no such properties were observed for trimipramine[48-50] or iprindole.[51] Doxepin[52,53] and desipramine[54,55] have also demonstrated milder REM suppressing effects.

2.2 Noradrenergic and Specific Serotonergic Antidepressants

Noradrenergic and specific serotonergic antidepressant (NaSSA), such as venlafaxine and mirtazapine, have been designed to enhance both noradrenergic and serotonergic neurotransmission with the least possible affinity for receptors mediating TCA-like adverse effects, such as muscarinic, α-adrenergic or histaminergic receptors. REM sleep has been shown to be completely suppressed in depressed patients after single-dose administration of venlafaxine (Stefos G, personal communication). Another polysomnographic study suggests that this compound mediates a sustained REM suppressant effect in depressed patients, since after both 1 week and 1 month of treatment venlafaxine induces an important increase in the onset latency of REM sleep and a decrease in REM sleep duration.[56] In the same way, a single dose of mirtazapine has shown some REM suppressant effects in healthy volunteers.[57]

2.3 Monoamine Oxidase Inhibitors

Monoamine oxidase inhibitors (MAOIs) induce comparable alterations in REM sleep to those observed with TCAs or NaSSAs in depressed patients, i.e. an initial large REM suppression occurs that persists for weeks and is followed by a rebound after withdrawal. This EEG sleep profile has been demonstrated for the nonselective agent phenelzine[58,59] as well as for the MAOI-A selective agent clorgiline.[60] These effects seem to be somewhat less marked with the reversible inhibitors of MAOI-A moclobemide[61,62] and toloxatone.[63]

2.4 Selective Monoamine Reuptake Inhibitors

Studies in healthy volunteers have clearly demonstrated that selective serotonin (5-hydroxytryptamine; 5-HT) reuptake inhibitors (SSRIs) such as zimeldine, fluvoxamine, fluoxetine and paroxetine increase REM latency and decrease REM sleep.[64,65] Maprotiline, oxaprotiline and viloxazine, three selective noradrenaline (norepinephrine) reuptake inhibitors (SNRIs), also decrease REM sleep in healthy individuals.[64,66]. In studies involving patients with depression, single-dose administration of both SSRIs and SNRIs have shown these REM suppressant properties.[67-69] The effects on REM sleep of 3 to 6 weeks treatment with fluvoxamine, sertraline, citalopram or paroxetine were comparable with those induced by most TCAs, i.e. a sustained REM suppression followed by a rebound after withdrawal.[55,70-72]

2.5 Other Antidepressant Drugs

Mianserin, a tetracyclic compound devoid of monoamine reuptake abilities but which has antagonist properties at a variety of monoamine receptors, including serotonin 5-HT_2, histamine H_1 and α_1- and α_2-adrenergic receptors,[73] increases REM latency during short and long term administration without changing REM duration either in healthy controls[74] or depressed patients.[75]

Trazodone has 5-HT_2 and α_1-adrenergic antagonism properties and weak serotonin reuptake blocking potency.[76] In healthy individuals and in those who sleep poorly, trazodone displays the usual REM suppressant profile of antidepressant drugs: it lengthens the onset of REM latency and reduces, in a sustained manner, the time spent in REM sleep with a rebound after withdrawal.[77,78] With one exception,[79] these alterations were found to be less marked in affectively disordered patients. Short or long term administration of trazodone did not affect REM sleep in dysthymic patients[80] and was shown to increase REM latency without affecting REM duration in patients with major depression.[81,82]

Nefazodone is chemically related to trazodone but lacks the α_1-adrenoceptor blocking properties of the latter compound. It is a potent 5-HT_2 antagonist and it possesses a modest ability to inhibit the reuptake of serotonin and noradrenaline.[83] Nefazodone has a pharmaco-sleep EEG profile that is distinct from that of other antidepressant drugs. This compound has demonstrated neutral or even enhancing effects on REM sleep. Short or long term administration of nefazodone does not seem to affect REM sleep duration or latency in either healthy individuals[78,84,85] or depressed patients,[86] although one study demonstrated an increase in total REM sleep time in depressed patients after long term nefazodone administration.[87]

Only one study has shown that an antidepressant drug could increase REM sleep: amfebutamone significantly increased REM sleep time and shortened its onset latency after long term administration in depressed patients.[88] The neuropharmacological basis of the antidepressant activity of amfebutamone is complex and incompletely understood.[89] It has no appreciable effect on the reuptake of serotonin and its most potent action is blockade of dopamine reuptake, although it also possesses some noradrenaline reuptake blocking properties.

Another dopamine reuptake blocker, amineptine, does not induce REM sleep changes in depressed patients.[90] Studies in healthy volunteers[91,92] or depressed alcoholic patients[93] suggest that tianeptine, an antidepressant drug that enhances serotonin reuptake, is also devoid of REM suppressant effect.

2.6 Pathophysiological Mechanisms

REM sleep neurophysiology has recently been reviewed by Hobson et al.[94] who concluded that noradrenergic and serotonergic influences impede REM sleep via anticholinergic mechanisms and that cholinergic mechanisms mediating REM sleep generation are fully expressed only when aminergic systems are inhibited. In this regard, it has been hypothesised that an imbalance between aminergic and cholinergic influences (increased cholinergic and/or decreased serotonergic/adrenergic influences) underlie REM sleep promotion (i.e. early onset of REM sleep) in depressive disorders.[95] Accordingly, some authors have proposed either a hypersensitivity of muscarinic receptors,[96] or an aminergic hyposensitivity[97] to explain REM sleep disturbances in patients with depression. Indeed, the ability of many antidepressant drugs to decrease REM sleep can be attributed to facilitation of noradrenergic and/or serotonergic function or to muscarinic cholinergic blockade. In some cases, as with the TCAs, all three mechanisms may be involved.

In this respect, the ability of amfebutamone to increase REM sleep in depressed patients, as well as the neutral or ambiguous effect of iprindole, trimipramine, trazodone, nefazodone, amineptine and tianeptine, are difficult to explain. A common characteristic of these compounds is that they do not, or only minimally, inhibit serotonergic reuptake.[98] Animal experiments using brain stem cells provide some compelling evidence that serotonergic neurons play a key role in the regulation of REM sleep; serotonergic dorsal raphe 'tone' has been found to be a potent determinant of the ultimate discharge pattern of upper brainstem cholinergic neurons that stimulate and maintain REM sleep.[99] Specifically, serotonin may inhibit REM sleep via 5-HT_{1A} receptors, since buspirone and ipsapirone, two 5-HT_{1A} agonists, have been shown to decrease REM sleep in healthy individuals,[78,100,101] an effect that seems to be mediated by post-synaptic receptors.[102] Moreover, there is some evidence for a down-regulation or a desensitisation of post-synaptic 5HT_{1A} receptors in depressive illnesses;[103] the resulting deficiency in serotonin transmission may play a role in the REM sleep disturbances seen in depression.

3. Effects of Antidepressant Drugs on Sleep Continuity and Non-REM Sleep

The reduction of nocturnal wakefulness and the concomitant increase in the duration of the various stages of non-REM sleep produced by antidepressants might also be of therapeutic importance. Nevertheless, reports of the effects of antidepressants on non-REM sleep variables in depression are much less consistent than their effects on REM sleep. Methods quantifying sleep EEG frequencies aimed at defining non-REM sleep microarchitecture, such as period amplitude analysis and power spectral analysis, could represent more accurate tools to investigate the clinical significance of drug-induced non-REM sleep alterations. The few studies using these techniques to characterise the effects of antidepressants are systematically discussed in sections 3.1 to 3.5.

3.1 Nonspecific Monoamine Reuptake Inhibitors

TCAs, particularly tertiary amines such as amitriptyline and trimipramine, have been shown to increase sleep continuity in healthy volunteers with[37] or without[50] concomitant increases in SWS, respectively. In depressed patients, TCAs that are sedative in nature (trimipramine, doxepin, amitriptyline) also increase sleep continuity[42,49,50,53] whereas imipramine[49] and nortriptyline[47] have no effect on this parameter. Desipramine, a less sedating TCA, has been shown to improve sleep continuity measures in depression.[55] Some TCAs have been reported to increase, decrease or have no effect on SWS, either in healthy volunteers or in depressed patients – for instance, amitriptyline increases SWS in healthy controls[37] but not in depressed patients.[41] In patients with major depression, imipramine was shown to decrease SWS[49] whereas an increase in SWS was observed with doxepin.[52]

Interestingly, a single dose of amitriptyline, clomipramine, imipramine or nortriptyline was found to strengthen the rate of production of delta-wave activity in the first non-REM period.[44,104-106] This redistribution of SWS in the first part of the night was observed without an increase in the total amount of SWS throughout the night. It remains essentially unchanged thereafter, even as long as 3 years into maintenance treatment.[104,107]

3.2 Noradrenergic and Specific Serotonergic Antidepressants

In healthy volunteers a single dose of mirtazapine has been shown to improve sleep continuity measures and to increase time spent in SWS.[57] Conversely, the other NaSSA, venlafaxine, seems to impair sleep continuity without significantly affecting SWS duration, at least in depressed patients. After 1 month of treatment, wake after sleep onset (WASO) [the duration of wake time after the first 30 seconds of stage 2 sleep] was found to be increased when venlafaxine was compared with placebo.[56] The power spectral analysis revealed that venlafaxine decreased the power of the delta–theta-waves and increased fast beta-activities during non-REM sleep, suggesting that this compound could lighten sleep intensity. Interestingly, venlafaxine, like TCAs, shifts delta power in the first part of the night.[56]

3.3 Monoamine Oxidase Inhibitors

In patients with major depression, nonselective MAOIs such as phenelzine tend to impair sleep continuity without producing consistent changes in SWS.[58,59] Moclobemide was shown to improve sleep continuity in depressed patients by decreasing awakenings in one study[61] but these findings were not confirmed elsewhere.[62] In the two studies, time spent in SWS appeared to be unchanged by the treatment.

3.4 Selective Monoamine Reuptake Inhibitors

SSRIs generally exhibit alerting effects (i.e. tend to enhance vigilance and therefore to induce arousal during sleep) on sleep continuity measures either in healthy controls or patients with depression. In healthy volunteers SSRIs such as fluoxetine, paroxetine, zimeldine and fluvoxamine reduce total sleep time and sleep efficiency and increase wakefulness.[64,65,84] Impairment of sleep continuity has also been observed in depressed patients over short or long term (up to 6 weeks) treatment with zimeldine,[67] fluvoxamine,[55] fluoxetine,[69] citalopram[70] and paroxetine.[71] However, a preliminary report suggested that 8 weeks' treatment with sertraline did not alter sleep continuity,[72] an effect that can be related to its sigma binding potency.[108] Indeed, the sigma ligand panamesine has recently been shown to decrease wake time after sleep onset and therefore to increase sleep efficiency in healthy controls.[109] No effects on SWS duration were evidenced for SSRIs either in healthy volunteers[64,65,85] or in patients with depression.[55,67,69-72]

The effects of paroxetine and citalopram on the non-REM sleep microarchitecture have been investigated. In healthy controls, 4 weeks of paroxetine administration did not alter any of the EEG spectral power values, but significantly increased, during non-REM sleep, the correlations between the powers of delta- and theta-waves and between delta and beta powers.[110] In depressed patients, 5 weeks of citalopram treatment significantly decreased the EEG power of the non-REM mainly in the 8 to 9Hz range (lower alpha-waves) without changing the power of the delta frequency range.[70]

The effects of SNRIs on non-REM sleep have been less widely reported than those observed with SSRIs. In patients with major depression, oxaprotiline produced a nonsignificant deterioration in sleep continuity without altering SWS,[83] whereas in healthy patients maprotiline increased the duration of stage 2 sleep.[64] Viloxazine has been shown to both decrease sleep continuity and SWS duration.[66]

3.5 Other Antidepressant Drugs

In depressed patients, mianserin improves sleep continuity measures both during short and long term treatment without affecting SWS,[75] which is in contrast with the SWS enhancement observed in healthy controls.[74]

Trazodone lessens the number of awakenings in healthy individuals and those who are poor sleepers.[77,78] In depressed or dysthymic patients, this molecule has been shown to improve sleep continuity and increase SWS.[80-82] However, these findings were questioned by Van Bemmel et al.,[79] who did not find effects on sleep continuity measures or SWS in depressed patients; further investigations of the non-REM sleep microstructure using spectral analysis revealed a significant decrease of the EEG power in the 13 to 14Hz range (lower beta-waves) without any change in the power of the delta-frequency range.[110]

In healthy volunteers, nefazodone did not affect either sleep continuity or SWS.[78,85] This same neutral effect was also found in patients with depression,[86] with one study showing a beneficial effect of the drug on sleep efficiency and number of awakenings.[87] Tianeptine shares with nefazodone its neutral profile on non-REM sleep.[91-93] Amfebutamone and amineptine significantly lessen SWS without affecting sleep continuity in patients with major depression.[88,90]

3.6 Pathophysiological Mechanisms

In summary, the reports on the effects of antidepressants on sleep continuity and non-REM sleep are inconsistent. Sleep continuity is found to be improved with sedating antidepressants such as most TCAs, whereas SSRIs, SNRIs, venlafaxine, amfebutamone and phenelzine exhibit alerting effects on sleep continuity measures. SWS is also variously affected by antidepressants: some compounds have been reported to increase it, others to decrease it or to leave it unchanged.

A fact worth mentioning in this context is that evidence supports the notion that serotonin, and in particular the 5-HT_2 receptor, plays a critical role in the regulation of SWS. The 5-$HT_{2A/2C}$ antagonist ritanserin produces a large dose-dependent increase in SWS in healthy controls[112-114] and in patients with major depressive disorders.[115] At present, it is not clear whether the 5-HT_{2A} or the 5-HT_{2C} receptor subtype is more involved in SWS regulation. A study in human volunteers comparing the effects of ritanserin and ketanserin (a 5-HT_{2A2C} antagonist with a significantly lower affinity for 5-HT_{2C} receptors than ritanserin) on SWS suggested a more important role for the 5-HT_{2C} receptor subtype.[116] Drugs with 5-HT_{2C} receptor agonist properties such as meta-chlorophenylpiperazine (mCPP) also appear to lower SWS in a dose-dependent manner in healthy volunteers.[117] However, a recent study demonstrated a clear SWS enhancement after the administration of SR46349B, a potent and selective 5-HT_{2A} receptor antagonist.[118] It can still be suggested that the ability of antidepressant drugs to enhance SWS reflects both their 5-HT_{2A} and 5-HT_{2C} antagonist properties. The effects of nefazodone or trazodone on SWS result from their dual action at 5-HT_{2C} receptors, the parent compound being an antagonist while the common metabolite, mCPP, being an agonist at these receptors. The fact that 5-HT_2 receptors seem to be upregulated in major depression[103,115] could explain why some antidepressants such as amitriptyline[37,41] and mianserin[74,75] elicit SWS enhancement in healthy controls but not in patients with major depression.

Studies investigating sleep microarchitecture are difficult to compare since different methodologies were used to record and analyse data. The Pittsburgh group[44,104-107] consistently reported that TCAs induce a redistribution of slow-wave activity in the first part of the night, a finding replicated with venlafaxine in our laboratory.[56] Other studies using power spectral analysis did not directly address the issue of the delta-shift hypothesis. Conversely, Kupfer and colleagues[44,104-107] have not focused on period-analysed EEG in anything other than the delta-frequency. It can be concluded, from data on citalopram,[70] paroxetine,[110] trazodone[111] and venlafaxine,[56] that antidepressants produce dissimilar EEG spectral response patterns, perhaps attributable to differences in their pharmacological actions.

4. Therapeutic Implications

Antidepressant-induced sleep EEG disturbances have been shown to predict the clinical response to various antidepressant therapies. For instance, the amount of REM sleep suppression observed after the first dose of antidepressant drugs may predict the ultimate clinical response.[40,41,43] Gillin et al.[41] noted that patients who improved during treatment with amitriptyline exhibited a clear REM sleep rebound during withdrawal, whereas patients who did not improve showed no such REM sleep rebound. In the same way, Kupfer et al.[119] demonstrated that the antidepressant response to 2 consecutive days of pulse loading of clomipramine followed by placebo was positively correlated with the amount of REM rebound. Induction of cytokine synthesis and fever have been shown to suppress REM sleep and improve mood in patients with major depression.[120] Finally, some studies showed that an increased REM activity identifies depressive patients who do not respond to psychotherapy and may warrant somatic treatment.[121,122] Recent data suggest that effective long term pharmacotherapy of recurrent major depression with imipramine[104] or nortriptyline[107] is associated with a higher REM activity than that observed in patients relapsing while receiving these drugs. Other studies were unable to demonstrate a consistent relationship between REM decreases and the alleviation of depression during treatment with antidepressants.[49,71,111] The REM suppressant effect may thus play an important role in the mechanism underlying treatment response to antidepressants, but cannot soley explain response to treatment.

It is also not clear whether changes in non-REM sleep, including SWS, are related to the improvement of depression. Quantification of non-REM sleep changes by visual scoring of sleep EEG in terms of changes in duration or proportion may be insufficient to detect such a relationship. For instance, the number of stage 2 microarousals (i.e. transient polysomnographic activation suggestive of an awake state) observed after the first doses of doxepine was found to be positively associated with antidepressant response.[123] Preliminary studies using spectral analysis methods have demonstrated that high pretreatment delta-activity, irrespective of sleep staging, may be related to clinical responsiveness to antidepressants;[44,124] another study suggests that redistribution of slow-wave activity to the earlier part of the night may predict the ultimate clinical response.[125]

With regard to the predictive value of observed sleep EEG changes after antidepressant administration, it has to be pointed out that there have not been methodologically sound studies using sleep EEG to assign treatments and assess outcome. Although a clearcut polysomnographic marker predicting clinical response to antidepressants is still lacking, knowledge of the sleep EEG effects of an antidepressant is useful in determining treatment strategies for major depression. Thus, drugs with sedative effects, such as TCAs, trazodone or mianserin, which tend to improve sleep continuity, may be helpful in some depressed patients experiencing severe insomnia; however, decrements in daytime alertness have been described with some sedative antidepressants at the beginning of the treatment. MAOIs and SSRIs have variable effects on daytime functioning and alertness that are difficult to predict; these may be due to the effects of age, dose and duration of therapy.[126]

5. Future Research

As is already the case with research on hypnotic drugs,[127] clinical research on the influence of antidepressant drugs on sleep microarchitecture will become increasingly important for interpreting the effects of these agents on sleep physiology. In this regard, Buysse et al.,[128] on the basis of fundamental studies by Steriade et al.,[129] have recently proposed that depression may differentially effect slow oscillations in non-REM sleep (primarily regulated by cortico-thalamo circuits) and traditional delta-activity (generated in thalamic nuclei). They demonstrated that higher delta-activity (2 to 3Hz) was more related to the acute depressive state while the lowest frequencies (0.5 to 1Hz) were linked to risk of recurrence.

Another promising direction for future research is the study of changes in dynamic relationships, or coherence, between frequency ranges.[130] Coherence evaluates the strength of covariation between two frequency rhythms: if two frequencies have high coherence, they are likely to be controlled by the same or similar timing mechanism. In this context, Armitage et al.[131] reported that, compared with healthy controls, beta- and delta-rhythms were less coherent in depressed patients and the recent study by Röschke et al.[107] suggested that 4 weeks administration of paroxetine to healthy volunteers significantly increased coherence between beta- and delta-frequencies.

6. Conclusions

The studies reviewed in sections 2 to 5 do not provide clear evidence for a common and unique pharmaco-sleep EEG profile of antidepressant drugs that could account for their clinical efficacy in the treatment of major depression. Rather, the observed drug-induced alterations in sleep EEG merely reflected the particular psychopharmacological properties of the molecule, for instance its particular effects on serotonergic, noradrenergic or cholinergic transmission. It can be suggested that drugs affecting 5-HT_{1A} transmission may influence REM sleep propensity while those affecting 5-HT_2 are more likely to influence SWS. Whether this influence of antidepressant drugs on sleep is related to clinical changes occurring in depressed patients during treatment is still unclear. More fundamental research on pharmaco-sleep EEG in terms of physiological processes is needed to interpret the relevance of antidepressant drug effects on sleep in major depression.

References

1. Reynolds CF III, Kupfer DJ. Sleep research in affective illness: state of the art circa 1987. Sleep 1987; 10: 199-215
2. Ford DE, Kamerow DB. Epidemiologic study of sleep disturbances and psychiatric disorders: an opportunity for prevention? JAMA 1989; 162: 1479-84
3. Wu JC, Bunney WE. The biological basis of an antidepressant response to sleep deprivation and relapse: review and hypothesis. Am J Psychiatry 1990; 147: 14-21
4. Wehr TA. Sleep-loss as a possible mediator of diverse causes of mania. Br J Psychiatry 1991; 159: 576-8
5. Barbini B, Bertelli S, Colombo C, et al. Sleep loss, a possible factor in augmenting manic episode. Psychiatry Res 1996; 65; 121-5
6. Wirz-Justice A. Biological rhythms in mood disorder. In: Bloom FE, Kupfer DJ, editors. Psychopharmacology, the fourth generation of progress. New York: Raven Press, 1995: 999-1017
7. Lesch DR, Spire JP. Clinical electroencephalography. In: Thorpy MJ, editor. Handbook of sleep disorders. New York: Marcel Dekker Inc., 1990: 1-31
8. Benca RM, Obermeyer WH, Thisted RA, et al. Sleep and psychiatric disorders. A meta-analysis. Arch Gen Psychiatry 1992; 49: 651-68
9. Buysse DJ, Kupfer DJ. Diagnostic and research applications of electroencephalographic sleep studies in depression: conceptual and methodological issues. J Nerv Ment Dis 1990; 178: 405-14
10. Kupfer DJ, Bulik CM, Grochocinski V. Relationship between EEG sleep measures and clinical ratings of depression. J Affect Disord 1984; 6: 43-52
11. Hubain P, Van Veeren C, Staner L, et al. Neuroendocrine and sleep variables in major depressed inpatients: role of severity. Psychiatry Res 1996; 63: 83-92
12. Kerkhofs M, Kempenaers C, Linkowski P, et al. Multivariate study of sleep EEG in depression. Acta Psychiatrica Scand 1988; 77: 463-8
13. Knowles JB, McLean AW. Age-related changes in sleep in depressed and healthy subjects: a meta-analysis. Neuropsychopharmacology 1990; 3: 257-9

14. Fossion P, Staner L, Dramaix M, et al. Does sleep EEG data distinguish between UP, BPI or BPII major depressions? An age and gender controlled study. J Affect Disord 1998; 49: 181-7
15. Hubain P, Souery D, Jönck L, et al. Relationship between the Newcastle scale and sleep polysomnographic variables in major depression: a controlled study. Eur Neuropsychopharmacol 1995; 5: 129-34
16. Stefos G, Staner L, Kerkhofs M, et al. Shortened REM latency as a psychobiologic marker for psychotic depression? An age, gender and polarity controlled study. Biol Psychiatry 1998; 44: 1314-20
17. Insel TR, Gillin JC, Moore A, et al. The sleep of patients with obsessive-compulsive disorder. Arch Gen Psychiatry 1982; 39: 1372-7
18. Uhde TW, Roy-Byrne P, Gillin JC, et al. The sleep of patients with panic disorder. A preliminary report. Psychiatry Res 1984; 12: 251-9
19. Papadimitriou GN, Kerkhofs M, Kempenaers C, et al. EEG sleep studies in patients with generalised anxiety: a preliminary comparison with depressed outpatients. Psychiatry Res 1983; 8: 81-9
20. Walsch BT, Goetz R, Roose SP, et al. EEG-monitored sleep in anorexia nervosa and bulimia. Biol Psychiatry 1985; 20: 947-56
21. Levy AB, Dixon KN, Schmidt H. Sleep architecture in anorexia nervosa and bulimia. Biol Psychiatry 1988; 23: 99-101
22. Delvenne V, Kerkhofs M, Appelboom-Fondu J, et al. Sleep polygraphic variables in anorexia nervosa and depression: a comparative study in adolescents. J Affect Disord 1992; 25: 167-72
23. Snyder S, Karacan I. Sleep patterns of sober chronic alcoholics. Neuropsychobiology 1985; 13: 97-100
24. Gillin JC, Smith TL, Irwin M, et al. EEG sleep studies in 'pure' primary alcoholism during subacute withdrawal: relationship to normal controls, age, and other clinical variables. Biol Psychiatry 1990; 27: 477-88
25. Le Bon O, Verbanck P, Hoffmann G, et al. Sleep in detoxified alcoholics: impairment of most standard sleep parameters and increased risk for sleep apnea, but not for myoclonias – a controlled study. J Stud Alcohol 1997; 58: 30-6
26. Hiatt JF, Floyd TC, Katz PH, et al. Further evidence of abnormal non-rapid eye movement sleep in schizophrenia. Arch Gen Psychiatry 1985; 42: 797-802
27. Ganguli R, Reynolds III CF, Kupfer DJ. Electroencephalographic sleep in young never-medicated schizophrenics. Arch Gen Psychiatry 1987; 44: 36-44
28. Kempenaers C, Kerkhofs M, Linkowski P, et al. Sleep EEG variables in young schizophrenics and depressive patients. Biol Psychiatry 1988; 24: 828-33
29. Katz JL, Kuperberg A, Pollack CP, et al. Is there a relationship between eating disorder and affective disorder? New evidence from sleep recordings. Am J Psychiatry 1984; 141: 753-9
30. Moeller FG, Gillin JC, Irwin M, et al. A comparison of sleep EEGs in patients with primary major depression and major depression secondary to alcoholism. J Affect Disord 1993; 27: 39-42
31. Zarcone VC, Benson KL Berger PA. Abnormal rapid eye movement latencies in schizophrenia. Arch Gen Psychiatry 1987; 44: 45-8
32. Le Bon O, Staner L, Murphy JR, et al. Critical analysis of the theories advanced to explain short REM sleep latencies and other sleep anomalies in several psychiatric conditions. J Psychiatry Res 1997; 31: 433-50
33. Vogel GW, Buffenstein A, Minter K, et al. Drug effects on REM sleep and on endogenous depression. Neurosci Biobehav Rev 1990; 14: 49-63
34. Hartmann E. Reserpine: its effect on the sleep-dream cycle in man. Psychopharmacologia 1966; 9: 242
35. Bhatti T, Gillin JC, Selfritz E, et al. Effects of a tryptophan-free amino acid drink challenge on normal human sleep electroencephalogram and sleep. Biol Psychiatry 1998; 43: 52-9
36. Moore P, Gillin JC, Bhatti T, et al. Rapid tryptophan depletion, sleep electroencephalogram, and mood in men with remitted depression on serotonin reuptake inhibitors. Arch Gen Psychiatry 1998; 55: 534-9
37. Hartmann E, Cravens J. The effects of long-term administration of psychotropic drugs on human sleep. III. The effects of amitriptyline. Psychopharmacologia 1974; 33: 185-202
38. Passouant P, Cadhilac J, Billiard M. Withdrawal of the paradoxical sleep by clomipramine. A electrophysiological, histochemical and biochemical study. Int J Neurol 1975; 10: 186-97
39. Herdman JRE, Cowen PJ, Campling GM, et al. Effect of lofepramine on 5-HT function and sleep. J Affect Disord 1993; 29: 63-72
40. Kupfer DJ, Foster FG, Reich L, et al. EEG sleep changes as predictors in depression. Am J Psychiatry 1976; 133: 622-6
41. Gillin JC, Wyatt RJ, Fram D, et al. The relationship between changes in REM sleep and clinical improvement in depressed patients treated with amitriptyline. Psychopharmacology 1978; 59: 267-72
42. Mendlewicz J, Kempenaers C, De Martelaer V. Sleep EEG and amitriptyline treatment in depressed inpatients. Biol Psychiatry 1991; 30: 691-702
43. Hochli D, Riemann D, Zulley J, et al. Initial REM sleep suppression by clomipramine: a prognostic tool for treatment response in patients with major depressive disorder. Biol Psychiatry 1986; 21: 1217-20
44. Kupfer DJ, Ehlers CL, Pollock BJ, et al. Clomipramine and EEG sleep in depression. Psychiatry Res 1989; 30: 165-80
45. Chen CN. Sleep, depression and antidepressants. Br J Psychiatry 1979; 135: 385-402
46. Kupfer DJ, Coble P, Kane J, et al. Imipramine and EEG sleep in children with depressive symptoms. Psychopharmacology 1979; 60: 117-23
47. Kupfer DJ, Spiker DJ, Rossi A, et al. Nortriptyline and EEG sleep in depressed patients. Biol Psychiatry 1982; 7: 535-46
48. Wiegand M, Berger M, Zulley J, et al. The effect of trimipramine on sleep in patients with major depressive disorder. Pharmacopsychiatry 1986; 19: 198-9
49. Ware JC, Brown FW, Moorad PJ Jr, et al. Effects on sleep: a double-blind study comparing trimipramine to imipramine in depressed insomniac patients. Sleep 1989; 12: 537-49
50. Feuillade P, Pringuey D, Belogou JL, et al. Trimipramine: acute and lasting effects on sleep in healthy and major depressive subjects. J Affect Disord 1992; 24: 135-46
51. Baxter BL, Gluckman MI. Iprindole: an antidepressant which does not block REM sleep. Nature 1969; 223: 750-2

52. Blackburn AB, Karacan I, Salis PJ, et al. The effects of doxepin HCl on sleep patterns of neurotically depressed patients with sleep disturbances [abstract]. Sleep Res 1975; 4: 90
53. Roth T, Zorick F, Wittig R, et al. The effect of doxepine HCl on sleep and depression. J Clin Psychiatry 1982; 43: 366-8
54. Shipley JE, Kupfer DJ, Griffin SJ, et al. Comparison of effects of desipramine and amitriptyline on EEG sleep of depressed patients. Psychopharmacology 1985; 85: 14-22
55. Kupfer DJ, Perel JM, Pollock BG, et al. Fluvoxamine versus desipramine: comparative polysomnographic effects. Biol Psychiatry 1991; 29: 23-40
56. Luthringer R, Toussaint M, Schaltenbrand N, et al. A double-blind, placebo-controlled evaluation of the effects of orally administered venlafaxine on sleep in inpatients with major depression. Psychopharm Bull 1996; 32: 637-46
57. Ruigt GS, Kemp B, Groenhout CM, et al. Effect of the antidepressant Org 3770 on human sleep. Eur J Clin Pharmacol 1990; 38: 551-4
58. Wyatt RJ, Fram DH, Kupfer DJ. Total prolonged drug-induced REM sleep suppression in anxious-depressive patients. Arch Gen Psychiatry 1971; 24: 145-55
59. Kupfer DJ, Bowers MB Jr. REM sleep and central monoamine oxidase inhibitions. Psychopharmacologia 1972; 27: 183-90
60. Cohen RM, Pickar D, Garnett, et al. REM sleep suppression induced by selective monoamine oxidase inhibitors. Psychopharmacology 1982; 78: 137-40
61. Monti JM, Alterwain P, Monti D. The effects of moclobemide on nocturnal sleep of depressed patients. J Affect Disord 1990; 20: 201-8
62. Minot R, Luthringer R, Macher JP. Effect of moclobemide on the psychophysiology of sleep/wake cycles: a neuroelectrophysiological study of depressed patients administered with moclobemide. Int Clin Psychopharmacol 1993; 7: 181-9
63. Minot R, Luthringer R, Toussaint M, et al. Sleep/wake study of a selective IMAO antidepressant: toloxatone [abstract]. Biol Psychiatry 1991; 29: 100
64. Nicholson AN, Pascoe PA. 5-hydroxytryptamine and noradrenaline uptake inhibitions. Studies on sleep in man. Neuropharmacology 1986; 25: 1079-83
65. Saletu B, Frey R, Krupka M, et al. Sleep laboratory studies on the single-dose effects of serotonin reuptake inhibitors paroxetine and fluoxetine on human sleep and awakening qualities. Sleep 1991; 14: 439-47
66. Brezinova V, Adam K, Chapman K, et al. Viloxazine, sleep and subjective feelings. Psychopharmacology 1977; 55: 121-8
67. Shipley JE, Kupfer DJ, Dealy RS, et al. Differential effects of zimelidine on the sleep electroencephalogram of depressed patients. Clin Pharmacol Ther 1984; 36: 251-9
68. Berger M, Emrich HM, Lund D, et al. Sleep EEG variables as course criteria and predictors of antidepressant therapy with fluvoxamine/oxaprotiline. Adv Pharmacother 1986; 2: 110-20
69. Kerkhofs M, Rielaert C, De Martelaer V, et al. Fluoxetine in major depression: efficacy, safety and effects on sleep EEG variables. Int Clin Psychopharmacol 1990; 5: 253-60
70. Van Bemmel AL, Beersma DGM, Van Den Hoofdakker RH. Changes in EEG power density of NREM sleep in depressed patients during treatment with citalopram. J Sleep Res 1993; 2: 156-62
71. Staner L, Kerkhofs M, Detroux D, et al. Acute, subchronic, and withdrawal sleep EEG changes during treatment with paroxetine and amitriptyline: a double-blind randomized trial in major depression. Sleep 1995; 18: 470-7
72. Winokur A, 'Lexow N, Allen K, et al. Sertraline administered for 8 weeks to depressed patients did not alter sleep architecture: a preliminary report. [abstract]. 22nd Annual Physician Assistant Conference. 1994 25 May, San Antonio, Texas, pp. 24-5
73. Montgomery SA, Bullock T, Pinder RM. The clinical profile of mianserine. Nord Psykiatr Tidsskr 1991; 45: 24-35
74. Tormey WP, Buckley MP, O'Kelly DA, et al. A Sleep-endocrine profile of the antidepressant mianserin. Curr Med Res Opin 1980; 6: 456-60
75. Mendlewicz J, Dunbar GC, Hoffman G. Changes in sleep EEG architecture during the treatment of depressed patients with mianserine. Acta Psychiatrica Scand 1985; Suppl. 320: 26-9
76. Brodgen RN, Heel RC, Speight TM, et al. Trazodone: a review of its pharmacologic properties and therapeutic use in depression and anxiety. Drugs 1981; 21: 401-29
77. Montgomery I, Oswald I, Morgan K, et al. Trazodone enhances sleep in subjective quality but not in objective duration. Br J Clin Pharmacol 1983; 16: 139-44
78. Ware JC, Rose FV, McBrayer RH. The acute effects of nefazodone, trazodone and buspirone on sleep and sleep-related penile tumescence in normal subjects. Sleep 1994; 17: 544-50
79. Van Bemmel AL, Havermans RG, van Diest R. Effects of trazodone on EEG sleep and clinical state in major depression. Psychopharmacology 1992; 107: 569-74
80. Parrino L, Spaggiari MC, Boselli M, et al. Clinical and polysomnographic effects of trazodone CR in chronic insomnia associated with dysthymia. Psychopharmacology 1994; 116: 389-95
81. Mouret J, Lemoine P, Minuit MP, et al. Effects of trazodone on the sleep of depressed subjects - a polygraphic study. Psychopharmacology 1988; 95: S37-S43
82. Scharf MB, Sachais BA. Sleep laboratory evaluation of the effects and efficacy of trazodone in depressed insomniac patients. J Clin Psychiatry 1990; 51 Suppl.: 13-7
83. Taylor DP, Carter RB, Eison AS, et al. Pharmacology and neurochemistry of nefazodone, a novel antidepressant drug. J Clin Psychiatry 1995; 56 Suppl. 6: 3-11
84. Vogel G, Cohen J, Mullis D, et al. Nefazodone and REM sleep: how do antidepressant drugs decrease REM sleep? Sleep 1998; 21: 70-7
85. Sharpley AL, Williamson DJ, Attenburrow ME, et al. The effects of paroxetine and nefazodone on sleep: a placebo controlled trial. Psychopharmacology 1996; 126: 50-4

86. Armitage R, Rush AJ, Trivedi M, et al. The effects of nefazodone on sleep on sleep architecture in depression. Neuropsychopharmacology 1994; 10: 123-7
87. Rush JA, Armitage R, Gillin JC, et al. Comparative effects of nefazodone and fluoxetine on sleep in outpatients with major depression. Biol Psychiatry 1998; 44: 3-14
88. Nofzinger EA, Reynolds CF III, Thase ME, et al. REM sleep enhancement by bupropion in depressed man. Am J Psychiatry 1995; 152: 274-6
89. Ferris RM, Cooper BR. Mechanism of antidepressant activity of bupropion. J Clin Psychiatry Monogr 1993; 11: 2-14
90. Di Perri R, Mailland F, Bramanti P. The effects of amineptine on mood and nocturnal sleep of depressed patients. Progr Neuropsychopharm Biol Psychiatry 1986; 11: 65-70
91. Macher JP, Luthringer R, Toussaint M, et al. Brain mapping and psychoactive drugs. In: Hindmarch I, Stonier PD, editors. Human psychopharmacology: methods and measures. Vol 3. New York: John Wiley & Sons, 1990: 1-20
92. Staner L, Mendlewicz J. Effect of a single dose of tianeptine in healthy volunteer on sleep electrophysiological parameters [abstract]. Eur Psychiatry 1994; 9 Suppl. 1: 141
93. Macher JP, Minot R, Duval F, et al. Neuro-electrophysiologic studies in abstinent and depressed alcoholic patients treated with tianeptine. Presse Med 1991; 20: 1853-7
94. Hobson AJ, Stickgold R, Pare-Schott EF. The neuropsychology of REM sleep dreaming. Neuroreport 1998; 9: R1-R14
95. McCarley RW. REM sleep and depression: common neurobiological control mechanisms. Am J Psychiatry 1982; 139: 565-70
96. Gillin JC, Sitaram N, Mendelsohn WB. Acetylcholine, sleep and depression. Hum Neurobiol 1982; 1: 211-9
97. Schittecatte M, Charles G, Machowski R, et al. Reduced clonidine rapid eye movement sleep suppression in patients with primary affective illness. Arch Gen Psychiatry 1992; 49: 637-42
98. Seeman R. Receptor tables vol 2: dissociation constants for neuroreceptors and transporters. Toronto: SZ Research, 1993
99. Rye DB. Contributions of the pedunculopontine region to normal and altered REM sleep. Sleep 1997; 20: 757-88
100. Driver HS, Flaningan MJ, Bentley AJ, et al. The influence of ipsapirone, a 5-HT_{1A} agonist, on sleep pattern of healthy subjects. Psychopharmacology 1995; 117: 186-92
101. Gillin JC, Jernajczyk W, Valladares-Neto DDC, et al. Inhibition of REM sleep by ipsapirone, a 5-HT_{1A} agonist in normal volunteers. Psychopharmacology 1994; 116: 433-6
102. Tissier MH, Lainey E, Fattaccini CM, et al. Effects of ipsapirone, a 5-HT1A agonist on sleep/wakefulness cycles: probably a post-synaptic action. J Sleep Res 1993; 2: 103-9
103. Maes M, Meltzer HY. The serotonin hypothesis of major depression. In: Bloom FE, Kupfer DJ, editors. Psychopharmacology, the fourth generation of progress. New York: Raven Press, 1995: 933-44
104. Kupfer DJ, Ehlers CL, Franck E, et al. Persistent effects of antidepressants: EEG sleep studies in depressed patients during maintenance treatment. Biol Psychiatry 1994; 35: 781-93
105. Kupfer DJ, Shipley JE, Perel JM, et al. Antidepressants and sleep EEG: Search for specificity. In: Dahl SG, Gram LF, Paul SM, et al., editors. Clinical pharmacology in psychiatry: selectivity in psychotropic drugs action – promises or problems? New York: Springer-Verlag, 1987: 167-73
106. Reynolds CF III, Hoch CC, Buysse DJ, et al. Sleep in late-life recurrent depression: changes during early continuation therapy with nortriptyline. Neuropsychopharmacology 1991; 5: 85-96
107. Reynolds CF III, Buysse DJ, Brunner D, et al. Maintenance nortriptyline effects on electroencephalographic sleep in elderly patients with recurrent major depression: double-blind, placebo- and plasma-level-controlled evaluation. Biol Psychiatry 1997; 42: 560-7
108. Schmidt A, Lebel L, Koe BK, et al. Sertraline potently displaces [3H]3-PPP binding to sigma site in rat brain. Eur J Pharmacol 1989; 165: 335-6
109. Frieboes RM, Murck H, Antonijevic I, et al. Characterization of the sigma ligand panamesine, a potential antipsychotic, by immune response in patients with schizophrenia and by sleep EEG changes in normal controls. Psychopharmacology 1999; 141: 107-10
110. Röschke J, Kögel P, Schlössser R, et al. Analysis of sleep EEG microstructure in subchronic paroxetine treatment of healthy subjects. Psychopharmacology 1997; 132: 44-7
111. Van Bemmel AL, Beersma DGM, Van Den Hoofdakker RH. Changes in EEG power density of non-REM sleep in depressed patients during treatment with trazodone. J Affect Disord 1995; 35: 11-9
112. Idzikowski C, Mills FJ, Glennard R. 5-hydroxytamine-2 antagonist increases human slow wave sleep. Brain Res 1986; 378: 164-8
113. Sharpley AL, Solomon RA, Fernando AI, et al. Dose-related effects of selective 5-HT2 receptor antagonists on slow wave sleep in humans. Psychopharmacology 1990; 101: 568-9
114. Brandenberger G, Luthringer R, Muller G, et al. 5-HT2 receptors are partially involved in the relationship between renin release and relative delta power. J Endocrinol Invest 1996; 19: 556-62
115. Staner L, Kempenaers C, Simonnet MP, et al. 5-HT2 receptor antagonism and slow wave sleep in major depression. Acta Psychiatr Scand 1992; 86: 133-7
116. Sharpley AL, Elliott JM, Attenburrow MJ, et al. Slow wave sleep in humans: the role of 5-HT_{2A} and 5-HT_{2C} receptors. Neuropharmacology 1994; 13: 467-71
117. Katsuda Y, Walch AE, Ware CJ, et al. Meta-chlorophenylpiperazine decreases slow wave sleep in humans. Biol Psychiatry 1993; 33: 49-51
118. Landolt HP, Meier V, Burgess HJ, et al. Serotonin-2 receptors and human sleep: effect of a selective antagonist on EEG power spectra. Neuropsychopharmacol 1999; 21: 455-66
119. Kupfer DJ, Pollock BG, Perel JM, et al. Effect of pulse loading with clomipramine on EEG sleep. Psychiatry Res 1994; 54: 161-75

120. Bauer J, Hohagen F, Gimmel E, et al. Induction of cytokine synthesis and fever suppresses REM sleep and improves mood in patients with major depression. Biol Psychiatry 1995; 38: 611-21
121. Thase ME, Simons AD, Reynolds CF III. Abnormal electroencephalographic sleep profiles in major depression. Association with response to cognitive behavior therapy. Arch Gen Psychiatry 1996; 53: 99-108
122. Buysse DJ, Tu XM, Cherry CR, et al. Pretreatment REM sleep and subjective sleep quality distinguish depressed psychotherapy remitters and nonremitters. Biol Psychiatry 1999; 45: 205-13
123. Staedt J, Hunerjager H, Ruther E, et al. Sleep cluster arousal analysis and treatment response to heterocyclic antidepressants in patients with major depression. J Affect Disord 1998; 49: 221-7
124. Luthringer R, Minot R, Toussaint M, et al. All-night spectral analysis as a tool for the prediction of clinical response to antidepressant treatment. Biol Psychiatry 1995; 38: 98-104
125. Ehlers CL, Havstad JW, Kupfer DJ. Estimation of time course of slow-wave sleep over the night in depressed patients: effects of clomipramine and clinical response. Br J Psychiatry 1996; 39: 171-81
126. Neylan TC. Treatment of sleep disturbances in depressed patients. J Clin Psychiatry 1995; 56 Suppl. 2: 56-61
127. Borbely AA, Akerstedt T, Benoit O, et al. Hypnotics and sleep physiology: a consensus report. Eur Arch Psychiatry Clin Neurosci 1991; 241: 13-21
128. Buysse DJ, Frank E, Lowe KK, et al. Electroencephalographic sleep correlates of episode and vulnerability to recurrence in depression. Biol Psychiatry 1997; 41: 406-18
129. Steriade M, McCormick DA, Sejnowski TJ. Thalamocortical oscillations in the sleeping and aroused brain. Science 1993; 262: 679-85
130. Armitage R. Microarchitectural findings in sleep EEG in depression: diagnostic implications. Biol Psychiatry 1995; 37: 72-84
131. Armitage R, Roffwarg H, Rush A, et al. Digital period analysis of EEG in depression: periodicity, coherence, and interhemispheric relationships during sleep. Prog Neuropsychopharmacol Biol Psychiatry. 1993; 17: 363-72

Correspondence: Dr *Luc Staner*, FORENAP, Centre Hospitalier, 27 rue du 4éme R.S.M., F-68250 Rouffach, France.
E-mail: luc.staner@forenap.asso.fr

Measuring Quality of Life in Patients with Depression or Anxiety

Diane Whalley and *Stephen P. McKenna*

Galen Research, Manchester, England

1. Introduction

1.1 Depression

Major depression is characterised by such symptoms as depressed mood, poor appetite, weight loss or weight gain, insomnia, agitation, lethargy, loss of interest, fatigue, negative self-concept and recurrent thoughts of death or suicide.[1] The most commonly used classes of antidepressants are tricyclic antidepressants (TCAs), monoamine oxidase inhibitors (MAOIs) and the newer selective serotonin (5-hydroxytryptamine; 5-HT) reuptake inhibitors (SSRIs).

1.2 Anxiety

Five main anxiety states have been identified:[1] (i) panic disorder; (ii) generalised anxiety disorder; (iii) obsessive-compulsive disorder; (iv) phobic disorders; and (v) post-traumatic stress disorder. The literature concerning well-being and quality of life in patients with anxiety concentrates mainly on generalised anxiety and panic disorders with or without agoraphobia, as does this review. Some patients experience one short episode, while others may have recurrences for several years.[2] Panic disorder and generalised anxiety disorder often occur together.

Panic disorder is characterised by symptoms such as sudden attacks of laboured breathing, heart palpitations, chest pain, feelings of smothering, dizziness and feelings of intense terror. Many of the anxiety disorders are accompanied by panic attacks. Antidepressants and benzodiazepines can be effective treatments.

Patients with generalised anxiety disorder can be chronically and persistently anxious about everyday life situations. Benzodiazepines are commonly used to treat patients with this disorder.

1.3 Concurrent Anxiety and Depression

The distinction between anxiety and depression is not straightforward. This is partly because they have symptoms in common. For example, generalised anxiety disorder and major depression both induce symptoms of dysphoric mood, agitation, sleep disturbance and poor concentration. These symptoms are diagnostic criteria for both conditions.

Anxiety and depression are also difficult to distinguish because they frequently occur together. Between 20 and 30% of patients presenting with major depression also have panic disorder,[3,4] and an average of 40 to 50% of patients with panic disorder will have had at least one episode of major depression at some time in their lives.[5,6]

The original aim of this article was to review the research conducted into the effect of pharmacological treatment on quality of life in patients with anxiety and depression. However, a literature search on 'Medline' identified very few studies in which quality of life was assessed, so the scope of the search was widened to include related areas of health status such as well-being. These areas are frequently referred to as quality of life by the authors of the articles. Studies that address economic analyses of anxiety and depression are also reviewed.

Within this field there is considerable overlap in the content of measures of symptom severity, well-being and quality of life. This review includes the most widely used instruments of each type, and comments on the suitability and psychometric properties of the quality-of-life (QOL) and well-being instruments.

2. Severity Rating Scales for Depression and Anxiety

There are many scales available to assess the severity of depression, both patient- and clinician-completed. The most commonly used patient-completed scales are the Self-Rating Depression Scale (SDS),[7] Beck Depression Inventory (BDI),[8] Carroll Rating Scale (CRS)[9] and Center for Epidemiologic Studies Depression Scale (CES-D).[10,11] The Hamilton Depression Rating Scale (HDRS)[12,13] and the Montgomery-Åsberg Depression Rating Scale (MADRS)[14] are the most widely used observer-completed scales.

Fewer rating scales are available for evaluating the severity of anxiety. The most commonly used are the Hamilton Anxiety Rating Scale (HARS)[15] and the Clinical Anxiety Scale (CAS),[16] which are both observer rated. Neither of these scales cover panic attacks, which is a serious limitation. Although the developers of the CAS make suggestions for such an item, it is not included in the main scale. The Beck Anxiety Inventory (BAI)[17] is a patient-completed rating scale.

The main scales available to assess the presence and severity of both depression and anxiety are patient-completed: (i) the Symptom Checklist 90-R [SCL-90-R];[18] (ii) the General Health Questionnaire (GHQ);[19] and (iii) the Hospital Anxiety and Depression Scale (HAD).[20] The HAD contains two subscales: one each for anxiety (HAD-A) and depression (HAD-D).

The scales listed in this section are concerned with the presence and/or severity of symptoms. They provide no information on the impact of the illness and its treatment on the patients' lives.

3. Quality of Life

As pressure grows on health service expenditure throughout the world, more questions are being asked about the effectiveness of treatments. The new generation of antidepressants (i.e. the SSRIs) are becoming the preferred treatment for depression because they have fewer adverse effects than older drugs such as the TCAs and, consequently, produce better compliance. Without considering the relative benefits of treatments to patients' quality of life, a move to new treatments would be unlikely. The SSRIs are considerably more expensive than the older products and have few additional benefits in terms of symptom alleviation.[21]

There is a lack of consensus on a definition of quality of life. This is compounded by researchers' tendency to interchange the terms 'health status', 'well-being' and 'quality of life'.

For the purpose of this review, 'health status instruments' are those that measure aspects of impairment, disability and handicap. They tend to be confined to symptoms and function. 'Well-being' is usually used in the context of psychological or emotional well-being. As such, it covers only some of the aspects that are encompassed in quality of life.

Authors rarely define what they mean by quality of life. A common method of QOL measurement is the components approach, which assumes that certain areas of function, well-being and symptoms should be measured. Specific areas are often identified from the literature and/or from discussions with clinicians. Consequently, many instruments reflect the areas of importance to researchers and clinicians, rather than patients.

Recently, the term 'health-related quality of life' has been introduced. Patrick and Erickson[22] defined health-related quality of life as 'the value assigned to duration of life as modified by the impairments, functional states, perceptions, and social opportunities that are influenced by disease, injury, treatment, or policy'. However, the term 'health-related quality of life' is inappropriate because it suggests that patients should be able to attribute how they feel and how they behave to different causes.

For example, the Medical Outcomes Study (MOS) Short-Form General Health Survey (SF-36)[23] asks: 'During the *past 4 weeks*, have you had any of the following problems with your work or other regular daily activities *as a result of your physical health*?' This question is then asked again, but in relation to 'any emotional problems'. In reality, this kind of attribution is rarely possible. Furthermore, it is not possible to ignore other important influences on health and quality of life. For example, McKenna et al.[24] found that employed depressed patients responded better to treatment with fluoxetine than unemployed patients, as measured by the General Well-Being Index (GWBI)[25] and MADRS.[14]

A needs-based model of quality of life has recently been developed.[26] The theory underlying the approach is that a condition will have a detrimental effect on quality of life if it prevents the patient from fulfilling his or her needs. Under this approach, quality of life is seen as going beyond health status and HRQL, in that such factors (in addition to others) are seen as influences on, rather than being an integral part of, the construct.[27] Many disease-specific instruments have been produced on the basis of this model. They have been shown to be highly acceptable and relevant to patients and to have excellent psychometric properties.[28-36]

Any QOL measure must be based on a theory or model of the construct (i.e. the attribute that the instrument is intended to measure). Only then can it be shown to have construct validity.[37] However, most instruments that claim to measure quality of life have no theoretical basis, listing areas or components considered to be important by the authors.[23]

It is argued that patients and clinicians differ in their assessment of the severity of illness and the effect of treatment.[24,38] In the area of quality of life, the patient is the only valid source of information.[39] Consequently, the items included in measures should be derived from relevant patients rather than other sources.[25] Where the items for a questionnaire are derived from relevant patients through in-depth interviews, the face and content validity of the measure is ensured.

The result of not developing a measure in this way is exemplified by Rost and associates.[40] These authors designed an outcomes module for major depression and dysthymia that focused on diagnosis and severity. This rather complex and long package was created by members of an expert panel, who selected parts of existing measures and reduced the length of others considered to be too long. The measure has poor reliability and was unable to show differences between patients who had received pharmacological treatment for 8 weeks and those who had not. The poor psychometric performance of this instrument reflects its method of development.

All measures must be shown to be reliable, internally consistent and valid before they are used in clinical trials. Test-retest reliability is expressed as a correlation, and the currently recommended minimum value is 0.85.[41] Values below this level indicate too high a proportion of measurement error, and low levels of reliability also limit the instrument's validity.[37]

The internal consistency of an instrument is an estimate of the extent to which its items are inter-related. It is usually represented by Cronbach's α coefficient and values below 0.7 are indicative of individual items not contributing to the overall scale.[37] Internal consistency is often quoted in place of test-retest reliability. However, authors have argued recently that internal consistency is an inappropriate and insufficient estimate of reliability.[37,42] Furthermore, α is also often used as evidence for the undimensionality of a scale. Again, use of the statistic in this way has been shown to be incorrect.[42,43]

Proving the validity of a measure is more complex. It cannot be done in a single study, but rather evidence grows over time with use. Test developers often correlate scores on the new measure with those obtained on an established measure. Where this is done, the comparator measure must be reliable and valid and assess a relevant construct.

4. Quality-of-Life Instruments for Depression and Anxiety

Hunt and McKenna[26] used their model of quality of life as a basis for developing the Quality of Life in Depression Scale (QLDS). They defined quality of life as the extent to which a person's needs are met. An impairment will have a detrimental effect on quality of life if it prevents, or interferes with, a person's ability to fulfil his or her needs. Hunt and McKenna[26] argued that deriving items for an instrument from in-depth interviews with many relevant patients ensures that the areas of concern to them are covered in the questionnaire. In addition, using the actual words of the patients enhances the questionnaire's acceptability to respondents.

The QLDS was developed in this way, and proved to have excellent reliability (test-retest correlation = 0.94 for patients with stable depression; n = 37) and internal consistency (Cronbach's $\alpha = 0.95$; n = 74). Construct validity was shown by correlating QLDS scores with scores on the GWBI (n = 65).[28]

A Dutch version of the measure was developed in parallel with the UK version, and was shown to have equally good psychometric properties.[44] This version has been used in a general practitioner (GP)-based study of depression in The Netherlands.[44] The measure was found to be acceptable to patients and to show clear improvements in quality of life with treatment. Median scores on the QLDS were 22, 14, 8 and 6 at baseline and after 4 weeks, 8 weeks and 6 months of treatment with fluoxetine, respectively (scores on the QLDS can range from zero to 34, with a high score indicating poor quality of life). Thus, the measure is responsive to effective treatment of depression. Evidence of the validity of the Dutch version has also been provided from studies in depressed patients over the age of 60 years.[45]

Validated versions of the QLDS are available for the UK, The Netherlands, Canada (French and English), Denmark, France, Germany/Austria, Italy, Morocco, Spain and the US.[28,44-48] Further adaptations are in preparation for Australia, Brazil, Finland, Israel, Norway, Russia, South Africa (English and Afrikaans) and Sweden.

The SmithKline Beecham Quality of Life Scale (SBQOL)[49] was designed for use in patients with affective disorders. The basis of the measure was the broad definition put forward by Joyce:[50] that is, quality of life is 'what the patient says it is'. The authors argued that the Repertory Grid Technique[51] is the ideal method of utilising this rather imprecise definition. However, such a technique is impractical in the clinical situation and makes comparisons between patients difficult. To overcome these problems, they used predefined elements and constructs identified from the literature. Thus, the content of the measure was not derived from patients, a basic requirement of all QOL measures. Furthermore, respondents are asked to make many hypothetical judgements, raising questions about the validity of the measure.

The reliability and validity of the SBQOL were tested on 110 patients with generalised anxiety disorder or major depression.[49] The test-retest reliability coefficients (with an interval of only 2 days between administrations) ranged from 0.66 to 0.83,[49] indicating inadequate reliability. The Cronbach's α coefficients ranged from 0.85 to 0.95, indicating adequate internal consistency. The HDRS, HARS, HAD, GHQ and the Sickness Impact Profile (SIP)[52] were used to validate the SBQOL, but all have limitations as validation instruments for QOL measures.

Although the SBQOL demonstrates adequate internal consistency, it has poor test-retest reliability. In addition, its scoring is somewhat cumbersome, yielding three total scores (self now, sick self and ideal self), two total distances (self now/sick self and self now/ideal self) and other more complex scores, such as flexigrid distances.

Revicki et al.[53] developed a health-related QOL battery for the evaluation of antidepressant therapy. The authors used literature searches and discussions with clinicians to identify areas that should be covered in the Depression-Specific Quality of Life Battery (DQOLB). The instrument is made up of scales taken from the MOS[54] (health perceptions, energy and vitality, and cognitive function) and the SIP (alertness behaviour, work behaviour and home management). Social activity and interaction were assessed with a Social Behaviour scale.[55] In addition, two single items were included: number of disability days[56,57] and life satisfaction.[58]

Test-retest reliability was assessed by intraclass correlation coefficients, three of which were below the required level of 0.85 [cognitive function (MOS), work behaviour (SIP) and social behaviour; n = 28]. The authors reported that all the scales apart from work behaviour were responsive to changes in depression severity, as measured by the MADRS.

However, only three of the scales showed a statistically significant change after 21 days of antidepressant treatment, despite a substantial improvement in MADRS score. These three scales were the MOS-cognitive function, social behaviour and life satisfaction scales, two of which were among the least reliable. The authors point out that all the change scores were in the expected direction, but only the MOS-energy change scores approached statistical significance (p = 0.098). From these results it cannot be concluded that the DQOLB is responsive to change in depression severity, especially as the assertion is based on only 12 patients. Furthermore, as the instrument is not founded on a theory of quality of life, it is not possible to establish whether it has construct validity.[37]

Endicott et al.[59] developed the Quality of Life Enjoyment and Satisfaction Questionnaire (Q-LES-Q), which covers areas of daily functioning and is intended for use with many medical and psychiatric conditions. It has 93 items, 91 of which make up eight subscale scores, and two of which are single items. The Q-LES-Q was shown to have adequate internal consistency with all Cronbach's α values above 0.90 (n = 83). However, test-retest reliability was very poor, with only the school/course work scale having a coefficient value of above 0.85. This section was only completed by 6 of the 54 patients included in the study.

Other scales used in studies of depression include the SF-36,[23] the Salamon-Conte Life Satisfaction in the Elderly Scale (LSES)[60] and the Social Adjustment Scale (SAS).[61] The SF-36 assesses function and limited aspects of well-being, the LSES assesses life satisfaction, and the SAS addresses social and interpersonal relationships. Although they are often mistakenly referred to as such, none of these fulfil the requirements for a measure of quality of life.

No measures of quality of life specific to anxiety were identified in the literature.

Care must be taken to ensure that the content is appropriate when selecting instruments to assess the severity of condition and health status in elderly patients. For example, the applicability of the HDRS[12,13] to elderly patients has been questioned,[62] particularly since its validity was tested in young patients. The SF-36 has been shown to be inappropriate for use in elderly patients.[63-65] In contrast, Mesters et al.[66] used the QLDS in elderly patients and found it to be well accepted. The Nottingham Health Profile[67] is currently used with elderly depressed patients to assess their physical, emotional and social distress.

5. Studies of Quality of Life in Depression and Anxiety

Little work has focused on the quality of life of patients with depression and anxiety. There has been research in related areas of health status, such as well-being and function.

Massion, Warshaw and Keller[68] conducted a study of the quality of life of patients with panic disorder and generalised anxiety disorder. To assess quality of life, they used the Modified Short Form Health Survey[69] and items from the Longitudinal Interval Follow-Up Evaluation.[70] The authors reported on co-morbidity, overall functioning, emotional health, suicide and hospitalisations, severity of panic, and role, marital and social functioning. However, most of the data presented were frequencies; for example, the percentage of patients reporting that they were unable to get along with their spouses very well.

Markowitz et al.[71] took quality of life to include physical and emotional health, alcohol and drug abuse, suicide attempts, social and marital functioning, financial dependency and use of treatment. Separate measures for each area were used but no detailed descriptions of them were given. Patients with panic disorder and major depression were at risk from poor physical and emotional health, abuse of alcohol or drugs, attempted suicide, financial dependence, spending less time on their hobbies and having poor marital relations. In addition, they found that such patients used clinicians (general medicine and psychiatric) and hospital emergency departments more frequently. The study suggested that patients with anxiety and depression place a great burden on care providers.

Fifer and coworkers[72] found that primary care patients with untreated anxiety had reduced functioning and well-being compared to those without anxiety. Although they claimed to have measured quality of life, they actually used the SF-36.

6. Effect of Drug Treatment on Quality of Life in Patients with Depression

Very few published studies are available on the effect of drug treatment on quality of life in depression.

Mesters et al.[66] conducted an open multicentre study on the effect of treatment with fluoxetine on the quality of life of depressed patients over the age of 60 years. The Dutch version of the QLDS was used to assess quality of life. There was an improvement in depression (as measured by the HDRS) after 2 weeks' treatment. Symptoms continued to improve over the 8-week study period and the frequency of adverse events decreased. Mean QLDS scores changed from 23.1 at baseline to 8.4 after 8 weeks' treatment,[45] indicating a substantial improvement in quality of life.

Lonnqvist and colleagues[73] conducted a double-blind study, which was designed to evaluate clinical efficacy and quality of life, of moclobemide (a reversible inhibitor of monamine oxidase) and fluoxetine. Both drugs have been shown to be effective in placebo-controlled trials in patients with depression.[74,75] However, to assess quality of life, the authors used the MOS Short-Form General Health Survey (SF-20),[69] an instrument that was replaced by the SF-36 in an attempt to increase precision of measurement.[23] They also used the 15D Measure of Quality of Life.[76] This consists of 15 items, including breathing, mental function, sight, movement, working, hearing, sleep, social participation and perceived health. It concentrates on symptoms and function rather than quality of life.

At the 2-week evaluation, moclobemide was found to be better than fluoxetine in the role and physical functioning subscales of the SF-20, and in the 15D score. However, there were no differences between the treatments after 6 weeks. The authors reported that the dimension scores of the SF-20 correlated well with the 15D total scores, and that most of the dimension scores correlated with the HDRS scores. However, the correlations were not reported. It was concluded that moclobemide was preferable in these evaluations. Care should be taken when evaluating studies that employed unreliable measures of function and well-being, particularly where change with treatment is being assessed.

The GWBI[25] was used by McKenna and associates[24] to assess the well-being of depressed patients. They reported an improvement in well-being with fluoxetine treatment, and that this was accompanied by an improvement in the severity of depression as measured by the MADRS.

Evans et al.[77] found that cancer patients with major depression or depressive symptoms, who were adequately treated with imipramine or similar therapy, showed better psychosocial adjustment to their cancer, as measured by the Psychosocial Adjustment to Illness Scale,[78] compared with patients who did not receive adequate antidepressant treatment. Although this was a pilot study, it has important implications. If patients can cope better with their physical illness when associated secondary depression is treated, then their quality of life might be expected to improve.

Patients are often excluded from clinical trials if they have concomitant medical conditions. However, patients with a psychiatric disorder often have another medical condition.[79]

The studies discussed earlier in this section all involved patients in psychiatric settings. It has been argued that pathophysiology, severity, history and causation are different in patients with major depressive syndromes seen in the medical setting, compared with those seen in the psychiatric setting.[80] If this is so, it raises doubts about whether findings from trials in psychiatric environments can be applied to primary medical care. This is an important concern, because it has been estimated that 90 to 95% of patients with diagnosed depression are treated by GPs.[81,82]

There is also the problem of drug compliance in the primary care setting. Katon et al.[83] found that a number of patients did not receive an adequate dosage or duration of treatment with antidepressants. Between 20 and 60% of primary care patients cease taking antidepressants within 3 weeks of starting them because of adverse effects, early recovery or worsening of symptoms.[84,85] However, it is recommended that antidepressants are taken for at least 4 months after the acute symptoms have been treated.[86-88]

7. Effect of Drug Treatment on Quality of Life in Patients with Anxiety

Few studies have been conducted into the effects of treatment on quality of life in patients with anxiety. In our literature search, no clinical trials assessing quality of life were identified. Most studies reported on alleviation of symptoms and adverse effects only.

Benzodiazepines provide safe and effective short term anxiolytic therapy. However, with long term use, they have negative effects such as dependence, problems with withdrawal, and sedation.[89-91] Alprazolam is a benzodiazepine that is used in the treatment of panic disorder, anxiety associated with depression, and mild reactive depression. In a review of 84 controlled studies, Jonas and Cohon[92] concluded that alprazolam was at least as effective as the active comparator drugs used in the studies (e.g. imipramine and diazepam). The authors found that the most commonly reported adverse effects of the benzodiazepines were drowsiness, sedation, light-headedness and headache. The serious adverse events that had previously been associated with the benzodiazepines, such as suicide, hostility and depression, occurred rarely with any of the drugs in the studies reviewed. It was concluded that these adverse effects could be attributable to the psychiatric disorder itself rather than to its treatment.

Buspirone has been shown to be as clinically effective as the benzodiazepines in anxiety, and has many advantages over other treatments. It is less likely than other anxiolytics to cause drowsiness and sedation[93,94] and does not appear to cause dependence[95] or problems with withdrawal.[93,96]

Given the emphasis in these studies on the adverse effects of treatment, there is a clear need for QOL studies using anxiety-specific instruments.

8. Costs of Depression and Anxiety

Because clinicians have to work under increasingly tight budgetary restraints within the UK National Health Service and in other health organisations around the world, it is no longer sufficient to prove the merits of new drug treatments simply in terms of clinical efficacy and tolerability. QOL measures have a vital part to play in economic analyses.

Feighner[97] has argued that only 12% of the cost of depression results from diagnosis and treatment of the disorder. Patients with depression miss more work days, have more bed disability days and more illness days than nondepressed patients.[57,98] In 1992, Kind and Sorensen[99] estimated the annual direct cost of depression in England and Wales to be £420 million (£1 ≈ $US1.60, July 1995). They reported that drugs account for only a small percentage of this figure, with admissions to mental hospitals accounting for the highest proportion. Similarly, Souêtre et al.[100] found hospitalisation to be a major cost in patients with generalised anxiety disorder, although drugs contributed only a small part of the total cost.

Our literature search failed to locate studies that have addressed quality of life as part of economic analyses of depression and anxiety.

9. Discussion

Although major depression is common and information is readily available to the clinician, it has been shown that one-third to one-half of primary care patients with major depression in the USA are not diagnosed correctly.[56,79] Even if correctly diagnosed, patients are often not adequately treated.[101] Similarly, Fifer and associates[72] found that only 44% of primary care patients with anxiety were recognised as such and treated accordingly.

Henry[102] described the Depression Cascade. In this hypothetical model, only five out of 100 depressed people in the community will benefit from treatment. This is based on reported recognition rates,[103,104] adequate treatment rates,[105] compliance rates[106] and positive response to appropriate treatment.[107] Even after diagnosis and after drug treatment is prescribed, the Depression Cascade suggests that 50% of patients will not benefit from treatment because of noncompliance and a lack of positive response. These two factors are directly related to the choice of drug and its effect on quality of life. Therefore, it is vital that clinicians, both in the psychiatric and general medical setting, are provided with accurate information about the effects of available drugs on quality of life.

At present, the main distinguishing feature between various antidepressants and anxiolytics is their adverse effect profile. These are sometimes difficult to identify[108] and constitute only one influence on quality of life. At its best, QOL assessment will provide an accurate picture of the overall impact of the illness and its treatment on the patient, including the impact of adverse effects of the treatment.

Henry[102] reported that at any one time 3 to 5% of the UK population have depression, and that 1.9% of the total UK drug bill in 1990 was spent on antidepressants. With prevalence rates and treatment costs as high as these, effective and optimal therapy is vital.

10. Conclusions

With the wide choice of treatments available for depression and anxiety, QOL assessment should be accompanied by well designed economic analyses. While the newer treatments are more expensive, they have advantages in terms of acceptability to patients, quality of life and tolerability.

It is surprising that so little work has been carried out to establish the economic benefits of the treatment of anxiety and depression. In some countries, such studies are likely to be required in support of reimbursement and pricing submissions for new pharmaceutical products.

Depression and anxiety both have a detrimental effect on quality of life. Studies have shown that effective treatment can do much to improve the quality of life of patients with depression. However, the amount of research conducted in the area is very limited, especially in the case of anxiety. Indeed, our literature search failed to identify a measure of quality of life that was suitable for use in anxious patients. Given the prevalence of anxiety and its distressing and debilitating nature, there is an urgent need for such an instrument.

References

1. American Psychiatric Association. Diagnostic and statistical manual of mental disorders. 3rd rev. ed. Washington, DC: American Psychiatric Association, 1987
2. Rickels K. Antianxiety therapy: potential value of long-term treatment. J Clin Psychiatry 1987; 48 Suppl.: 7-11
3. Leckman JF, Weissman MM, Merikangas KR, et al. Panic disorder and major depression: increased risk of depression, alcoholism, panic and phobic disorders of depressed probands in families of depressed probands with panic disorder. Arch Gen Psychiatry 1983; 40: 1055-160

4. Robinson DS, Kayser A, Corcella J, et al. Panic attacks in outpatients with depression: response to antidepressant treatment. Psychopharmacol Bull 1985; 21: 562-7
5. Clancy J, Noyes Jr R, Hoenk PR, et al. Secondary depression and anxiety neurosis. J Nerv Ment Dis 1978; 166: 846-50
6. Breier A, Charney DS, Heninger GR. Major depression in panic disorder. Arch Gen Psychiatry 1984; 41: 1125-39
7. Zung WWK. A self-rating depression scale. Arch Gen Psychiatry 1965; 12: 63-70
8. Beck AT, Ward CH, Mendelson M, et al. An inventory for measuring depression. Arch Gen Psychiatry 1961; 4: 561-71
9. Carroll BJ, Feinberg M, Smouse PE, et al. The Carroll rating scale for depression: I. Development, reliability and validation. Br J Psychiatry 1981; 138: 194-200
10. Radloff LS. The CES-D scale: a self report depression scale for research in the general population. Appl Psychol Measurement 1977; 1: 385-401
11. Weissman MM, Sholomskas D, Pottenger M, et al. Assessing depressive symptoms in five psychiatric populations: a validation study. Am J Epidemiol 1977; 106: 203-14
12. Hamilton M. A rating scale for depression. J Neurol Neurosurg Psychiatry 1960; 23: 56-62
13. Hamilton M. Development of a rating scale for primary depressive illness. Br J Soc Clin Psychol 1967; 6: 276-96
14. Montgomery SA, Åsberg M. A new depression scale designed to be sensitive to change. Br J Psychiatry 1979; 134: 382-9
15. Hamilton M. The assessment of anxiety states by rating. Br J Med Psychol 1959; 32: 50-5
16. Snaith RP, Baugh SJ, Clayden AD, et al. The Clinical Anxiety Scale: a modification of the Hamilton Anxiety Scale. Br J Psychiatry 1982; 141: 518-23
17. Beck AT, Epstein N, Brown G, et al. An inventory for measuring clinical anxiety: psychometric properties. J Consult Clin Psychol 1988; 56: 893-7
18. Derogatis LR. SCL-90-R: administration, scoring and procedures manual II. Towson (MD): Clinical Psychometrics Research, 1983
19. Goldberg D. The detection of psychiatric illness by questionnaire. London: Oxford University Press, 1972
20. Zigmond AS, Snaith RP. The hospital anxiety and depression scale. Acta Psychiatr Scand 1983; 67: 361-70
21. Rudorfer MV, Potter WZ. Antidepressants: a comparative review of the clinical pharmacology and therapeutic use of the 'newer' versus the 'older' drugs. Drugs 1989; 37: 713-38
22. Patrick DL, Erickson P. Health status and health policy. New York: Oxford University Press, 1993
23. Ware JE, Sherbourne CD. The MOS 36-Item Short-Form Health Survey (SF-36): 1. Conceptual framework and item selection. Med Care 1992; 30: 473-83
24. McKenna SP, Hunt SM, Tennant A. Psychological well-being in depressed patients. Int J Methods Psychiatr Res 1993; 3: 245-51
25. Hunt SM, McKenna SP. A British adaptation of the General Well-Being Index: a new tool for clinical research. Br J Med Econ 1992; 2: 49-60
26. Hunt SM, McKenna SP. The QLDS: a scale for the measurement of quality of life in depression. Health Policy 1992; 22: 307-19
27. McKenna SP, Whalley D, Doward LC. Which outcomes are important in schizophrenia? Int J Methods Psych Res. In press
28. McKenna SP, Hunt SM. A new measure of quality of life in depression: testing the reliability and construct validity of the QLDS. Health Policy 1992; 22: 321-30
29. Holmes SJ, McKenna SP, Doward LC, et al. Development of a questionnaire to assess the quality of life of adults with growth hormone deficiency. Endocrinol Metab 1995; 2: 63-9
30. McKenna SP, Doward LC, Alonso J, et al. The QoL-AGHDA: an instrument for the assessment of quality of life in adults with growth hormone deficiency. Qual Life Res 1999; 8: 373-83
31. Wagner TH, Patrick DL, McKenna SP, et al. Cross-cultural development of a quality of life measure for men with erection difficulties. Qual Life Res 1996; 5: 443-9
32. Whalley D, McKenna SP, de Jong Z, et al. Quality of life in rheumatoid arthritis. Br J Rheumatol 1997; 36: 884-8
33. de Jong Z, van der Heijde D, McKenna SP, et al. The reliability and construct validity of the RAQoL: a rheumatoid arthritis-specific quality of life instrument. Br J Rheumatol 1997; 36: 878-83
34. Doward LC, McKenna SP, Kohlmann T, et al. The international development of the RGHQoL: a quality of life measure for recurrent genital herpes. Qual Life Res 1998; 7: 143-53
35. McKenna SP, Doward LC, Mackenzie Davey K. The development and psychometric properties of the MSQOL; a migraine-specific quality-of-life instrument. Clin Drug Invest 1998; 15: 413-23
36. McKenna SP, Whalley D, Renck-Hooper U, et al. The development of a quality of life instrument for use with post-menopausal women with urogenital atrophy in the UK and Sweden. Qual Life Res 1999; 8: 393-8
37. Streiner DL, Norman GR. Health measurement scales: a practical guide to their development and use. Second Edition. New York: Oxford University Press, 1995
38. Prusoff B, Klerman G, Paykel E. Concordance between clinical assessments and patients' self report in depression. Arch Gen Psychiatry 1972; 26: 546-52
39. Berzon R, Hays RD, Shumaker SA. International use, application and performance of health-related quality of life instruments. Qual Life Res 1993; 2: 367-8
40. Rost K, Smith GR, Burnman MA, et al. Measuring the outcomes of care for mental health problems: the case of depressive disorders. Med Care 1992; 30 (5 Suppl.): MS266-73
41. Weiner E, Stewart B. Assessing individuals. Boston: Little Brown, 1984
42. Cortina JM. What is coefficient alpha? An examination of theory and applications. J Appl Psychol 1993; 78: 98-104
43. Green SB, Lissitz RW, Mulaik SA. Limitations of coefficient alpha as an index of the test unidimensionality. Educ Psychological Measure 1977; 37: 827-38

44. Tuynman-Qua H, de Jonghe F, McKenna SP. Quality of Life in Depression Scale (QLDS). Development, reliability, validity, responsiveness and application. Eur Psychiatry 1997; 12: 199-202
45. Grégoire J, de Leval N, Mesters P, et al. Validation of the Quality of Life in Depression Scale in a population of adult depressive patients aged 60 and above. Qual Life Res 1994; 3: 13-9
46. Mercier C, Piat M, McKenna SP. Cultural adaptation and validation of the Quality of Life in Depression Scale in Canada. Qual Life Res 1995; 4: 462-3
47. Cervera-Enguix S, Ramírez N, Girala N, et al. The development and validation of a Spanish version of the Quality of Life in Depression Scale (QLDS). Eur Psychiatry 1999; 14: 392-8
48. McKenna SP, Doward LC, Kohlmann T, et al. International development of the Quality of Life in Depression Scale. J Affect Disord. In press
49. Stoker MJ, Dunbar GC, Beaumont G. The SmithKline Beecham 'quality of life' scale: a validation and reliability study in patient with affective disorder. Qual Life Res 1992; 1: 385-95
50. Joyce CRB. Report from the European Standard for Clinical Trials (ESCT) meeting in Strasbourg 23-24 May 1991, on issues of concern in the standardization and harmonization of drug trials in Europe: health-related quality of life session. Qual Life Newsletter 1992; 3: 10
51. Kelly GA. The psychology of personal constructs. New York: WW Norton, 1955
52. Bergner M, Bobbitt RA, Carter WB, et al. The sickness impact profile: development and final revision of a health status measure. Med Care 1981; 19: 787-805
53. Revicki DA, Turner R, Brown R, et al. Reliability and validity of health-related quality of life battery for evaluating outpatient antidepressant treatment. Qual Life Res 1992; 1: 257-66
54. Stewart AL, Ware JE. Measuring functioning and well-being: the Medical Outcomes Study approach. Durham (NC): Duke University Press, 1992
55. Omvik P, Thaulow E, Herland OB, et al. Double-blind, parallel, comparative study on quality of life during treatment with amlodipine or enalapril in mild or moderate hypertensive patients: a multicenter study. J Hypertens 1993; 11: 103-13
56. Wells KB, Stewart A, Hays RD, et al. The functioning and well-being of depressed patients: results from the medical outcomes study. JAMA 1989; 262: 914-9
57. Broadhead WE, Blazer DG, George LK, et al. Depression, disability days, and days lost from work in a prospective epidemiologic survey. JAMA 1990; 264: 2524-8
58. Campbell A, Converse PE, Rogers WL. The quality of American life. New York: Russell Sage Foundation, 1976
59. Endicott J, Nee J, Harrison W, et al. Quality of life enjoyment and satisfaction questionnaire: a new measure. Department of Psychiatry, Columbia University and New York State Psychiatric Institute. Psychopharmacol Bull 1993; 29: 321-6
60. Salamon MJ, Conte VA. The life satisfaction in the elderly scale. Odessa (FL): Psychological Assessment Resources, 1984
61. Schooler N, Hogarty G, Weissman MM. Social Adjustment Scale II (SASII). In: Hargreaves WA, Attkisson CC, Sorensen JE, editors. Resource materials for community health program evaluators. Publ. No. (ADM) 79-328. Washington, DC: US Department of Health, Education and Welfare, 1979: 290-330
62. Gershon S. The conduct of clinical trials in the impaired elderly. Psychopharmacol Bull 1981; 17: 108-16
63. Hill S, Harries U. Assessing the outcome of health care for older people in community settings: should we use the SF-36? Outcomes Briefing 1994 Aug; 4: 26-7
64. Brazier J, Harper R, Jones N, et al. Validating the SF-36 health survey questionnaire: new outcome measure for primary care. BMJ 1992; 305: 160-4
65. Jenkinson C, Coutler A, Wright L. Short form 36 (SF 36) health survey questionnaire: normative data for adults of working age. BMJ 1993; 306: 1437-40
66. Mesters P, Cosyns P, Dejaiffe G, et al. Assessment of quality of life in the treatment of major depressive disorder with fluoxetine, 20 mg, in ambulatory patients aged over 60 years. Int Clin Psychopharmacol 1993; 8: 337-40
67. Hunt SM, McEwen J, McKenna SP. Measuring health status. London: Croom Helm, 1986
68. Massion AO, Warshaw MG, Keller MB. Quality of life and psychiatric morbidity in panic disorder and generalized anxiety disorder. Am J Psychiatry 1993; 150: 600-7
69. Stewart AL, Hays RD, Ware JE. The MOS Short-Form General Health Survey: reliability and validity in a patient population. Med Care 1988; 26: 724-35
70. Keller MB, Lavori PW, Friedman B, et al. The longitudinal interval follow-up evaluation: a comprehensive method for assessing outcome in prospective longitudinal studies. Arch Gen Psychiatry 1987; 44: 540-8
71. Markowitz JS, Weissman MM, Ouellette R, et al. Quality of life in panic disorder. Arch Gen Psychiatry 1989; 46: 984-92
72. Fifer SK, Mathias SD, Patrick DL, et al. Untreated anxiety among adult primary care patients in a health maintenance organization. Arch Gen Psychiatry 1994; 51: 740-50
73. Lonnqvist J, Sintonen H, Syvalahti E, et al. Antidepressant efficacy and quality of life in depression: a double-blind study with moclobemide and fluoxetine. Acta Psychiatr Scand 1994; 89 (6): 363-9
74. Silverstone T. Moclobemide placebo-controlled trials. Int Clin Psychopharmacol 1993; 7 (3-4): 133-6
75. Hall J. Fluoxetine: efficacy against placebo and by dose – an overview. Br J Psychiatry 1988; 153 (3 Suppl.): 59-63
76. Sintonen H, Pekurinen M. A generic 15 dimensional measure of health-related quality of life (15D). J Social Med 1989; 26: 85-96
77. Evans DW, McCartney CF, Haggerty JJ, et al. Treatment of depression in cancer patients is associated with better life adaptation: a pilot study. Psychosom Med 1988; 50 (1): 72-6
78. Derogatis LR. The psychosocial adjustment to illness scale (PAIS). J Psychosom Res 1986; 30 (1): 77-91
79. Katon W, Sullivan M. Depression and chronic medical illness. J Clin Psychiatry 1990; 51 (6 Suppl.): 3-14
80. Schulberg H, Coulehan J, Block M, et al. Strategies for evaluating treatments for major depression in primary care patients. Gen Hosp Psychiatry 1991; 13: 9-18

81. Thompson C, Thompson CM. The prescribing of antidepressants in general practice: I. A critical review. Human Psychopharmacol 1989; 4: 190
82. Paykel ES, Freeling P, Hollyman JA. Are tricyclic antidepressants useful for mild depression? A placebo controlled trial. Pharmacopsychiatry 1988; 21: 15-8
83. Katon W, von Korff M, Lin E, et al. Adequacy and duration of antidepressant treatment in primary care. Med Care 1992; 30: 67-76
84. Johnson DAW. Treatment of depression in general practice. BMJ 1973; 2: 18-20
85. Thompson J, Rankin H, Ashcroft CW, et al. The treatment of depression in general practice. Psychol Med 1982; 12: 741-51
86. Doogan DP, Caillard V. Sertraline in the prevention of depression. Br J Psychiatry 1992; 160: 217-22
87. Klerman GL, Dimascio A, Weissman A, et al. Treatment of depression by drugs and psychotherapy. Am J Psychiatry 1974; 131: 186-91
88. Montgomery SA, Dunbar GC. Paroxetine is better than placebo in relapse prevention and the prophylaxis of recurrent depression. Int J Psychopharmacol 1993; 8: 189-95
89. Lader M. Dependence on benzodiazepines. J Clin Psychiatry 1983; 44: 121-7
90. Winokur A, Rickels K, Greenblatt DJ. Withdrawal reaction from long-term, low dosage administration of diazepam. Arch Gen Psychiatry 1980; 37: 101-5
91. Rickels K, Csanalosi I, Greisman P, et al. A controlled clinical trial of alprazolam for the treatment of anxiety. Am J Psychiatry 1983; 140: 82-5
92. Jonas JM, Cohon MS. A comparison of the safety and efficacy of alprazolam versus other agents in the treatment of anxiety, panic, and depression: a review of the literature. J Clin Psychiatry 1993; 54 Suppl.: 25-48
93. Goa KL, Ward A. Buspirone: a preliminary review of its pharmacological properties and therapeutic efficacy as an anxiolytic. Drugs 1986; 32: 114-29
94. Rickels K, Cohen D, Csanalosi I, et al. Alprazolam and imipramine in depressed outpatients: a controlled study. Curr Ther Res 1982; 32 (6): 157-64
95. Cole JO, Orzack MH, Beake B, et al. Assessment of the abuse liability of buspirone in recreational sedative users. J Clin Psychiatry 1982; 43 (12 Sect. 2): 69-74
96. Murphy SM, Owen RT, Tyrer PJ. Withdrawal symptoms after six weeks treatment with diazepam [abstract]. Lancet 1984; 2: 1389
97. Feighner JP. A double-blind comparison of paroxetine, imipramine and placebo in depressed outpatients. In: Ashcroft GW, editor. Depression – a once in a lifetime event? Oxford: Clinical Neuroscience Publishers, 1991
98. Johnson J, Weissman MM, Klerman GL. Service utilization and social morbidity associated with depressive symptoms in the community. JAMA 1992; 267: 1478-83
99. Kind P, Sorensen J. The costs of depression. Third international symposium: RIMAs in subtypes of depression: focus on moclobemide; 1992: Vienna. Int Clin Psychopharmacol 1993; 7 (3-4): 191-5
100. Souêtre E, Lozet H, Cimarosti I. Cost of anxiety disorders: impact of comorbidity. J Psychosom Res 1994; 38 (1 Suppl.): 151-60
101. Keller MB, Shapiro RW, Lavori PW, et al. Relapse in major depressive disorder: analysis with life table. Arch Gen Psychiatry 1982; 39: 911-5
102. Henry JA. Debits and credits in the management of depression. Br J Psychiatry 1993; 163 Suppl. 20: 33-9
103. Murphy GRE. The physician's responsibility for suicide: 1. An error of commission; and 2. Errors of omission. Ann Intern Med 1975; 82: 301-9
104. Katon W, Roy-Byrne PP. Antidepressants in the medically ill: diagnosis and treatment in primary care. Clin Chem 1988; 34 (5): 829-36
105. Prescott LF, Highley MS. Drugs prescribed for self-poisoners. BMJ 1985; 290: 1633-6
106. Weissman MM. The epidemiology of suicide attempts, 1960-1971. Arch Gen Psychiatry 1974; 30: 737-46
107. Gerner R, Estabrook W, Steuer J, et al. Treatment of geriatric depression with trazodone, imipramine and placebo: a double-blind study. J Clin Psychiatry 1980; 41: 216-20
108. Henry JA. The safety of antidepressants. Br J Psychiatry 1992; 160: 439-41

Correspondence: *Diane Whalley*, Galen Research, Enterprise House, Manchester Science Park, Lloyd Street North, Manchester M15 6SE, England.

Constraints on Antidepressant Prescribing and Principles of Cost-Effective Antidepressant Use

Part 1: Depression and its Treatment

John A. Henry and *Carol A. Rivas*

St Mary's Hospital, London, England

Society is increasingly concerned about the impact of depression on public health. Following campaigns in the US and UK directed towards primary-care physicians, the treatment of depression has become a high priority in the last decade.[1,2] By focusing on awareness of the illness, the campaigns ultimately aimed to increase the number of patients who receive suitable treatment.

However, at first glance, this objective appears to be incompatible with the worldwide focus on the costs of healthcare. The situation has been compounded by the introduction and promotion, in the last few years, of clinically attractive, but more expensive, antidepressants. As a result, there is a need for accurate and relevant analyses of the cost effectiveness of antidepressant treatment. Such analyses must ultimately make it possible to reliably compare the burden of untreated illness, the effects of various treatments, and the human and clinical benefits of using these different treatments.

This is the approach followed by this review. Part 1 gives an overview of the economic and human burden of depression, and how treatment affects this. The antidepressants are considered from a clinical perspective, with consideration of influences on prescribing, as well as measures adopted in various countries to control treatment costs. Part 2 (page 195) takes the data one step further, and considers the way that cost-effectiveness and cost-utility studies are developed, how they have been used to compare the different antidepressants, and the conclusions that can be drawn. There is also discussion of the costs associated with different treatments, which are often omitted from costings studies, but are important.

1. The Burden of Depression

Depression is a common disorder. Each year, 2 to 3 million people in the UK experience depression that requires medical care.[3-5] In England and Wales, this is equivalent to a 12-month prevalence rate of 30 to 50 per 1000 individuals,[3-5] with a lifetime prevalence of 50 to 100 per 1000.[6,7] Estimates of the 12-month prevalence rate in the US range from 20 to 250 per 1000 individuals;[2,8] for example, Stoudemire et al.[9] reported a 6-month prevalence rate of 22 to 32 per 1000 for major depression. Precise figures depend on the types of depression included in the estimate. With such a high prevalence, it is clear that treatment options for patients with depression deserve careful consideration because of the magnitude of the cost implications.

Depression is not only common, but tends to have a chronic time course. Untreated episodes of depression often last several months (20% can last at least 2 years). They subsequently recur, and 30% of patients report depressive symptoms between acute episodes.[10] This chronicity amplifies the negative effects that depression has on quality of life. A depressed person often withdraws from social and employment activities, with days spent at home or in bed or with impaired functioning.[11-13] This may be the result of physical as well as emotional and psychological symptoms.[2,14] Many depressive symptoms are somaticised,[15-17] leading to a similar level of physical impairment to that observed in patients with severe chronic medical disorders.[13,14,18-20] This is true even of milder depressive disorders, which have fewer symptoms and a less-consistent potential for disability;[21,22] even though symptoms come and go, they are usually present for at least 2 weeks at a time.

The damage done to a patient's employment and domestic life by the psychological, emotional and physical problems of depression may be irreparable, even when the disease has remitted or responded to treatment. There are significant cost implications for both the individual and society, but they are difficult to assess accurately in cost analyses. Moreover, patients with depression also have more physical illnesses (considering only those that are apparently unrelated to the depression) than do other patients in the primary-care setting.[8,23] This adds 'hidden' costs to the healthcare budget. Both the psychological and physical functional impairments of depression lead to increased healthcare utilisation. 25% of patients seen in general practice are depressed[8] (often undiagnosed), but they account for 40 to 50% of the consultations.[24,25] This means that more effective diagnosis and treatment of depression could have a major impact on the workload in general practice. The potential cost benefits are clear.

The precise cost burden of the illness depends on the type of depression considered, and is likely to be lower for milder forms. Greenberg et al.[26] estimated that in 1990, about 5 million people in the US had major depression, and 1.8 million had bipolar disorder, with 2 million of these individuals having concomitant dysthymia. These authors[26] considered that a further 4.1 million people had dysthymia alone. In practice, some patients who are diagnosed with dysthymia may have inadequately treated, or inadequately diagnosed, major or resistant depression.[27] Moreover, about 50 to 94% of patients with dysthymia also have major depression.[28,29] Thus, dysthymic patients may be considered to be among the most severely debilitated of depressed patients. However, the cost implications of dysthymia have received little attention and although they may be greater than those of depression, we are not at present able to consider them further.

Apart from being a disabling disorder, depression can also have a fatal outcome, with a 10 to 15% mortality rate from suicide for major depression.[30-32] 60 to 70% of suicides are carried out by depressed individuals,[33-35] and in both the US[36] and the UK,[37] suicide is the eighth most common cause of death, with a rate in England and Wales in 1994 of 30 per million women and 111 per million men.[38] 82% of these patients were less than 65 years old,[37,38] so suicide has important economic repercussions. It is notoriously hard to predict which depressed individuals will commit suicide.[39-45]

Although adequate documentation is lacking, it is widely assumed that effective treatment of depression can and does prevent suicide. However, there is no evidence that the suicide rate has decreased since the introduction of antidepressants. The reasons for this are complex and the subject of much discussion, although the inadequate use of these drugs may be a factor. The diagnosis and management of depression can be represented by a cascade, in which a series of events culminates in only a small percentage of people with depression – perhaps only 5% in the UK – benefiting from antidepressant therapy. The majority of individuals with depression are not even diagnosed,[8,46] and fewer than one-third of those diagnosed as depressed may be prescribed antidepressants.[47,48] Of the patients who are treated, about one-third do not comply with therapy,[49] and one quarter do not respond to treatment, sometimes because they are prescribed inadequate dosages.[50,51]

2. Putting Monetary Values on the Burden of Depression

Depressive illness clearly has important cost implications. But the ways in which these can be determined (and used to evaluate the cost-effectiveness of treatment) are not as simple as they may first seem. Estimates by different authors[3,9,21,22,52-59] vary widely. Typically, indirect costs (which are usually measured in terms of effects on functioning or productivity, or earnings lost as a result of the illness) are less accurately determined than direct costs.

It may not be feasible to consider all the direct or indirect costs of illness that may possibly accrue, and the end requirements of evaluations have dictated which were chosen for study. They have often been restricted to the most significant costs, or to those that were relevant to one budget holder, such as the UK National Health Service (NHS),[3] US Medicaid[60] or primary-care physicians.[58,61] Studies of the cost-effective use of antidepressants that incorporate these data are similarly restricted in their implication and interpretation. One thing on which all authors agree is that the costs of depressive illness form a considerable proportion of any healthcare budget.

2.1 Direct Costs

To be costed, the burden of depression must be broken down into a list of items (table I). This is easier for direct costs (those incurred in the prevention, detection, diagnosis and treatment of the illness). Direct costs are payments that are actually made, and it is usually fairly straightforward to assign values to them from budgets, prices and salary lists, and to have confidence in the accuracy of

Table I. Breakdown of factors that incur costs in the treatment of patients with depression

Health service
Variable direct costs:
staff time [community physician, community psychiatric care, psychosocial services, social services, hospital nonmedical staff (e.g. administration), information services, pharmacy]
medical supplies (drugs for depression, other drugs, treatment for adverse effects of drugs, needles, equipment)
outpatient visits
hotel component of hospital care
procedures [investigations (biochemical/haematological), tests, therapeutic monitoring, x-ray, ECG, etc.]
electroconvulsive therapy
Fixed direct costs:
other staff (administration, cleaners, etc.)
overheads (heating, lighting etc.)
capital equipment, premises etc.
Patient
Direct costs:
self (travel)
family (travel, care)
treatment (prescription costs)
insurance (subscriptions, reimbursement)
Indirect costs:
self (loss of income and quality of life)
death (life lost by suicide)
treatment adverse effects (loss of income and quality of life)
family (loss of income and quality of life)
emotional (stress, family breakdown)
Other
Direct costs (staff: salaries of legal and social professionals, and clergy)
Indirect costs (staff: time of legal and social professionals, and clergy)

these values.[9,21,58,59,62-68] However, some direct costs that may be particularly pertinent to depression, such as for social services and community nursing, are especially hard to quantify and their value is less absolute.[58]

Costs of prescribing, dispensing, administering and monitoring the use of a drug (e.g. ECGs and plasma drug concentrations) are rarely itemised separately. They are often implicitly included in the costs of visits to healthcare professionals,[21] rather than as part of the cost of drugs. Rice et al.[69] are the only authors identified in this review who have included support costs, such as expenditure for research and training in all associated fields; they estimated these to be 8% of direct costs.

Items that are not used uniquely because of the illness, such as hospital ward overheads, pose a particular problem for a list of costs. This problem is inadequately dealt with by most retrospective studies, such as the Burden of Illness Study by Kind and Sorensen.[3] Drummond et al.[70] have attempted to define methodology that copes with this.

Stoudemire et al.,[9] in one of the most important studies of the cost burden associated with major depression, considered 1980 US data. They gave a figure for direct costs of $US2.1 billion for major depression (updated to $US26 billion in 1990 $US terms by Greenberg et al.[26]), including travel to receive medical care. Greenberg et al.,[26] in another careful analysis of the burden of depression, included the costs of bipolar disorders and dysthymia, and obtained a direct cost total for 1990 of $US12.4 billion. Neither study considered secondary direct costs.

Subsequently, Kind and Sorensen,[3] in a similar study, considered the costs of depression to the UK NHS, but made broader and less well substantiated assumptions, perhaps because of brevity requirements. Their, somewhat lower, estimate of 417 million pounds sterling (£) for the direct costs of depression may reflect this. For example, they suggested a value for local authority social services spending on depressed elderly patients, even though such specific apportionment of UK social services spending in costings analyses is very inaccurate.[11] To put a value on the cost of a depressed patient being treated in a psychiatric hospital, Kind and Sorensen[3] used the average amount for all types of mental hospital patients. Nevertheless, different illnesses require different levels of resource commitment, and time spent in hospital is a factor in this. The daily costs for an inpatient are likely to be highest in the first few days of hospital stay, particularly if the admission was precipitated by an acute episode.

Depression in 1986 to 1987 accounted for 18% of hospital admissions in the UK, and West,[52] with a similar approach to Kind and Sorensen,[3] made the crude assumption that it, therefore, accounted for 18% of all mental health costs. Adjusted to 1990 prices, this totalled £250 million. To this, West[52] added £28 million for general practice visits for patients with neurotic depression and £55 million for antidepressant sales, giving a total of £333 million for the direct costs of neurotic-type depression.

While several authors, including Kind and Sorensen[3] and West[52] have put a broad figure on the cost of hospitalisation for depression, all have ignored the ‘hidden’ direct hospital costs caused by independent physical illnesses that coincide with the depression. The prevalence of depression for medical inpatients in the US has been estimated as 15%, compared with 5 to 10% in outpatients.[8] Depressed individuals who are admitted for a physical complaint are rarely considered in statistics of depression. However, they can make a significant contribution to costs, and a goal should be to include them in future cost analyses.[26] For example, days spent in hospital by physically ill patients with depression are nearly double those of nondepressed individuals matched for severity, type and extent of physical disease;[71] hospital costs are 35% greater for the depressed patients.[35]

Hertzman[59] estimated the direct cost of psychosis in Sweden in 1975 to be 2157 million Swedish kronor (SKr). Most of the cost was accounted for by inpatient care. His estimate of total direct and indirect costs of affective psychoses was 4% of the total cost of psychoses (or SKr176 million), and the cost for neuroses was 7% of the total (SKr308 million).[59] The data were not broken down into individual items, and so should be used with caution.

Croft-Jeffreys and Wilkinson[58] circumvented the problem of establishing hospital costs, since they were irrelevant to their study. They considered the cost of neurotic disorder (including anxiety and neurotic depression) associated with patients who were treated entirely in UK general practice. Only consultations made specifically for neurotic disorders were considered, even though the authors acknowledged that patients with mental disorders are more likely to also consult for a physical illness. Although the study[58] restricted itself to one type of budget holder within the UK NHS, it also evaluated the cost to the individual (patient and carer). The study authors concluded that the direct costs of neurotic disorders in UK general practice in 1985 were £120 million, accounted for by consultation costs of £75 million, psychotropic drug costs of £38 million and patient prescription charge costs of £7 million[58] (the latter should arguably not be included). Their final total, which combined the costs to general practice and to the individual, accidentally included drug cost twice, that is both the cost to patients' budgets of £2 per prescription plus the doctors' budgetary cost of retail drug price per prescription.

2.2 Indirect Costs

Indirect costs, measured in terms of effects on functioning or productivity, or earnings lost on account of illness (table I), receive much less attention than direct costs, even though they probably account for 72 to 88% of the total cost of depression.[9,26,54] The disproportionate neglect of indirect costs is partly because they are of less immediate concern to most budget-holders, tending to be a cost to society. Moreover, they are more difficult to determine accurately than direct costs (section 2.1). However, different antidepressant drugs may be associated with vastly different indirect costs. For example, an overdose with a tricyclic antidepressant (TCA) is far more likely to result in death than an overdose with one of the apparently more expensive selective serotonin (5-hydroxytryptamine; 5-HT) reuptake inhibitors (SSRIs), with a greater relative burden of productivity loss to society.

2.2.1 Suicide

Most premature deaths in patients with depression are the result of suicide. Depression is associated with a risk of suicide between 13 and 30 times higher than that in the rest of the population.[72] In one study, 8% of 67 patients with diagnosed neurotic depression had committed suicide within 10 years of their index admission to a university teaching hospital in Australia.[73] It has been estimated that 25% of patients who are actually diagnosed as having major depression attempt suicide in their lifetime and 15% of patients with major depression ultimately die by suicide.[30-32,74] Suicide attempts are twice as frequent in patients with recurrent brief depression as in those with major depressive disorders.[75]

The indirect cost of successful suicide in the US has been evaluated by Weinstein and Saturno,[76] who calculated that a suicide in the 15- to 24-year-old age group resulted in a loss of productivity of $US432 000 per person, with a total annual cost of suicides from all causes in this group of $US2.26 billion. (The accuracy of their 'human capital' approach is discussed in section 2.3.1.) Given that 60 to 70% of suicides are the result of depression,[33-35] we can crudely estimate that the cost of depression-related suicide in this age group is $US1.5 billion. However, this assumes that suicides from depression are evenly spread across all age groups, which is not correct. In the US in 1985, the cost of mortality associated not just with depression, but with mental illness overall, was determined to be less than our figure, at $US9265 million, with productivity losses per death of $US233 337.[69] However, these estimates were considered to be conservative.[69]

2.2.2 Failed Suicide

Failed suicide attempts also result in a productivity loss to society, which is additional to that caused by the morbidity of the illness itself. The indirect cost of these attempts is rarely evaluated in detail, but was considered by Weinstein and Saturno[76] for the US situation, along with concomitant direct costs, such as medicolegal liability. As with suicide, their subject was not depression itself, but failed suicide from all causes. They considered reduced quality of life associated with failed suicide (independent of the morbidity of depressive disease itself). Weinstein and Saturno[76] estimated that the total economic cost of failed suicide attempts among 15- to 24-year-olds in the US, including direct and indirect costs, was $US3.19 billion (a mean of $US609 826 per attempt a year), and so was greater than the productivity loss associated with completed suicide in the same group. It is not clear how many suicide attempts are the result of depression, so these figures cannot be broken down further.

2.2.3 Mortality from Physical Illness

Individuals with major depressive disorder may also be more likely to die from seemingly unrelated causes, since increased mortality is apparent even when suicide and accidents are taken into account.[77] The increased risk, compared with nondepressed patients, has been put at 25% in medical inpatients matched for age, sex and physical health.[78] Untreated depression may compromise resistance to tumour growth and microbial infection.[79] Cardiovascular mortality is higher in elderly men who have been inadequately treated for depression than in those who have received adequate therapy,[80] and in elderly depressed women who were not given electroconvulsive therapy compared with those who did receive it.[81] The residents of one nursing home had a 59% increase in risk of death in the first year after admission if they had major depressive disorder.[82] However, the evidence that affective disorder increases the risk of death from physical illness is inconclusive.[83]

2.2.4 Morbidity of Depression

Indirect costs are particularly neglected when they are related to short and long term lack of functioning, rather than the premature death of the depressed individual. However, since depression rarely results in death, morbidity is the larger component of indirect costs, with big financial implications.

The morbidity of depression, and effects on quality of functioning, can result in significant production losses to society. In Belgium,[55] Germany,[68] Sweden[68] and the US,[9,26,68] 21%, 69%, 98% and 70 to 85%, respectively, of the indirect cost to society of depression, or of mental illness overall, has been estimated to be incurred because of morbidity, with the remaining (generally smaller) portion resulting from mortality.

Psychiatric disorders led to the loss of 71 million working days in the UK in 1989.[24] This accounted for 17% of all absences from sickness and cost £4 billion in lost working days and £6.8 million in UK NHS treatment.[84] For the individual, the sickness rate attributable to mild psychiatric morbidity, when other sickness is allowed for, has been put at 5.8 days per year.[85]

Psychiatric morbidity can affect work output, even when it is not severe enough to result in sick leave. Recurrent brief depressive disorder may account for short episodes (3 to 7 days) of impaired functioning 6 to 10 times a year.[86] These rates encompass both those who are effectively treated and those who are not. One study[18] has quantified the effect of treatment on incapacitating psychiatric morbidity. It found that among 145 high utilisers of healthcare, those with severe depression that did not improve with treatment had a mean 134.1 disability days per year at baseline and 128.8 days at 1 year follow-up; however, those who improved showed a change from 79.2 to 50.6 days per year; for individuals with improved moderate depression, the change was from 61.6 days to 17.5 days.[18]

It would be a simple matter to attach costs to such data, although this has rarely been attempted. The Stoudemire et al.[9] study is one of the few exceptions. As well as direct costs of major depression, it evaluated the indirect costs of lost productivity resulting from absence from work related to morbidity and mortality. Stoudemire et al.[9] costed morbidity at $US10 billion in 1980, which others have updated to $US16 billion for 1990[26] and to $US18 billion for 1991.[53] Stoudemire et al.[9] assumed that two-thirds of depressed patients received treatment, and that treated patients spent 16 days in hospital per year, while untreated ones spent 32 days at home in bed.

Broadhead et al.[12] criticised Stoudemire et al.,[9] because the latter group only considered major depression and may have excluded patients who appear to have minor depression, but who are in fact suffering from major depression at an attenuated stage in its periodicity.[12] In their own study,[12] which did not put an actual price on lost productivity, they calculated the number of days per 90-day period in which normal functioning was affected in depressed patients. The study considered both disability days (when the person spent at least part of a day in bed or was kept from their usual activities because of their depression) and days lost from work, in a prospective epidemiological survey. Data were controlled for psychiatric and medical comorbidity, social support and life stress. Results were compared with those expected for asymptomatic individuals. The proportion of extra disability days was 5.6% in patients with major depression, 0.6% in those with dysthymia and 8.5% in those with minor depression. Similarly, for employed people, the excess days lost from work expressed as a percentage of all days lost from work were 2% for major depression, 2% for dysthymia, 7.4% for minor depression with mood disturbance, and 10.8% for minor depression without mood disturbance.

Greenberg et al.[26] based their study on that of Stoudemire et al.,[9] but acknowledged Broadhead et al.'s criticisms.[12] They went one stage further than Broadhead et al.[12] by including patients with bipolar disorder or dysthymia in their costings of absenteeism and of reduced functioning while at work. Greenberg et al.[26] took into account that individuals with dysthymia often also have either major depression or bipolar disorder. Dysthymia was assumed to affect the untreated individual every workday throughout the year (which contrasts with Broadhead et al.[12]), but bipolar disorders and major depression were only considered during the active episode. For their measure of the costs of absenteeism, Greenberg et al.[26] assumed the same proportion of untreated patients and number of hospital or home bed-days as Stoudemire et al;[9] however, they also assumed that treated patients spent one-quarter of the rest of their episode in outpatient care and that untreated patients were incapacitated for one-third of the rest of their episode.[26]

The estimate of Greenberg et al.,[26] which they stressed should only be considered as indicating the magnitude of the problem, is not strictly comparable with that of Stoudemire et al.,[9] partly because Greenberg and colleagues[26] considered all types of depression. However, Greenberg et al.[26] compared their findings with those of Stoudemire et al.[9] by expressing the results of the earlier study in 1990 $US and deducting from their own figures the costs of reduced capacity at work, since Stoudemire et al.[9] did not calculate this. This gave a total in Greenberg et al.'s study[26] of $US31.6 billion, with 39% from direct costs, 24% from mortality and 37% from morbidity, compared with the revised Stoudemire et al.[9] value of $US26 billion, with 13% from direct costs, 26% from mortality and 61% from morbidity. Unlike Stoudemire et al.,[9] Greenberg et al.[26] did not place a value on homemakers, which, together with the different types of depression considered, may explain some of the differences in the breakdown of their figures.

Greenberg et al.[26] used published estimates for mental disorder overall to derive a measure of reduced functioning while at work for a depressed individual, which was 20% of their potential. Annual potential output was valued at $US44.73 billion for dysthymic patients and $US9.03 billion for patients with major depression or bipolar disorders. Greenberg et al.'s[26] final total for morbidity costs was $US23.8 billion, broken down into 49.2% from absenteeism and 50.8% from impaired capacity while at work.

A recent study has shown that the cost of lost earnings because of depression may be fully offset against the cost of treating the depression.[86a]

2.3 Valuing an Indirect Cost

Clearly, it is no easy task to put a value on indirect costs. They do not have a set market price and there is no standardisation in methodology or assumptions. The studies we have considered so far have been based on the so-called 'human capital' method, which measures loss of productivity in terms of pay. More recent cost analyses have assessed quality of life or used the willingness-to-pay approach.

2.3.1 Human Capital Method

There are several problems with the human capital method. Assumptions based on the employed may exclude large numbers of depressed individuals. Homemakers have only been valued by a few authors,[58,59,69,76] using the mean wage for their age group. No studies have valued the unemployed, those past retirement age or children. In theory, life expectancy and its changes over the years, potential earnings, and rates of participation in the labour force at each age for each sex, should be incorporated in calculations, but only a few authors[26,59,69,76] have done so. The use of such actuarial data should be established and standardised. Inaccurate figures emerge whenever they are not used, as occurs when one rate is assumed for all ages for mean participation in the labour market, and then used (as some authors[3,9] have) to determine days of lost productivity.

Short term absences from work will normally be covered by sickness benefits, sick pay, and temporary accommodation by colleagues, but at present, calculations of lost productivity cannot be reduced to allow for this. Nor can the effect of premature death from any cause or a fall in an individual's earnings as a result of depression be used to reduce calculations. The association of unemployment or reduced financial circumstances and consequent depression is never taken into account.

Relevant effects on a depressed patient's carers or dependents have not been considered in evaluations. These might increase the final cost. For example, a man may have to give up work or pay for childcare as a result of his wife's depression and its consequences, while a woman with a depressed husband may become the main or only breadwinner, even though she is likely to command a lower salary. The financial implications to society of the long term effects of depression, such as divorce, are especially difficult to quantify, and have until now been invariably ignored in studies of healthcare costs.

2.3.2 Quality of Life

Quality of life is measured in terms of the ability to perform and derive satisfaction from life tasks and social roles.[25] However, there are many problems in assessing quality of life, particularly for psychiatric patients.[3,25,87,88]

Quality of life provides a subjective measure of the effects of depression and their modification by treatment, and doctors and patients put very different values on the chosen parameters.[88] This subjectivity may reduce the reliability of cross-comparisons and repeated measures, although in practice, this does not seem to be too much of a problem. Also, in most comparisons, a treatment programme that provides a large number of quality-adjusted life-years (QALYs) to a few patients is as good as one that gives a smaller number to a larger number of people.[89] In fact, outcome may be as important as the number of people affected. Various weights – for example, depending on patient group, and measures such as illness, age, race and sex – or time discounts may be employed; this is because it has been shown that individuals do not give a constant quality of life value to each successive year of poor health and that there is a maximum time that people can cope with an illness.[89]

There has been little real research into the effect of depressive illness and its treatment on quality of life *per se*. Often, quality-of-life (QOL) considerations are omitted from a cost study, because the data cannot be obtained retrospectively. Wells et al.[11,14] found that depressed patients had much poorer quality of life, whether or not they had a depressive disorder. They reported worse physical and social functioning, more pain and worse current health, and spent more days in bed than many patients with chronic medical conditions such as diabetes mellitus, arthritis and hypertension. Measures of effect were given on a scale of 1 to 100, which equates with percentage of the best outcome (100%); scores for depression of 77.6% for physical well-being, 81.2% for social well-being, 58.7% for current health and 64.5% for freedom from pain were thus derived from the study. Patients had spent an average of 1.4 days in bed in the previous 30 days.

Sackett and Torrance[90] assigned a utility value (a measure of satisfaction) of 44% to quality of life for patients in a depressive state. This was worse than for tuberculosis, dialysis, or having a kidney transplant or a mastectomy. Kaplan and Anderson[91] determined a value of 68% for depressed outpatients and 61% for depressed inpatients. These differing evaluations make it clear that it is difficult to determine quality of life objectively, and that some psychometrically derived measures of quality of life may not be easily incorporated into cost-effectiveness analyses. Standardisation is increasingly recognised as necessary, since quality of life can be measured using a number of different methodologies. These are not directly comparable or interchangeable.

Typical QOL measures are similar to measures used in the diagnosis and assessment of depression. This suggests that QOL differences between depressed individuals are affected primarily by the severity of the depression. A relatively new battery of tests, specifically designed for health-related – as opposed to emotional-functioning – measures of quality of life,[92] has been used in several studies of depressed patients. These have indicated that the antidepressant sertraline has a beneficial effect on lifespan and quality of life.

2.3.3 Willingness-to-Pay

The willingness-to-pay method puts a value on what society, or an individual, is prepared to pay in order to lessen the effects of morbidity of an illness on quality of life. Thus, it can be employed for direct cost comparisons of the effects on morbidity of different antidepressants, and can take into account differences in the adverse effects of treatment.

The concept has been used to compare the use of moclobemide and TCAs.[93] Patients valued differences in adverse effects based on clinical trials data. They were shown, in graphic form, the relative reduction from using moclobemide and were asked whether they would take the new drug in preference to a TCA, given a range of possible cost implications. Their own abilities to pay were taken into account. The net benefit (willingness-to-pay minus costs) of moclobemide relative to the TCAs could then be calculated. The study considered confounding factors such as income, education and patients' previous experience of the adverse effects. However, the study did not consider any negative effects of moclobemide use, and all patients had used TCAs for at least 6 weeks in the previous year, to ensure that they would understand the concept of the adverse effects more meaningfully; the more experience an individual had of a particular adverse effect, the more they tended to rate it as bothersome. The study considered each adverse effect separately but this is not realistic and an aggregate willingness-to-pay may have given very different results. Indirect costs of lost productivity and the costs of treating adverse effects were not considered, but would only have influenced the magnitude of effect.

The final results of the study[93] showed that when between-treatment differences in cost were considered, there may be a negative benefit for moclobemide compared with amitriptyline and imipramine, but a positive net benefit compared with desipramine and clomipramine. Interestingly, only 77 to 86% of the 95 respondents would switch to moclobemide even when they did not have to pay anything, despite the fact that the adverse-effect profile was presented to them as being better. Individuals' willingness-to-pay also varied widely with each adverse effect.

The authors[93] concluded that there is some way to go before the willingness-to-pay approach can be used as a valid tool for health policy decisions. Further studies should also take into account societal willingness-to-pay, which includes the views of current nonusers.

3. Reducing the Burden of Depression

Studies of the direct and indirect costs of depression show, despite their inadequacies, that the illness is of great human and economic importance. However, the cost burden of depression may be greatly reduced by effective treatments, at a small cost relative to the cost burden of the illness itself.

Jonsson and Bebbington[21] gave some limited consideration to the relative importance of the more popular approaches to treating depression that are currently used in the UK. Their figures are notional, being derived from a model based on the value judgements of a panel of experts. They estimated the overall direct cost of treating depression to be £222 million in 1990; £6.6 million of this was for electroconvulsive therapy, £62.4 million for general practitioner visits, £8.75 million for outpatient visits, £48 million for drug purchase, £2.7 million for psychotherapy and £93.8 million for inpatient treatment.[21]

Antidepressants are generally accepted to be the most effective treatment for depression. However, there is a large number of clinically differing patient subgroups and this affects the choice of antidepressant and whether other approaches to treatment may be required.

3.1 Pharmacotherapy

Antidepressants are well established: the TCAs and the monoamine oxidase inhibitors (MAOIs) have now been available for over 40 years. The early MAOIs are now rarely used, largely because of the need for concomitant dietary care to prevent interaction with tyramine in food – the so-called 'cheese effect'. Between 1987 and 1992, the TCAs comprised 86% of all antidepressant prescriptions in Great Britain and, in 1990, 80% of such general practice prescriptions (UK Department of Health, personal communication). However, the development of newer classes of antidepressant means that the tricyclic share of general practice prescriptions in the UK had fallen to 47.5% by 1998 (UK Department of Health, personal communication).

The SSRIs (citalopram, fluoxetine, fluvoxamine, paroxetine and sertraline) became available in the 1980s, and proved to be especially popular in the US, where they have even been taken simply as a mood enhancer. As a result, fluoxetine became the most frequently prescribed antidepressant in the world; between 1988, when it was introduced in the US, and late 1993, fluoxetine had been used by 5 million individuals in the US and 10 million people worldwide.[94] More recently, 2 combined serotonin and noradrenaline (norepinephrine) reuptake inhibitors (venlafaxine and nefazodone) became available, and were termed SNRIs (serotonin-noradrenaline reuptake inhibitors). Mirtazapine, a noradrenaline and selective serotonin reuptake inhibitor (known as a NASSA), is one of the newest antidepressants, along with reboxetine, a selective inhibitor of noradrenaline uptake.

A fourth, pharmacologically heterogeneous, group of drugs comprises the so-called 'atypical' antidepressants. These have been introduced at varying intervals since the early 1970s, and include mianserin, trazodone, viloxazine and maprotiline (a bridged tricyclic that is sometimes included among the TCAs).

Another new group comprises the reversible inhibitors of monoamine oxidase (RIMAs), which have lower potential for interactions with foodstuffs and other drugs than the older MAOIs. Two RIMAs, toloxatone and moclobemide, are available in Europe and others are under study. Because of the relatively limited use of the older MAOIs and the lack of cost data on RIMAs, we have not considered either in detail in this article.

3.1.1 Maintenance Therapy

The final purchase cost of a drug will depend not only on its acquisition cost, but also on its dosage and length of time in use. In the acute phase of treatment, this may be highly variable, depending upon when the individual shows a clinical effect (section 5.3.1). The same may not be true of maintenance therapy, since by then the treatment should be relatively fixed (although the maintenance dosage should be dictated by the dosage that was effective in the acute phase).

There is some argument for considering acute and long term treatment of depression separately in any cost analysis.

The need for maintenance therapy of depression adds greatly to the final cost. Long courses of treatment are increasingly recognised as necessary to reduce relapse in what is a recurrent illness.[73,95] The World Health Organization[96] has recommended that all episodes of major depression should be treated for at least 4 to 6 months after the initial response is seen. Up to 50% of patients may otherwise have a recurrence of symptoms during this time, compared with 20 to 25% of patients who comply with the maintenance therapy.[97-99] It seems that many patients with moderate to severe unipolar recurrent depression should continue therapy for at least 2 years, if not indefinitely;[86,96,97,100-102] treatment lasting years is now recommended for elderly patients who recover from major depression.[103]

It has been estimated that 10% of patients will spontaneously discontinue treatment during the first year of maintenance therapy,[97] with a 65% relapse rate within the year for those who do.

There is a dearth of long term data, but some antidepressants may be more likely than others to reduce the relapse rate, including imipramine.[104] One analysis showed that sertraline therapy was associated with a relapse rate of 13%, compared with 45.7% for placebo.[105] Sertraline is the only antidepressant currently licensed in the UK for the prevention of relapse.

There is an increasing body of evidence to suggest that the dosage that produces remission in the acute phase should be continued through the maintenance period; previously, lower maintenance dosages had been preferred.

3.1.2 Improving Response

It is widely accepted that one-third of patients receiving antidepressants will not respond, with treatment success rates for antidepressant therapy of 65 to 80% in the hospital or clinic.[106,107] This may be improved by varying the treatment. In general practice, less than 24% of patients may be treated for a sufficiently long period at an adequate dosage,[108,109] so dosage and duration of therapy should be the first details to check in the case of poor response. Otherwise, the response rate can be improved by changing to a different antidepressant drug or using two drugs in combination. The second drug may be used to enhance the effects of the original medication, or it may have a different and complementary mechanism of action,[110] as with the combination of MAOIs and TCAs.

Combinations of a MAOI and a TCA work better in patients with treatment-resistant depression than in those who respond to other antidepressants, and in patients with endogenous, rather than neurotic, depression.[110] However, their effectiveness may diminish with time.[110] Such combinations have been used in the UK, the US and in Australia, where there has been some debate concerning their suitability.[111,112] This is because clinical trial data on the use of such combinations are sparse and mostly come from open trials or short term studies.[111,112] However, the combination is potentially hazardous, and not all permutations are suitable. Hence caution in the use of MAOI plus TCA combinations is recommended. In the same way, lithium has a limited use as monotherapy for depression and plasma concentrations must be monitored,[113] but it has been used in patients with refractory depression in combination with TCAs, and also with SSRIs and MAOIs.

When depression does not respond to any antidepressant, and lack of compliance and underdosing have been excluded as a possible cause, other drugs that may be tried are carbamazepine,[114] valproic acid (sodium valproate) and low-dose antipsychotic medication. Tryptophan and low doses of flupenthixol may be used for patients with mild depression.[115] Tryptophan is also used as adjunctive therapy.

3.2 Alternative Medicine

Only 12% of healthy people believe that they would be willing to take medication for clinical depression, but more than 70% would take medicine for a headache.[116] Although most patients do not reject prescriptions for antidepressants, some are reluctant to take medication on principle. Estimates of their number range from 6 to 34% in general practice,[116-121] while the figure may be around 2% in outpatient clinics.[117] Many of these patients turn to alternative medicine.

It has been suggested that in the UK, about £250 million was spent on nonorthodox medicine in 1985 (including £10 per consultation)[122] and the market is likely to have increased since then.[122] Similar trends are apparent in most Western countries. It is probable that a large proportion of this expenditure is accounted for by patients with diagnosed or undiagnosed depression.

3.3 Psychosocial Intervention

Depression often leads to job difficulties and withdrawal from social life. However, in many cases, mild depression results from difficulties within a person's life, including professional and interpersonal stresses, marital break-up and bereavement. If these problems are transient or readily overcome, nondirective counselling and social support may be effective treatments.[123,124] The assessments so far made may not be specific enough, or may be too limited or too small,[125] but it would seem that the most complete responses occur when pharmacological and psychosocial approaches are used concurrently, and this should be the rule.[126-129] Notwithstanding, few studies of the cost effectiveness of antidepressants consider concurrent psychosocial intervention.

3.4 Psychoanalysis

More directed, or analytically based, psychotherapy might be expected to have greater success than psychosocial methods. The two main psychotherapeutic approaches used for the type of depression encountered in primary care are interpersonal psychotherapy[127] and cognitive behavioural therapy.[130,131] The former concentrates on life events and past and present relationships whereas the latter is a structured attempt to impart to the individual a more positive attitude.

In one study of 50 patients, those given cognitive behavioural therapy did better than those on imipramine, and this difference was maintained at 3-month follow-up.[132] Although part of the effect was undoubtedly a result of the type of depression, another part may have resulted from the fact that there were fewer withdrawals from behaviour therapy. However, in another 3-year study in 128 patients, imipramine was more effective than psychotherapy.[133]

The US Agency for Healthcare Policy and Research's Depression Treatment Guidelines Panel considered the available evidence and concluded that patients treated with medication alone respond more quickly than those treated by psychotherapy alone.[134] From the point of view of costs, it is clear that person-to-person approaches such as counselling and psychotherapy tend to be labour-intensive and thus cost-intensive.

3.5 Other Forms of Therapy

Electroconvulsive therapy is considered to be the gold standard for treating patients with severe depression who are unresponsive to other treatments or are unable to take them.[134] It is often recommended for patients with major depression who experience psychomotor retardation, early morning waking or delusions, but is unlikely to lead to a response in those with hypochondriasis, hysteria, anxiety, emotional lability, crying and depersonalisation.[135]

Phototherapy is effective for seasonal affective disorder and, by altering sleep patterns, may be useful in some patients with unipolar and bipolar depression, usually in combination with antidepressant drugs.[136,137] Neither electroconvulsive therapy nor phototherapy is usually considered in cost models of treatment for depression.

4. Cost Burden of Treatment

Constraints on healthcare now operate in most western countries. Although they are effected in different ways, their aim is to control expenditure and to provide accountability for what is spent. Reimbursement on demand has been replaced with restrictions and limits, or fixed payments for healthcare providers, arrived at through competitive bidding and negotiation. The availability of drugs is controlled by limited lists, reference pricing, formularies, audit and global budgets.

4.1 National Trends

The situation in the UK is typical of this approach. There have been major reforms to the centrally funded NHS. The 1980s and 1990s saw the formation of self-governing hospital trusts and of fundholding schemes for general practice. In these schemes, the general practitioner managed his or her own defined budget and so became a direct purchaser of care. However, even nonfundholders were penalised if they did not stay within their indicative prescribing amounts. More recently, in 1999, geographical primary care groups (PCGs) were created in the UK, with the intention of evolving them into primary care trusts. In France, as in the UK, a system was introduced in the late 1990s whereby doctors' fees were cut if they exceeded the ceiling on growth in medical expenditure. This was 2.1% for 1996. In 1996, Belgium instigated less draconian measures to limit spending, even though it too set a ceiling. Sweden has been slower to introduce such schemes.[139] Measures to control expenditure within state-run healthcare systems are still in their infancy and are likely to be developed further, alongside the emergent discipline of evidence-based medicine.

Restrictions on the use of certain drugs are much easier for decision-makers to implement than institutional or structural changes, so they are a major focus of cost containment or cost-effectiveness policies. However, the cost benefits may be limited, not least because, correcting for inflation, the amount spent on drugs by the UK NHS has not even doubled in the last 25 to 30 years, and is small compared with other spending by the nation (it represents only 0.52% of the UK gross domestic product).[140] For the last 25 to 30 years, this has remained at about 10% of all NHS spending. The figures for other countries are similar, varying from 8.7% to over 20% of total healthcare expenditure, with an average of 14%.[141]

4.2 Effects of Focusing on Treatment Costs

An over-riding concern with the costs of treatment has several important effects.

It inevitably leads to treatment policies in which cost containment is achieved at the expense of managed care. There may be a need to refuse to treat some patients, or to avoid some therapies, in order to keep within budgets. Such a situation has occurred in the UK. In New Zealand, use of the SSRIs has been limited because of their high purchase cost; until September 1996, none could be prescribed in general practice without the recommendation of a specialist.[142] Even so, New Zealand regional health authority spending on antidepressants has increased by 40% annually in the last few years, with fluoxetine accounting for 44% of the antidepressant bill (and 150 000 prescriptions per year).[142] The number of prescriptions for new antidepressants rose by 38% in 1995 in New Zealand.

Centralisation of budgets should enable decisions to be made within the context of the overall budget, so that longer term implications of different therapies can be taken into account. This may be an advantage, but without fail-safe mechanisms in operation, decisions that are good for the budget may be bad for the community.

The recent cost-driven changes to healthcare mean greater accountability, clearly defined budgets and central audit. As a result, those who hold the purse-strings may restrict spending on items that have an immediate impact on their own budget – even if this means denying some forms of treatment – without considering the knock-on effects to other budgets.

Patients may increasingly be asked to pay for treatment. Private health insurance has assumed greater importance in the UK in the last few years. US Medicaid reimbursement rules have been revised. In France, there is more cost-sharing by patients than in any other European country; however, this has not affected use of ambulatory or of inpatient care in comparison with other countries, partly because of 'safety net' measures for the disadvantaged.[138]

In some countries, pharmaceutical companies have had to reduce or contain their profits. In Europe, the impact of this has been greatest in Italy and France, and may even have deleterious effects on the national pharmaceutical industries of these countries. There has been an effort to counterbalance this in the UK, with the Department of Health agreeing prices of drugs with pharmaceutical companies through the Pharmaceutical Price Regulatory Scheme. This may create conflict within the Department of Health, which also puts pressure on doctors to reduce drug costs.[143] It has been argued that in this way, doctors cannot be held responsible for UK national drug costs.[143]

In some European countries, pharmaceutical companies must carry out economic analyses of new drugs before they can receive government commendation or reference pricing. In the US, these economic analyses are necessary to obtain marketing and formulary approval. In 1993, it became mandatory in Australia (with Ontario, Canada, following the same route) for a drug company to prove that its product offers value for money before it can be considered for public reimbursement. In Spain in 1991, the Catalan Office for Health Technology Assessment was set up for the economic evaluation of drugs for inclusion in the local healthcare reimbursement system; in 1995, the Basque equivalent was set up. Belgium has also decided to consider the evaluation of drug treatment in terms of parameters such as efficacy and cost. One problem with this approach is that there are often insufficient data to prove the economic benefits of a drug when it is new, and so a useful pharmacotherapy may unjustly remain unused. In the late 1990s, the Swedish Industrial Association and the National Social Insurance Board set up an *ad hoc* group to evaluate the usefulness of pharmacoeconomics.

5. Formulary Considerations

An easy way to limit the availability of treatments to those that are effective, but relatively inexpensive (i.e. cost effective) – without excluding other treatments for difficult situations – is by the use of recommended lists and formularies. Such restrictions may operate at the level of the nation, the region or the prescribing budget-holder.

5.1 League Tables

League tables, which rank treatments by their relative cost effectiveness, are of increasing interest to healthcare decision-makers. They were implemented in the US state of Oregon in order to determine which procedures should be reimbursed under the state's Medicaid plan. Initial rankings were made in terms of overall cost per QALY and did not subdivide illness or treatment type. More recently, QALYs were only used in Oregon to rank items within disease categories, and costs were dropped from the consideration. League tables have also been used in a limited way in the UK, as a general guidance measure and with the acknowledgement that ranking may change with location.[144]

However, there is always the potential for the misuse of league tables. Some critics feel that they are being followed too rigorously and are used with the implicit aim of excluding some treatments, regardless of clinical demand, simply to keep healthcare within already stretched budgets.

This is unsound practice. League tables can never be truly accurate, for this would require a valuation for all existing and future treatments for all patient groups, in all their permutations of use, with each one calculated by the same standardised and comparable method.[144] Valuations would also need to take into account interactions between different types of treatment or illness. Technological advances and shifts in relative prices over time could also affect rankings, necessitating frequent revisions.[144]

Despite their drawbacks, Drummond et al.[144] consider league tables to be better than nothing, where 'nothing' means an informal, less-transparent assessment of relative value for money. League tables should be improved, not dismissed, but they will probably always need to be consulted with care, caution and intelligence.[143]

5.2 Drug Formularies

Drug formularies are used as a means of cost containment, but like league tables, they have been more appropriately described as 'pivotal tools for delineating and directing prescribing to the "drugs of choice"'.[145] They differ from league tables by their overt exclusion of some treatments and by the manner of their enforcement.

A good formulary should operate as a recommended list of therapeutic agents. It should be flexible, with frequent review by an expert panel and facilitated application by prescribers for the inclusion of other drugs. The use of alternative therapies should not be prohibited and rarely is, although it may incur penalties to the prescriber or patient.[146] A formulary may instead limit the way in which an agent is used, by restricting its availability to a few patients.

Thus, when considering a drug for inclusion in a formulary, treatment and usage guidelines should be determined,[147] and this information may be presented in the formulary. Newer drugs, such as the SSRIs, SNRIs and NASSAs, have the disadvantage of a relative lack of data and experience in use compared with the TCAs, and it may be difficult to determine a rationale for their inclusion.

The problems that have arisen in the compilation of formularies are made clear from the reports by Bochner et al.[147] and other commentators.[148-151]

5.3 Criteria for Inclusion of an Antidepressant Drug

The main requirements of a formulary drug are that it must produce the desired effect or treatment objective and have an acceptable tolerability profile, and it should also have the lowest cost among comparable drugs. However, there is much room for interpretation (or misinterpretation), and a wrong decision can have more far-reaching effects if it is perpetrated within a formulary than if it is made by an individual prescriber.

5.3.1 Treatment Objective

Clinical effectiveness should be one of the prime considerations in the selection of a drug for inclusion in a formulary,[152] although this is likely to be illness-dependent. Discrete and precise treatment end-points should in theory be formulated for evaluations of effectiveness,[147] but in practice, grades of treatment success may be considered – a drug that reduces morbidity, but that does not result in a cure, is better than no drug at all.

Taylor and McClean[153] have pointed out that when one drug is very effective in some patients and ineffective in others, while another drug is of moderate effectiveness in all cases, both drugs would have a similar efficacy when the data are pooled. This highlights the distinction that should be made between the efficacy of drugs in a trial and their effectiveness in the community. In efficacy comparisons, each drug is prescribed in identical conditions, with comparable doses and identical monitoring and patient types. In the community, an efficacious drug may not be effective in patients who differ from those of the clinical trial conditions, or when adverse effects are less acceptable to the patient because they receive less attention from the clinician. The antidepressants are all considered to have a similar efficacy, but the newer drugs may be more effective because of their wider applicability and high compliance rates.

5.3.2 Safety and Tolerability

Safety considerations should include the risk of overdose and the relative toxicity of drugs in overdose, both of which appear to be lower for the SSRIs than the TCAs.[72,154] Relative tolerabilities may be more important than a fixed-threshold exclusion tolerability profile, particularly since it is hard to define what is acceptable. Adverse effects may considerably increase the cost of treatment, decrease compliance and offset some of the benefits of treatment on quality of life. Although the newer antidepressant drugs have an advantage in this respect,[155] the TCAs have been in use for many years and there is a sense in which their adverse effects may therefore be said to be 'acceptable' or 'accepted'. This was shown by a study in which many patients said they were unlikely to switch from a TCA to a new drug, even when they were told it had fewer adverse effects (section 2.3.3).[93]

5.3.3 Cost

The retail price is often the most influential factor in the choice of drug for a formulary. However, unit retail price does not reflect a drug's actual immediate cost burden on the prescriber's budget; the dosage, duration of treatment and monitoring requirements will all affect this. The results of cost-effectiveness comparisons, which may have already taken these variables into account, should be evaluated.

When finite resources and different clinical indications compete for a given drug to be included in the formulary, there are arguments for choosing the least expensive one (in terms of acquisition cost) that has maximum health benefit overall for each indication.[147] However, one drug may be generally less effective or may have similar efficacy, but a higher retail cost, than another drug that is proposed for the formulary, but at the same time, it may be more cost effective for a specific subgroup of patients; this may apply to some of the SSRIs. It follows that a variety of drugs for the same indication should, in principle, be available in a formulary. Only then can appropriate clinical decisions be made without compromising the quality of patient care. This approach may not even result in greater overall or sustained expense,[156] although it often does.[157,158]

5.3.4 Familiarity

Practice formularies are a formal expression of the preference of a doctor for drugs with which he or she has more experience. Hospital formularies are developed by committees to reduce such bias, but cannot eliminate it, since it exists within each committee member. This means that older drugs tend to be favoured over newer ones, and that health-economic arguments have to be particularly powerful to get a drug into or out of a formulary. This may be one factor in the relatively rapid success of sertraline, which was the focus of more cost analyses than nefazodone. Sertraline was introduced in 1992 and within 6 months had been accepted by 44.9% of US hospital formularies. Nefazodone had a 28.7% acceptance rate 9 months after its US introduction in March 1995.[159]

By limiting choice, formularies increase the familiarity and expertise of the prescriber with all the drugs in the armamentarium, which might be thought to reduce prescribing problems.[160] However, despite greater medical experience with the TCAs, they are much more likely than SSRIs to be suboptimally prescribed.

A major disadvantage of formularies is that the possibility of developing familiarity with newer drugs is hindered. Newer antidepressants, such as the SSRIs, SNRIs and NASSAs, tend to have relatively high retail prices, which may be the basis of their exclusion from formularies. The lack of concordance in cost-analysis methodology means that their cost effectiveness is disputed, even when their potential usefulness and tolerability are generally agreed.

5.4 Factors Which Affect Antidepressant Use

Traditionally, formularies have been the domain of hospitals and, therefore, their effect on the treatment of depression has to be placed in context. Fewer than 18% of all 715 patients who were known to have depression in South Manchester, UK, in 1989 and 1990 were hospitalised,[161] and a panel of experts has suggested that an even lower figure of 5% should generally apply.[21] However, even when a depressed patient goes to hospital, the hospital physician may shift the burden of choice of treatment, as well as transferring the cost of pharmacotherapy onto another budget, by sending the patient back to primary care for their prescription.[163,164]

Thus, in the past, hospital prescribing policies have had only a minimal effect on patients with depression. However, the situation is now changing. UK government policies of the 1990s led to a shift towards community-based services and funding, which resulted, soon after implementation, in an increase in community service use of 122% for depression, and 549% for anxiety states, in South Manchester.[161]

Formularies for individual doctors and practices are increasingly being developed, especially in the UK, Canada, South America and New Zealand.[157] National Limited Lists are used in the UK, Ireland, Germany and Australia[157] as a means of cost containment.

Since most depressed patients are prescribed antidepressants by their primary-care physician, there is clearly a need to target any advice regarding the treatment of depression to such doctors. Generally speaking, the factors that should influence an individual prescriber are the same as those that determine whether a drug is selected for inclusion in a formulary.

5.4.1 Clinical Factors

Clinical influences on what is prescribed should be paramount. Data from conventional randomised clinical trials do not justify the general replacement of TCAs with newer antidepressants as first-line therapy. This is because there is no demonstrable difference in efficacy between the different antidepressants in clinical trials. However, this is an oversimplification. Some antidepressants may be more appropriate than others for particular subgroups of patients, both from the point of view of the illness – its symptom pattern and severity – and with regard to the limitations and contraindications of the drug.

For example, maprotiline and many TCAs, especially amoxapine, are proconvulsant and should be avoided in patients with epilepsy,[170] up to 60% of whom have depression or milder mood changes.[171] Antidepressants with a sedative effect, such as amitriptyline or mianserin, may be suitable for patients with concomitant insomnia (although this may only be helpful in the first few weeks and the benefits may then be outweighed by adverse effects on cognition), while stimulating drugs such as protriptyline or nomifensine may be better suited to somnolent or lethargic patients. Some doctors consider the lack of sedative effects in the SSRIs to be a problem,[171] but their use can nonetheless improve sleep patterns.[171] Alcohol abusers should be given the newer nonsedating drugs, although at minimal doses.[171] TCAs may promote bodyweight gain and SSRIs may cause bodyweight loss, and this should be borne in mind.

SSRIs may have a wider application than TCAs.[172,173] The age of the patient may be important; the SSRIs may become the treatment of choice in the elderly, who are particularly susceptible to the anticholinergic adverse effects of TCAs. It is possible that SSRIs may be prescribed to patients who are at greater risk of overdose; many studies have shown that they are more effective in reducing suicidal thoughts.[174-184] Apart from anecdotal reports concerning fluoxetine (which have been critically analysed[185-187]) only trazodone[185] and the older TCAs, including maprotiline,[188] desipramine, amoxapine, and nortriptyline,[185] have been implicated as able to precipitate or provoke suicidal ideation.[72,183,189] The SSRIs (e.g. paroxetine[27]) may also have a different role from TCAs in patients with treatment-resistant depression, and sertraline may be particularly useful for preventing relapse (section 3.1.1).

5.4.2 Adverse Effects

Influence on Compliance

The antidepressants differ in the relative incidence, type and severity of adverse effects and this has important clinical, and hence economic, implications. A large proportion of the cost of treating patients with depression is caused by consequences of noncompliance and treatment failure, resulting from adverse effects, on the health of patients – patients are more likely to

Table II. Available data on the percentage of patients filling prescriptions for antidepressants as treatment progresses.[54,109,117] This table assumes that each prescription is for one month

No. of months on treatment	SSRIs	TCAs
1		32-65
1.25		45
2	60-70	30
3		20
5	19.3	12

SSRIs = selective serotonin reuptake inhibitors; **TCAs** = tricyclic antidepressants

discontinue treatment early, or take ineffective dosages, when they experience adverse effects. The result may be a lengthening of the depressive episode, symptomatic relapse, reduced quality of life and productivity, and even a greater risk of death by suicide. There is also the more easily measured, but not yet quantified, cost of medical treatment and monitoring for certain adverse effects.

Dosage has a major effect on the incidence and the severity of adverse effects.[119] Doogan[190] observed that the rate of withdrawal from sertraline treatment because of adverse effects was significantly affected by the regimen used: 36% with a fixed dosage of 200 mg/day, 16% with forced rapid upward titration from 50 to 200 mg/day, and 6% with flexible titration. Doogan[190] commented that the last regimen most typifies everyday use.

Initial dosage recommendations were unnecessarily high for each of the SSRIs.[190,191] This means that in many studies, the existing data on the consequences of adverse effects is weighted in favour of the TCAs drugs, which have been in use for many years at dosages that have long been established. However, most studies concur that SSRIs, even when given in higher doses than are now deemed necessary, still have a tolerability advantage over TCAs.

The poorer tolerability profile of the TCAs has been observed in clinical trials. In a meta-analysis of 42 randomised controlled trials that compared SSRIs with TCAs in patients with major depression, the pooled rate of discontinuation because of adverse effects was 14.9% for SSRIs and 19% for TCAs ($p < 0.01$).[155] It is apparent from published data that the compliance rate for TCAs is no different than it was before the newer drugs became available.[192]

Correspondingly, there are indications from everyday use that treatment withdrawals related to adverse effects are more common with the older TCAs, although the figure may depend on the setting and duration of treatment. 32 to 36% of patients in general practice stopped TCA therapy within 4 weeks because of adverse effects,[117] compared with 64% of outpatients (see table II). The difference may be attributed to the intensity of monitoring and the degree of contact with health workers as well as effects on the patient's perception of medical care.

As we show in Part 2 of the article (page 195), the tolerability advantage of the SSRIs has important cost implications. It can mean the difference between cost effectiveness and cost ineffectiveness.

Influence on Dosage

Most of the common adverse effects of drugs are dosage-related. This often results in the tendency to use low dosages; the patient may never receive an adequate dosage, or the physician may lower the dosage as adverse effects appear. In one study this was true for 24% of outpatients on TCAs, who experienced anticholinergic adverse effects.[193] Johnson's experience[193,194] was that the dosage was not increased even if the patients failed to respond.

The end result is that 25 to 50% of the prescribed dose may not be taken by 70% of depressed patients given TCAs.[195] Thompson and Thompson[162] suggested that amitriptyline 75 mg/day or its equivalent dosages for other drugs should always be considered as subtherapeutic. In 33.8% of 6713 new episodes of major depression in US Medicaid patients, a minimum effective dosage was never achieved.[60] Similar figures were given by Thompson and Thompson[51] and in two UK surveys of depressed patients in general practice.[194,196] However, the figure may well vary with setting. 88% of patients with major depression treated at university medical centres did not receive an adequate dosage of imipramine or its equivalent.[197] This contrasts with an analysis of 119 'distressed' (presumably depressed) high utilisers of US healthcare services, in which only 16% were receiving an inadequate TCA dosage.[13] 25 to 50% of patients in UK general practice who were treated with antidepressants[194,196,198] and 42% of depressed patients in an outpatient psychiatric practice in the US[199] were found to be receiving what are usually considered to be inadequate dosages. However, some of these studies[13,198,199] may have included patients who were prescribed antidepressants for conditions other than depression, which could be a source of bias. Moreover, some community doctors have tried to establish that lower dosages may be effective.[200-202] However, this has not been demonstrated in a controlled study.

Underdosing has great cost implications. Lower doses mean lower costs of a drug, but also reduced effectiveness. Thus, in effect, the cost of treatment is transferred to other budgets and may well exceed any cost savings from decreasing the dose. For example, lower effectiveness means more money spent on medical care for depression and associated physical complaints,[11-13] hospitalisation, days off work, lack of functioning and even suicide attempts.[203]

5.4.3 Costs

An annual average of 510.67 million prescriptions were written for antidepressants between 1987 and 1992 (UK Department of Health, personal communication), or around 450 per UK general practice, so the primary-care physicians has a heightened awareness of their use and, with recent cost-constraint policies, their impact on his budget. A UK general practice may dispose of over £2000 annually in the management of depressive illness in expenditure on drugs, since 1.9% (£47.6 million) of the UK drug bill was spent on antidepressants in 1990 (UK Department of Health, personal communication).

There is a real danger that doctors may seek to limit costs by restricting the prescription of more expensive drugs or by prescribing fewer drugs in total, without considering the other factors that should influence prescribing decisions. This is exemplified by the finding that fundholding general practices in the Grampian region of Scotland were more cautious in their use of SSRIs than nonfundholders.[204] Nonfundholders had higher unit drug costs, with twice as many SSRI prescriptions (39.9% of all antidepressant prescriptions). In contrast, a study by Hux and Naylor[169] suggested that if doctors are given feedback on drug costs they may moderate their prescribing of expensive treatments, regardless of who pays, and that knowledge of the costs incurred is a greater moderator than knowledge that someone else will no longer pay. In support of this, the UK statistics for 1995 showed that while fundholders had lower prescribing costs, these rose faster than for nonfundholders.

Much of the contemporary interest in understanding the prescribing behaviour of doctors[165] has as its goal improved cost control. Several studies[166-5] have shown that using such knowledge to educate doctors can have the intended effect on prescribing. Given the impact of cost on prescribing decisions, it is important to educate doctors that a drug's purchase price is only a small part of its total cost. This has been demonstrated to be effective in the specific case of depression.[61] Educating general practitioners in Gotland, Sweden, led to a reduction in sick leave, inpatient care and numbers of suicides in patients with depression, while treatment became more appropriate, with larger dosages of antidepressants and less use of sedatives. However, the effect of alternative influences on prescribing could not be excluded.[61] Moreover, these beneficial effects diminished within 2 years of ceasing the campaign.[61]

5.4.4 Familiarity

Physicians tend to exhibit conservatism in their prescribing and demonstrate a tendency to prescribe drugs with which they are familiar. Most doctors who are currently practising have more familiarity with the older antidepressants (TCAs). Despite the acknowledged disadvantages of these, it may be hard to convince some to prescribe the newer drugs. In the UK and most western countries, although not in the US, the newer drugs are still relegated by some doctors to second-line therapy. This is despite the conclusions of the cost analyses of Boyer and Feighner,[97] Jonsson and Bebbington,[21,22] Kind and Sorensen[3,207] and Le Pen et al.[208] which are considered further in Part 2, page 195. These authors have each shown that the poorer compliance, and poorer response in general use, with TCAs as first-line therapy may in fact make the SSRIs more economical as the antidepressant of first choice.

6. Conclusions

The costs of depressive illness are high, but suitable treatments exist. However, the choice of treatment depends on a number of factors, some clinical, some economic. The current focus of attention on the price of things rather than their worth is to the disadvantage of the SSRIs, since they have a higher retail price than the longer-established antidepressants. For example, SSRIs, SNRIs and NASSAs are generally prescribed at low, but effective, daily doses, which can hardly be reduced to save on costs. Ironically, it is the (cheaper retail cost) TCAs that are more likely to be prescribed in subtherapeutic doses. This affects the real cost and value of treatment. Hence prescribing decisions should not be affected by retail cost alone.

References

1. Montgomery SA, Bebbington P, Cowen P, et al. Guidelines for treating depressive illness with antidepressants. J Psychopharmacol 1993; 7 (1): 19-23
2. Regier DA, Hirschfeld RMA, Goodwin FK, et al. The NIMH depression awareness, recognition and treatment program: structure, aims and scientific basis. Am J Psychiatry 1988; 145: 1351-7
3. Kind P, Sorensen J. The costs of depression. Int Clin Psychopharmacol 1993; 7: 191-5
4. Henry JA. Debits and credits in the management of depression. Br J Psychiatry 1993; 163 (20 Suppl.): 33-9
5. Hagnell O, editor. The incidence of mental illness over a quarter of a century. The Lundby longitudinal study of mental illness in a total population based on 42,000 observation years. Stockholm: Almkvist and Wiksell, 1990
6. Jablensky A. Prediction of the course and outcome of depression. Psychol Med 1987; 17: 1-9
7. Blacker CV, Clare AW. Depressive disorder in primary care. Br J Psychiatry; 150: 737-51
8. Katon W, Roy-Byrne PP. Antidepressants in the medically ill: diagnosis and treatment in primary care. Clin Chem 1988; 34 (5): 829-36
9. Stoudemire A, Frank R, Hedemark N, et al. The economic burden of depression. Gen Hosp Psychiatry 1986; 8: 387-94
10. Gold PW, Goodwin FK, Chrousos GP. Clinical and biochemical manifestations of depression: relation to the neurobiology of stress. N Engl J Med 1988; 319: 348-53
11. Wells KB, Stewart A, Hayes RD, et al. The functioning and well-being of depressed patients: results from the medical outcome study. JAMA 1989; 262 (7): 914-19
12. Broadhead WE, Blazer DG, George LK, et al. Depression, disability days and days lost from work in a prospective epidemiologic study. JAMA 1990; 264: 2524-8
13. Katon W, Von Korff M, Lin E, et al. Distressed high utilizers of medical care: DSM-III-R diagnoses and treatment needs. Gen Hosp Psychiatry 1990; 12: 355-62
14. Wells KB, Golding JM, Burnam MA. Psychiatric disorder and limitations in physical functioning in a sample of the Los Angeles general population. Am J Psychiatry 1988; 145: 712-7
15. Bridges K, Goldberg D. Somatic presentation of DSM-III psychiatric disorder in primary care. J Psychiatr Res 1985; 29: 563-9

16. Bridges K, Goldberg D. Somatic presentation of depressive illness in primary care. In: Freeling P, Downey LJ, Malkin JC, editors. The presentation of depression: current approaches. London: Royal College of General Practitioners, 1987
17. Goldberg D, Huxley P. Common mental disorders: a bio-social model. London: Routledge, 1992
18. von Korff M, Ormel J, Katon W, et al. Disability and depression among high utilizers of health care. Arch Gen Psychiatry 1992; 49: 91-100
19. Weissman MM, Leaf PJ, Tischler GL, et al. Affective disorders in five United States communities. Psychol Med 1988; 18 (1): 141-53
20. Weissman MM, Myers JK. Affective disorders in a US urban community: the use of research diagnostic criteria in an epidemiological survey. Arch Gen Psychiatry 1978; 35 (11): 1304-11
21. Jonsson B, Bebbington P. Economic studies of the treatment of depressive illness. In: Jonsson B, Rosenbaum J, editors. Health economics of depression. New York: John Wiley, 1993: 35-48
22. Jonsson B, Bebbington P. What price depression? The cost of depression and the cost-effectiveness of pharmacological treatment. Br J Psychiatry 1994; 164: 665-73
23. Coulehan JL, Schulberg HC, Block MR, et al. Medical comorbidity of major depressive disorder in a primary medical practice. Arch Intern Med 1990; 150 (11): 2363-7
24. Office of Population Censuses and Surveys. Series VS No 15. London: OPCS, 1990
25. Turner R. Quality of life: experience with sertraline. Int Clin Psychopharmacol 1994; 9: 27-31
26. Greenberg PE, Stiglin LE, Finkelstein SN, et al. The economic burden of depression in 1990. J Clin Psychiatry 1993; 54 (11): 405-18
27. Montgomery SA. Anxiety and depression. Petersfield: Wrightson Biomedical Publishing Ltd, 1990: 46, 59
28. Angst J, Vollrath M, Koch R. New aspects on epidemiology of depression. In: Angst J, Woggon B, editors. Lofepramine in the treatment of depressive disorders. Vieweg: Braunschweig, 1988: 1-14
29. Kocsis JH, Frances AJ, Voss C, et al. Imipramine treatment for chronic depression. Arch Gen Psychiatry 1988; 45: 253-7
30. Tsuang MT, Woolson JRF, Fleming JA. Premature deaths in schizophrenia and affective disorders. Arch Gen Psychiatry 1980; 37: 979-83
31. Guze SB, Robins E. Suicide and primary affective disorders. Am J Psychiatry 1970; 117: 437-8
32. Winokur G, Tsuang M. The Iowa 500: suicide in mania, depression and schizophrenia. Am J Psychiatry 1975; 132: 650-3
33. Barraclough BM, Bunch J, Nelson B, et al. A hundred cases of suicide: clinical aspects. Br J Psychiatry 1986; 125: 355-73
34. Paykel ES. The treatment of depression: the relevance of research for clinical practice. Br J Psychiatry 1989; 155: 754-63
35. Levenson JL, Hamer RM, Rossiter LF. A randomized controlled study of psychiatric consultation guided by screening in general medical inpatients. Am J Psychiatry 1992; 149: 631-7
36. Kellerman AL, Rivara FP, Somes G, et al. Suicide in the home in relation to gun ownership. N Engl J Med 1992; 327: 467-72
37. Office of Population Censuses and Surveys, series DH4. Mortality statistics – accidents and violence (England and Wales). London: Her Majesty's Stationery Office 1990, 1991, 1992
38. Office of Population Censuses and Surveys, series DH2. Mortality statistics – accidents and violence (England and Wales). London: Her Majesty's Stationery Office, 1990, 1991, 1992, 1993
39. Goldstein RB, Black DW, Nasrallah A, et al. The prediction of suicide: sensitivity, specificity, and predictive value of a multivariate model applied to suicide among 1906 patients with affective disorders. Arch Gen Psychiatry 1991; 48: 418-22
40. Hawton K. Assessment of suicide risk. Br J Psychiatry 1987; 150: 145-53
41. Kreitman N. How useful is the prediction of suicide following parasuicide? In: Wilmotte J, Mendlewicz J, editors. New trends in suicide prevention. Basel: Karger, 1982
42. McNamee JE, Offord DR. Prevention of suicide. Can Med Assoc J 1990; 142: 1223-30
43. Motto JA. An integrated approach to estimating suicide risk. Suicide Life Threat Behav 1991; 21: 74-89
44. Winokur G, Black DW. Suicide – what can be done? N Engl J Med 1992; 327: 490-1
45. Nordentoft M, Breum L, Munck LK, et al. High mortality by natural and unnatural causes: a 10 year follow up study of patients admitted to a poisoning treatment centre after suicide attempts. BMJ 1993; 306: 1637-41
46. Murphy GE. Suicide and substance abuse. Arch Gen Psychiatry 1988; 45: 593-4
47. Prescott LF, Highley MS. Drugs prescribed for self poisoners. BMJ 1985; 290: 1633-6
48. Weissman MM, Klerman GL, Prusoff BA, et al. Depressed outpatients: results one year after treatment with drugs and/or interpersonal psychotherapy. Arch Gen Psychiatry 1981; 38: 51-5
49. Weissman MM. The psychological treatment of depression: update of clinical trials. In: Williams JBW, Spitzer RL, eds. Psychotherapy research: where are we and where should we go? New York: Guilford Press, 1984: 89-105
50. Gerner R, Estabrook W, Steuer J, et al. Treatment of geriatric depression with trazodone, imipramine and placebo: a double-blind study. J Clin Psychiatry 1980; 41: 216-220
51. Thompson C, Thompson CM. The prescribing of antidepressants in general practice II. A placebo-controlled trial of low-dose dothiepin. Hum Psychopharmacol 1989; 4: 191-204
52. West R. Depression. London: Office of Health Economics, 1992
53. Abraham IL, Bryant Neese J, Westerman PS. Depression: nursing implications of a clinical and social problem. Nurs Clin North Am 1991; 26 (3): 527-36
54. Feighner JP. A double-blind comparison of paroxetine, imipramine and placebo in depressed outpatients. In: Ashcroft GW, editor. Depression – a once in a lifetime event? Oxford: Clinical Neuroscience Publishers, 1991
55. Mendlewicz J. The social burden of depressive disorders. Neuropsychobiology 1989; 22: 178-80

56. Rice DP. Conceptual and estimation issues related to cost of illness studies [abstract]. The Second Workshop of Cost and Assessment in Psychiatry: the costs of affective disorders. 1992 Oct 26-28; Venice
57. McGuire TG. Outcomes, costs and design of health insurance for depression. In: Jonsson B, Rosenbaum J, editors. Health economics of depression: perspectives in psychiatry, Vol 4. Chichester: Wiley, 1993: 77-96
58. Croft-Jeffreys C, Wilkinson G. Estimated costs of neurotic disorder in UK general practice 1985. Psychol Med 1989; 19: 549-58
59. Hertzman P. The economic costs of mental illness in Sweden 1975. Acta Psychol (Scand) 1983; 68: 359-67
60. McCombs JS, Nichol MB. The cost of treatment failure. In: Jonsson B, Rosenbaum J, editors. Health economics of depression: perspectives in psychiatry, Vol 4. Chichester: Wiley, 1993: 49-64
61. Walinder J, Carlsson P, Rutz W. The economic impact of an educational programme on diagnosis and treatment of depression in Sweden. In: Jonsson B, Rosenbaum J, editors. Health economics of depression: perspectives in depression, Vol 4. Chichester: Wiley, 1993: 97-110
62. Weiss KB, Gergen PJ, Hodgson TA. An economic evaluation of asthma in the United States. N Engl J Med 1992; 326: 862-6
63. Eisenberg JM, Glick H, Koffer H. Pharmacoeconomics: economic evaluation of pharmaceuticals. In: Strom BL, editor. Pharmacoepidemiology. New York: Churchill Livingstone, 1989: 325-50
64. Hartunian NS, Smart CN, Thompson MS. The incidence and economic costs of major health impairments. Lexington: Lexington Books, 1980
65. Weisbrod BA. Benefit-cost analysis of a controlled experiment treating the mentally ill. J Hum Resour 1981; 16: 523-48
66. Cooper BS, Rice DP. The economic cost of illness revisited. Soc Secur Bull 1976: 39: 21-36
67. Black DAK, Pole JD. Priorities in biomedical research: indices of burden. Br J Prevent Med 1975; 29 (4): 222-7
68. Weisbrod BA. Economics of mental illness: costs, benefits and incentives. In: Jonsson B, Rosenbaum J, editors. Health economics of depression: perspectives in psychiatry, Vol 4. Chichester: Wiley, 1993: 15-34
69. Rice DP, Kelman S, Miller LS. Estimates of economic costs of alcohol and drug abuse and mental illness, 1985 and 1988. Public Health Rep 1991; 106 (3): 280-92
70. Drummond MF, Stodden GL, Torrence G. Methods for the economic evaluation of healthcare programmes. Oxford: Oxford Medical, 1987
71. von Korff M, Ormel J, Katon W, et al. Disability and depression among high utilizers of health care. Arch Gen Psychiatry 1992; 49: 91-100
72. Montgomery SA. Suicide and antidepressants. Drugs 1992; 43 Suppl.: 24-31
73. Kiloh LG, Andrews G, Neilson M. The long-term outcome of depressive illness. Br J Psychiatry 1988; 153: 752-57
74. Bulik CM, Carpenter LL, Kupfer DJ, et al. Features associated with suicide attempts in recurrent major depression. J Affect Disord 1990; 18 (1): 29-37
75. Angst J, Stassen HH, Gross G, et al. Suicide in affective and schizoaffective disorders. In: Marneros A, Tsuang MT, editors. Affective and schizoaffective disorders. Berlin: Springer Verlag, 1990: 186-95
76. Weinstein MC, Saturno PJ. Economic impact of youth suicide and suicide attempts. In: US DHSS Publication: 1982-1989. Rockville: Department of Health and Human Services, 1989: ADM 89-1264
77. Wells KB. Depression as a tracer condition for the national study of medical care outcomes: background review. Rand Corporation 1985: R-3293-RWJ/HJK
78. Eaton WW, Holzer CE III, von Korff M, et al. The design of the Epidemiological Catchment Area surveys: the control and measurement of error. Arch Gen Psychiatry 1984; 41: 942
79. Pettito JM, Folds JD, Ozer H, et al. Abnormal diurnal variation in circulating natural killer cell phenotypes and cytotoxic activity in major depression. Am J Psychiatry 1992; 149: 694-6
80. Robinson RG, Starr LB, Price TR. A two year longitudinal study of mood disorder following stroke: prevalence and duration at six months follow-up. Br J Psychiatry 1984; 144: 256-62
81. Babigian HM, Guttmacher LB. Epidemiologic considerations in electroconvulsive therapy. Arch Gen Psychiatry 1984; 41: 246-53
82. Rovner BW, German PS, Brant LJ, et al. Depression and mortality in nursing homes. JAMA 1991; 265 (8): 993-6
83. Goodwin GM. The effects of treatment on mortality in affective illness. J Psychopharmacol 1992; 6: 312-7
84. Thompson D, Pudney M. Mental illness: the fundamental facts. London: Mental Health Foundation, 1989
85. Jenkins R. Minor psychiatric morbidity in employed young men and women and its contribution to sickness absence. Br J Ind Med 1985; 42: 147-54
86. Angst J. Epidemiology of depression. Psychopharmacology (Berl) 1992; 106 Suppl.: 71S-4S
86a. Zhang M, Rost KM, Fortney JC, et al. A community study of depression treatment and employment earnings. Psychiatr Serv 1999; 50: 1209-13
87. Bech P, Dunbar GC, Stoker MJ. The challenge of measuring quality of life in psychiatric patients. In: Jonsson B, Rosenbaum J, editors. Health economics of depression: perspectives in psychiatry, Vol 4. Chichester: Wiley, 1993: 111-28
88. Slevin ML, Plant H, Lynch D, et al. Who should measure quality of life, the doctor or the patient? Br J Cancer 1988; 57: 109-12
89. Olsen JA. Persons vs years: two ways of eliciting implicit weights. Health Econ 1994; 3: 39-46
90. Sackett DL, Torrance GW. The utility of different health states as perceived by the general public. J Chron Dis 1978; 31: 697-704
91. Kaplan RM, Anderson JP. A general health policy model: update and applications. J Health Serv Res 1988; 23: 203-35
92. Simon G, Wagner E, Von Korff M. Cost-effectiveness compari-sons using 'real world' randomized trials: the case of new antidepressant drugs. J Clin Epidemiol 1995; 48: 363-73

93. O'Brien BJ, Novosel S, Torrance G, et al. Assessing the economic value of a new antidepressant: a willingness-to-pay approach. Pharmacoeconomics 1995; 8: 34-45
94. Toufexis A. The personality pill. Time 1993 Oct 11; 76-7
95. Lee AS, Murray RM. The long-term outcome of Maudsley depressives. Br J Psychiatry 1988; 153: 741-51
96. WHO Mental Health Collaborating Centres, 1989
97. Boyer WF, Feighner JP. In: Jonsson B, Rosenbaum J, editors. Health economics of depression: perspectives in psychiatry, Vol. 4. Chichester: Wiley, 1993: 65-76
98. Mindham RH, Howland C, Shepherd M. Continuation therapy with tricyclic antidepressants in depressive illness. Lancet 1987; II: 854-55
99. Prien R, Kupfer D. Continuation drug therapy for major depressive episodes: how long should it be maintained? Am J Psychiatry 1986; 143: 18-23
100. Weissman MM, Klerman GL. Epidemiology of mental disorders: emerging trends in the United States. Arch Gen Psychiatry 1978; 35 (6): 705-12
101. Kupfer DJ, Frank E, Perel JM, et al. Five-year outcome for maintenance therapies in recurrent depression. Arch Gen Psychiatry 1992; 49: 769-73
102. Greden JF. Antidepressant maintenance medications: when to discontinue and how to stop. J Clin Psychiatry 1993; 54: 39-45
103. Old Age Depression Interest Group. How long should the elderly take antidepressants? Br J Psychiatry 1993; 162: 175-82
104. Prien RF, Klett CJ, Caffey EM. Lithium carbonate and imipramine in the prevention of affective episodes. Arch Gen Psychiatry 1973; 29: 420-25
105. Doogan DP, Caillard V. Sertraline in the prevention of depression. Br J Psychiatry 1992: 160: 217-22
106. Hirschfeld RMA, Goodwin FK. Mood disorders. In: Talbott JA, Yudowsky SC, editors. Textbook of psychiatry. Washington, DC: American Psychiatric Press, 1988
107. Baldessarini RJ. Current status of antidepressants: clinical pharmacology and therapy. J Clin Psychiatry 1989; 50: 117-26
108. McCombs JS, Nichol MB, Stimmel GL, et al. The cost of antidepressant drug therapy failure: a study of antidepressant use patterns in a Medicaid population. J Clin Psychiatry 1990; 51 (6): 60-72
109. Katon W, von Korff M, Lin E, et al. Adequacy and duration of antidepressant treatment in primary care. Med Care 1992; 30: 67-76
110. Berlanga C, Ortega-Soto HA. A 3-year follow-up of a group of treatment-resistant depressed patients with a MAOI/tricyclic combination. J Affect Disord 1995; 34: 187-92
111. Tiller J, Mitchell P, Burrows GD. Monoamine oxidase inhibitors (MAOI) or reversible inhibitors of monoamine oxidase (RIMA) tricyclic (TCA) combination therapy. Aust N Z J Psychiatry 1992; 26: 327-9
112. Grounds D. On combining TCAs and MAOIs. Aust N Z J Psychiatry 1993; 26: 327-9
113. Johnson FN. The evolution of lithium therapy. J Psychopharmacol 1992; 6: 325-9
114. Ballenger JC, Post RM. Carbamazepine in manic-depressive illness: a new treatment. Am J Psychiatry 1980; 137: 782-90
115. Robinson DS, Nies A, Ravaris L, et al. Clinical pharmacology of phenelzine. Arch Gen Psychiatry 1978, 35: 629-35
116. Roper Reports. Report to Medicaid: what people do for minor health problems. New York: Roper Organization, 1986: 86-8.
117. Johnson DAW. Non-compliance with antidepressant therapy: an underestimated problem. Intern Med 1986; 11 Suppl.: 14-7
118. Waters WH, Gould NV, Lunn JE. Undispensed prescriptions in a mining general practice. BMJ 1976; 1: 1062-3
119. Begg D. Do patients cash prescriptions? An audit in one practice. J R Coll Gen Pract 1984; 34: 272-4
120. Rashid A. Do patients cash prescriptions? BMJ 1982; 284: 24-6
121. Beardon PH, McGilchrist MM, McKendrick AD, et al. Primary non-compliance with prescribed medication in primary care. BMJ 1993; 307: 846-8
122. Murray J, Shepherd S. Alternative or additional medicine? A new dilemma for the doctor. J R Coll Gen Pract 1988; 38: 511-4
123. Corney RH. Marital problems and treatment outcome in depressed women: a clinical trial of social work intervention. Br J Psychiatry 1987; 151: 652-9
124. Freeling P, Harris CM. The doctor/patient relationship. London: Churchill Livingstone, 1984
125. Hawton K. Controlled studies of psychosocial intervention following attempted suicide. In: Kreitman N, Platt S, editors. Current research on suicide and parasuicide. Edinburgh: Edinburgh University Press, 1989
126. Rosenberg NK. Psychotherapy of the suicidal patient. Acta Psychiatr Scand 1993; 371 Suppl.: 54-6
127. Elkin I, Shea MT, Watkins JT, et al. National Institute of Mental Health treatment of depression collaborative research program: general effectiveness of treatments. Arch Gen Psychiatry 1989; 46: 971-82
128. Paykel ES, Dirlascio A, Haskell D, et al. Effects of maintenance amitriptyline and psychotherapy on symptoms of depression. Psychol Med 1975; 5: 67-77
129. Sturm R, Wells KB. How can care for depression become more cost-effective? JAMA 1995; 273: 51-8
130. Blackburne IM, Bishop S, Glen IM, et al. The efficacy of cognitive treatment in depression: a treatment trial using cognitive therapy and pharmacotherapy, each alone and in combination. Br J Psychiatry 1981; 139: 181-9
131. Teasdale JD, Fennell MJV, Hibbert GA, et al. Cognitive therapy for major depressive disorders in primary care. Br J Psychiatry 1984; 144: 400-6
132. Rush AJ, Beck AT, Kovacs M, et al. Comparative efficacy of cognitive therapy and pharmacotherapy in the treatment of depressed outpatients. Cognit Ther Res 1977; 1: 17-37

133. Frank E, Kupfer DJ, Perel JM, et al. Three-year outcomes. for maintenance therapies in recurrent depression. Arch Gen Psychiatry 1990; 47: 1093-9
134. Agency of Health Care Policy and Research – Depression Guideline Panel. Depression in Primary Care, vol. 2. Treatment of major depression. Clinical practice guideline 5. Rockville (MD): US Dept of Health and Human Services, 1993; ACHPR Publication 93-0551
135. Avery D, Winokur G. The efficacy of electroconvulsive therapy and antidepressants in depression. Biol Psychiatry 1977; 12: 507-23
136. Sack DA, Nurnberger J, Rosenthal NE, et al. The potentiation of antidepressant medications by phase advance of the sleep-wake cycle. Am J Psychiatry 1985; 142: 606-8
137. Schligen B, Tolle R. Partial sleep deprivation as therapy for depression. Arch Gen Psychiatry 1980; 37: 267-71
138. Glaser WA. The politics of paying physicians. Health Aff 1989; 8: 129-46
139. Jonsson B. The pharmaceutical market. In: Bourdet, editor. Internationalisation, market power and consumer welfare. London: Routledge, 1992
140. Association of the British Pharmaceutical Industry. Pharma Facts and Figures. London: ABPI, 1992
141. European Federation of Pharmaceutical Industries' Associations. The pharmaceutical industry in Europe 1990-1991. EFPIA, 1992
142. Coney S. NZ's Pharmac tackles antidepressant bill. Lancet 1994; 344: 463-4
143. McLeod AJ. Rational prescribing [letter]. BMJ 1994; 308: 1573
144. Drummond M, Torrance G, Mason J. Cost-effectiveness league tables: more harm than good? Soc Sci Med 1993; 37: 33-40
145. Rucker TD, Schiff G. Drug formularies: myths-in-formation. Med Care 1990; 28 (10): 928-42
146. Shepherd MD, Salzman RD. The formulary decision-making process in a health maintenance organisation setting. Pharmacoeconomics 1994; 5 (1): 29-38
147. Bochner F, Martin DE, Burgess NG, et al. Drug rationing in a teaching hospital: a method to assign priorities. BMJ 1994; 308: 901-5
148. Donaldson C. Formulate, don't formularise. BMJ 1994; 308: 905-6
149. Petrie JC. First consider the overall process of care [letter]. BMJ 1994; 308: 906
150. Chadwick R. Fairness is at issue [letter]. BMJ 1994; 308: 907-8
151. Drummond MF. The economics of drug formularies. Pharm J 1989; 15: 451-2
152. Hanson ES, Shepherd MD, Pleil A, et al. How P&T committee members in HMSOs make formulary decisions. PT 1992; 17: 247-54
153. Taylor S, McLean P. Outcome profiles in the treatment of unipolar depression. Behav Res Ther 1992; 31 (3): 325-30
154. Henry JA, Alexander CA, Sener EK. Relative mortality from overdose of antidepressants. BMJ 1995; 310: 221-4
155. Montgomery SA, Henry JA, McDonald G, et al. Selective serotonin reuptake inhibitors: meta-analysis of discontinuation rates. Int Clin Psychopharmacol 1994; 9: 47-54
156. Sloan FA, Gordon GS, Cocks DL. Hospital drug formularies and use of hospital services. Med Care 1993; 31 (10): 851-67
157. Pearce MJ, Begg EJ. A review of limited lists and formularies. Pharmacoeconomics 1992; 1(3): 191-202
158. Hazlet TK, Hu TW. Association between formulary strategies and hospital drug expenditure. Am J Hosp Pharm 1992; 49 (9): 2207-10
159. Scrip 26 Mar 1996
160. Raisch DW. Relationship among prescription payment methods and interactions between community pharmacists and prescribers. Ann Pharmacother 1992; 26 (7-8): 902-6
161. Goldberg D. Gater R. Estimates of need. Psychiatr Bull 1991; 15: 593-5
162. Thompson C, Thompson CM. The prescription of antidepressants in general practice: a critical review. Hum Psychopharmacol 1989; 4: 91-102
163. Bradlow J, Coulter A. Effect of fundholding and indicative prescribing schemes on general practitioners' prescribing costs. BMJ 1993; 307: 1186-9
164. Bligh J, Walley T. The UK Indicative Prescribing Scheme. Pharmacoeconomics 1992; 2 (2): 137-52
165. Bradley C. Decision making and prescribing patterns: a literature review. Fam Prac 1991; 8 (3): 276-87
166. Avorn J, Soumerai SB. Improving drug-therapy decisions through educational outreach: a randomized control trial of academically based 'detailing'. N Engl J Med 1983; 308: 1457-63
167. Gehlbach SH, Wilkinson WE, Hammond WE, et al. Improving drug prescribing in a primary care practice. Med Care 1984; 22: 193-201
168. Harris CM, Jarman B, Woodman E, et al. Prescribing: a case for treatment. London: Royal College of General Practitioners, 1984: occasional paper no. 24
169. Hux JE, Naylor CD. Drug prices and third party payment: do they influence medical selection? Pharmacoeconomics 1994; 5 (4): 343-50
170. Jabbari B, Bryan GE, Marsh EE, et al. Incidence of seizures with tricyclic and tetracyclic antidepressants. Arch Neurol 1985; 42 (5): 480-1
171. Hale AS. New antidepressants: use in high-risk patients. J Clin Psychiatry 1993; 54 (8 Suppl.): 61-70
172. Overall JE. Efficacy of nomifensine in different depressive syndromes. J Clin Psychiatry 1984; 45 (4): 85-8
173. Boyer WF. Potential indications for the SSRIs. Int Clin Psychopharmacol 1992; 53: 61-6
174. Wakelin JS, Coleman BS. The influence of the 5-HT specific antidepressant, fluvoxamine maleate, on suicidal behaviour [abstract]. Int J Neurosci 1986; 31: 216

175. Mullin JM, Pandita-Gunawardena VR, Whitehead AM. A double-blind comparison of fluvoxamine and dothiepin in the treatment of major affective disorder. Br J Clin Prac 1988; 42 (2): 51-5
176. Sacchetti E, Vita A, Guarneri L et, al. The effectiveness of fluoxetine, clomipramine, nortriptyline and desipramine in major depressives with suicidal behaviour: preliminary findings. In: Casano GB, Akiskal HS, editors. Serotonin-related psychiatric syndromes: clinical and therapeutic links. London: Royal Society of Medicine, 1991 (International Congress and Symposium Series; 165)
177. Feldman HS, Denber HC. Long-term study of fluvoxamine: a new rapid-acting antidepressant. Int Pharmacopsychiatry 1982; 17: 114-22
178. Henry JA, Martin AJ. The risk-benefit assessment of antidepressant drugs. Med Toxicol 1987; 2: 445-62
179. Muijen M, Roy D, Silverstone T, et al. A comparative clinical trial of fluoxetine, mianserin and placebo with depressed outpatients. Acta Psychiatr Scand 1988; 78: 384-90
180. Wakelin J. The role of serotonin in depression and suicide. Adv Biol Psychiatry 1988; 17: 70-83
181. de Wilde JEM, Doogan DP. Fluvoxamine and clomipramine in endogenous depression. J Affec Disord 1982; 4: 249-59
182. Martin AJ, Tebbs VM, Ashford JJ. Affective disorders in general practice: treatment of 6000 patients with fluvoxamine. Pharmatherapeutica 1987; 5: 40-8
183. Montgomery SA, Pinder RM. Do some antidepressants promote suicide? Psychopharmacology 1987; 92: 265-6
184. Montgomery SA, McAulay R, Rani SJ. A double blind comparison of zimelidine and amitriptyline in endogenous depression. Acta Psychiatr Scand 1981; 63: 314-27
185. Damluji NF, Ferguson JM. Paradoxical worsening of depressive symptomatology caused by antidepressants. J Clin Psychopharmacol 1988; 8 (5): 347-9
186. Beasley CM, Dornseif BE, Bosomworth MES, et al. Fluoxetine and suicide: a meta-analysis of controlled trials of treatment of depression. BMJ 1991; 303: 665-92
187. Fava M, Rosenbaum JF. Suicidality and fluoxetine – is there a relationship? J Clin Psychiatry 1991; 52: 108-11
188. Rouillon R, Philips R, Serrurier D, et al. Rechutes du depression unipolaire et efficacite de la maprotiline. L'Encephale 1993; XV: 527-34
189. Feuerstein TJ, Jakisch R. Why do some antidepressants promote suicide [letter]? Psychopharmacol 1986; 90: 422
190. Doogan DP, Caillard V. Sertraline in the prevention of depression. Br J Psychiatry 1992; 160: 217-22
191. Wernicke JF, Bosomworth JC, Ashbrook E. Fluoxetine at 20 mg per day: the recommended and therapeutic dose in the treatment of depression. Int Clin Psychopharmacol 1989; 4 Suppl. 1: 63-7
192. Weissman MM. The epidemiology of suicide attempts, 1960-1971. Arch Gen Psychiatry 1974; 30: 737-46
193. Johnson DAW. Depression: treatment compliance in general practice. Acta Psychiatr Scand 1981; 63: 447-53
194. Johnson DAW. Antidepressant treatment observed: some problems of compliance by doctors and patients. In: Sims, Ottofson, editors. Antidepressants: progress in problem areas. London: Franklin Scientific Projects, 1984
195. Canino GJ, Bird HR, Shrout PE, et al. The prevalence of specific psychiatric disorders in Puerto Rico. Arch Gen Psychiatry 1987; 44 (8): 727-35
196. Blacker CVR, Clare AW. The prevalence and treatment of depression in general practice. Psychopharmacol 1988; 95: 14-17
197. Keller MB, Klerman GL Lavori PW, et al. Treatment received by depressed patients. JAMA 1982; 248 (15): 1848-55
198. Tyrer P. Drug treatment of psychiatric patients in general practice. BMJ 1978: 2: 1008-10
199. Kass F, Charles E, Walsh T, et al. Quality review of outpatient psychopharmacological practice with APA Task Force criteria. Am J Psychiatry 1983; 140 (2): 221-4
200. Fish D. What is an effective dose [letter]? BMJ 1997; 314: 826
201. Gill D. Systematic review of all pertinent trials is required to establish guidelines [letter]. BMJ 1997; 314: 826-7
202. Tan RS. Low dose tricyclic antidepressants are effective in treating major depression [letter]. BMJ 1997; 314: 827
203. Gorham PN. Who bears the cost of antidepressants in Australia? Med J Aust 1995; 162: 162-3
204. Maxwell M, Heaney D, Howie JGR, et al. General practice fundholding: observations on prescribing patterns and costs using the defined daily dose method. BMJ 1993; 307: 1190-4
205. Griffin JP, Griffin TD. The economic implications of therapeutic conservatism. J R Coll Physicians Lond 1993; 27 (2): 121-6
206. Goldstein AO, Ives TJ. Depression treatment. J Fam Pract 1994; 38: 49-57
207. Kind P, Sorensen J. Modelling the cost-effectiveness of the prophylactic use of SSRIs in the treatment of depression. Int Clin Psychopharmacol 1995; 10: 41-8
208. Le Pen C, Levy E, Ravily V, et al. The cost of treatment dropout in depression: a cost-benefit analysis of fluoxetine vs tricyclics. J Affect Disord 1994; 31: 1-18

Correspondence: Prof. *John A. Henry*, Accident and Emergency, St Mary's Hospital, London W2, England.

Constraints on Antidepressant Prescribing and Principles of Cost-Effective Antidepressant Use

Part 2: Cost-Effectiveness Analyses

John A. Henry and *Carol A. Rivas*

St Mary's Hospital, London, England

International attempts to control expenditure in healthcare have focused on the cost of drugs and constraints on what is prescribed. Acquisition cost is an increasingly important influence on clinical decisions. However, the use of drug costs alone in determining healthcare policies at the level of a nation, region or individual prescriber inevitably overlooks the other direct costs of treating the disease, which may also be attributable to the same budget. Hence, not only can restriction of spending on drugs have unwanted effects on other budgets, but it may also fail to achieve its goal. It also hinders research and development of new drugs.

In Part 1 of this review (see page 167),[1] we discussed the relative clinical merits of the different treatments, and how economic policies that reduce the use of indisputably cost-ineffective treatments should preserve the availability of a range of choices. Pharmacoeconomic studies enable a more structured comparison and evaluation of different treatments that may not be adequately compared by clinical or purchase cost considerations alone. They enable efficacy and tolerability to be considered when targeting resources, as well as other clinical and pharmacological factors.

This is important, since the final overall cost of treatment can vary greatly for each patient, not just with the drug chosen, but with the initial and final dosages, how long the patient needs to be treated and how many therapies have to be tried before a satisfactory response occurs. When compliance is taken into account, economic studies that compare the different antidepressant treatments may demonstrate marginally greater benefits from the newer antidepressants.[2-5] Lower direct costs arise because relapse and consequent hospitalisation is less likely,[5-7] although the advantages may be cancelled out if the interpretation and assumptions are only slightly changed.[8-10]

1. Data Used in Pharmacoeconomic Studies

Pharmacoeconomic studies must draw from a large pool of diverse clinical, epidemiological, cost and pharmacological data. These data come from a number of sources.

1.1 Clinical Trials

Clinical trials provide most of the source data on the effectiveness and outcome of antidepressant therapy. They are designed to minimise confounding and make results as unambiguous as possible. Unfortunately, these design features ironically mean that clinical trials are relatively artificial, a problem that many authors recognise.[7,11] Their generalisability to usual clinical practice is severely limited.[12] Moreover, many elements may weight clinical trial data against the newer antidepressant drugs and towards the tricyclic antidepressants (TCAs).

For example, patients receiving clinical trial therapies have higher compliance rates and higher dosages than in the naturalistic setting. It is common in the community for TCAs to be taken at below the usually recommended dosages, often in order to minimise their adverse effects.[11,13-16] This is not so for the selective serotonin (5-hydroxytryptamine; 5-HT) reuptake inhibitors (SSRIs), which are better tolerated and have a larger range of effective dosages. Thus in a trial, TCAs will have more adverse effects, but be more effective than in the naturalistic setting, and SSRIs will have more adverse effects without any useful compensating increase in effectiveness.

Complex or demanding treatment regimens also have an advantage in clinical trial conditions. Blinding necessitates that patients assigned to different treatments receive identical care, in terms of such parameters as drug administration schedules, clinic visits and laboratory monitoring. Since care must be designed around the most demanding treatment, for ethical reasons, the advantages of a drug with less frequent administration, less monitoring or fewer dosage adjustments will be obscured.[12,17] These advantages might potentially tip the economic scales in favour of a new drug, but would not be picked up in a clinical trial.

Other features that may favour the TCAs include the selection of patients with major depressive disorder or those from tertiary-care psychiatric clinics, and the common exclusion of 'complicated patients', patients at risk of adverse effects[18] and those who are already suicidal. Patients in the naturalistic setting may experience common diseases such as epilepsy, diabetes and hypertension, which would be exclusions from a clinical trial and might constrain the choice of antidepressant drug. Clinical trial participants differ from patients in the average general practice not only in terms of illness,[11,19,20] but also with regard to motivation and willingness to accept placebo.[11] Simon et al.[12] concluded that patients in the community could not be more poorly matched to clinical trial patients, being clinically heterogeneous rather than homogeneous, mildly rather than severely ill, more likely to discontinue treatment, showing a high rate of spontaneous remission, and often experiencing co-morbid medical conditions.

Hence, there are many parameters that might bias data from clinical trials in favour of the TCAs. Against this, some authors believe that, in general, new drugs may be favoured in a clinical trial.[21] However, the factors they list to support this notion relate mainly to (sometimes intentional) prestudy bias or to poor methodology, which should be relatively easy to monitor and guard against, rather than inherent features. Factors include generally poor trial design,

Table I. Differences in the ratio of direct to indirect costs for depression and mental illness from different studies

Country	Subject	Ratio of direct to indirect costs
US[32]	Mental illness	1.35
US[33]	Mental illness	0.21
Germany[33]	Mental illness	0.55
Sweden[33]	Mental illness	2.09
US[36]	Major depression	6.76
UK[30]	Depression	7.19
US[37]	Depression	6.14
US[38]	Depression	7.33
US[39]	Depression	2.52
Belgium[40]	Depression	1.59
Sweden[35]	Psychotic depression	0.84
UK[34]	Neurotic depression	0.50
Sweden[35]	Neurotic depression	5.11
US[41]	Youth suicide	2.73

poor choice of dosages used and variables studied, misuse or misunderstanding of statistics, poor handling of patient withdrawals and other exclusions, and selective reporting.[21] These failings should be detectable in any report.

Despite their disadvantages, clinical trials provide the strongest causal link between drug use and outcome,[22] and such 'hard' data make for more clear-cut results in assessments. There are insufficient available data from everyday medical practice that can serve as a basis for cost studies. Such research is highly expensive and few studies of this nature exist at present.

1.2 'Real World' Trials

An alternative to clinical trials, a 'real world randomised trial', has been advocated by Simon et al.[12] Treatments are randomly assigned under conditions of everyday clinical practice. Clinicians are not blind to the choice of treatment and are free to determine its dosage and duration. They are also told to keep to clinical decisions that they would normally make, and that they can withdraw the patient or switch to an alternative treatment of their choice if they wish, according to their normal practice. Only the data collators are blind to the drug used, and data collection is totally separate from treatment.

Simon et al.[12] recommend a multifactorial assessment of outcome after antidepressant use in 'real world' trials, and measures of cognitive and functional impairment as well as a traditional depression rating scale. This has important benefits, but makes any analysis more complex. This, together with the presence of many confounding factors that are normally excluded in a clinical trial and the need for a larger sample size to allow for biases, makes such a study better suited as a complement to clinical trial data rather than an alternative.

1.3 Pharmacoeconomic Arms in Clinical Trials

Perhaps the most convenient and accurate source of data is the pharmacoeconomic analysis incorporated into clinical trials *ab initio*. This has important benefits: data collection can be prospective and can focus on the most appropriate parameters, and standard statistical tests can be used. However, the necessary sample size may be larger than that needed to show differences in clinical effectiveness. This creates an ethical dilemma, as it may be argued that a clinical trial should only be continued until a drug's efficacy or inefficacy, and clinical superiority or inferiority, has been demonstrated. Thus, the accuracy of pharmacoeconomic arms of clinical trials may need to be compromised to at least some degree.[10]

1.4 Healthcare Databases

Many studies concentrate on insurance claims databases such as the US Medicaid database, or other so-called 'observational' (or 'real world') databases compiled for administrative or billing purposes. Since these consider actual use, they avoid the problems of generalising from clinical trial data. They enable ready access to a large community sample of patients and are reasonably comprehensive, with detailed patient-level and longitudinal data on treatment delivered, as well as built-in charge figures.[23] These data provide useful indices of adherence to treatment and intermediate outcome measures, such as rates of hospital admission, although constraints on treatment utilisation, such as ceilings to claims, must be taken into account.

The major problem with Medicaid data is that there are sociodemographic and health differences from the general population. Other problems with such databases are that only the services and items reimbursed by insurance will be included, treatment will be affected by claims constraints, and indirect costs cannot be derived. Diagnoses tend to be hard to validate, clinical bias concerning the use of treatments cannot be measured, and chronic conditions may be under-reported.[23] Detailed data on clinical severity or functional outcomes, and other important clinical information, may be lacking. Charges made may need to be converted to give the true cost.[23] Breaks in the eligibility of patients may be interpreted as illness-free periods and variations in dosage cannot be measured. Thus, such data often cannot be used to determine differences in clinical effectiveness between treatments.

2. Limitations in Comparing Studies

In cost analyses of treatment, the aim is usually to quantify the effects on specific budgets of using specific treatments for specific patients. It is important to understand how this limits the way in which data are generalised to other budgets, healthcare settings or countries. Differences in basic assumptions and clinical practice, and the lack of a standardised methodology for cost analyses, increase the problems.

2.1 Setting

The severity and management of depression may vary considerably between areas with differing cultures and different diagnostic criteria, and between primary care and hospitals. Such differences exist not only between countries, but between neighbouring regions in a given country, especially those that are relatively independent, such as the states of the US. In the UK, for example, the various regional health authorities differ in funding priorities, patient and disease demographics (which are well documented, with a clear north-south divide), and local shared-care protocols.

Variations in parameters such as the availability of different healthcare resources with setting and time, their relative use, local clinical practice, and the relative prices of the resources mean that consideration of one budget or setting in isolation can give a false impression of cost effectiveness or degree of benefit. When applied to a different setting, the same stratagem may cease to be cost effective. This was shown by an analysis that compared use of the same drug, using identical methodology, in 4 countries.[24,25] Even though the drug was 36% more expensive to buy in the US, its overall use was more cost effective in that country than in the 3 European countries also considered.[24,25] However, other experience from the US has suggested that differences between healthcare settings in health and mental health status may not be a problem in cost analyses.[26]

2.2 Dosage

Minimum dosages tend to differ considerably with setting, particularly for the TCAs, and this affects the purchase prices quoted in studies. Johnson[15,16,27,28] considered 75 mg/day to be the typical dosage for the older TCAs dothiepin and amitriptyline actually prescribed in UK general practice, but in Boyer and Feighner's model,[7] hypothetical minimum dosages were 150 mg/day for amitriptyline, and – a more reliable – 20 mg/day for fluoxetine. The older TCAs when given at a dosage of less than 75 mg/day are often ineffective, and may be associated with more treatment failures[28] and, ultimately, increased costs, which exceed the savings made from the purchase of lesser amounts of drug. Even when long term therapy is considered, it cannot be assumed that a low maintenance dosage will be adequate, since evidence is now accumulating that the dosage that induced remission is also the dosage that is most likely to prevent relapse.[29]

Just how big an effect discordance over dose can have on cost studies may be partially examined using Boyer and Feighner's[7] own sensitivity analysis of the retail drug cost per patient, assuming a standard 6-month course, with full compliance. For example, a more realistic comparison of equivalent dosages, namely their 'low-dosage' amitriptyline (150 mg/day) and 'high-dosage' fluoxetine (80 mg/day) or paroxetine (50 mg/day), can be made. When this is done it suggests that, all other factors being equal, the two SSRIs are at least 2 to 3 times more expensive to buy than branded amitriptyline. This contrasts sharply with Boyer and Feighner's[7] claim that amitriptyline is slightly more expensive, based on a comparison of their proposed minimum-dosage figures for all three drugs.

However, their model produced little cost difference between 'high-dosage' sertraline (200 mg/day) at $US655.06, and 'low-dosage' branded desipramine (150 mg/day) at $US505.28. The arguably unfair dosage comparisons which Boyer and Feighner[7] made may in fact only alter the power of their argument in other settings and not their conclusions; in their overall model of a 6-month acute treatment course, TCAs were less economical than SSRIs with an 85% cost discount. This is greater than the 50% discount that would be needed to allow for the discrepancy between the cited minimum dosage of 150 mg/day for amitriptyline and the commonly used 75 mg/day.

2.3 Methodology

When two different authors consider the same location and setting at the same time, they may still provide different figures for the same items. Authors' estimates differ for the cost of depression in the UK,[2,30,31] using published statistics. The relative values of direct costs (that is, prices actually paid) and indirect costs (usually measures of lost productivity) differ with author when considering mental illness in the US[32,33] and also neurotic depression[34,35] (table I). There is greater concordance with regard to the relative value of direct and indirect costs of depression in the US and UK,[30,36-38] although Greenberg et al.[39] in the US and Mendlewicz[40] in Belgium provide a different figure (table I).

Such differences are the result of alternative methodology or assumptions. This was demonstrated by a study which estimated the cost of paroxetine therapy as similar to that of imipramine therapy using one outcome measure, and as cheaper using another measure (outcome measures are discussed in more detail in section 2.3.5).[2]

2.3.1 Top-Down Studies versus Bottom-Up Decision Trees

Existing data can be considered retrospectively or 'top-down', or they can be evaluated 'bottom-up'. With top-down analyses, the authors work backwards from published official figures or the results of published studies.[2,30,31] The main advantage is that all values originate from facts that can be taken as established. There is an automatic testing of any assumptions that are made, as they have to be constrained to fit the facts. However, original data that are taken as a premise often have marked shortcomings,[2] and will have been gathered with different and perhaps conflicting objectives.

Many statistics that are collated independently (such as national data) do not separately itemise an illness such as depression; also, patient numbers may need to be extrapolated from prescription numbers. Thus, data often have to be transformed to suit the requirements of the cost analysis, introducing relatively subjective assumptions.

Data collated from a number of sources may also introduce uncontrolled systematic sampling error. For any one year, data are frequently not available for all of the items under evaluation, but older and more recent data are often not compatible; a number of criteria may have changed over the years, such as definitions of long term efficacy, response and relapse.[42] There is also a trend towards shorter hospital stays, which will affect older costings, and also treatment rationalisation. Recent recommendations that maintenance therapy should continue for longer than hitherto,[18,43] and at an adequate dosage, will affect the interpretation of older data, as well as clinical trial data, since almost all of the standard clinical trials last for only a few weeks. This causes problems for all cost-effectiveness studies that are not *de novo*.

Some authors have designed bottom-up models, by generating algorithms known as decision trees or event trees, each branch being an alternative decision that leads to a different event. A treatment protocol defines how depression is treated, and the model then incorporates the probability of success and failure of each drug at each stage. All possible events or outcomes in a treatment sequence should ideally be included. Each is assigned both a probability and a utility (a measure of satisfaction with it), suggested by a panel of experts (sometimes known as a Delphi panel). The panel also approves and validates the synthesis of data. These models aim to combine the best of the data from real-life databases and clinical trials. Original data may sometimes be generated *de novo* from a study of patients.

However, decision trees typically rely on binary choices. So they can only describe discrete outcomes that are either irreversible or are time-limited,[12] and not those clinical measures that are continuous variables in the subject population or over time. Many branches of the decision tree cannot be determined because data are not available, such as the outcomes of patients who discontinue therapy; since patients experiencing more severe adverse effects or a lack of efficacy are more likely to discontinue, this can be an important problem. The experience of expert panels is biased towards patients who are seen more often, so expert estimates typically overestimate resource utilisation and hence 'real world' costs.

The top-down and bottom-up approaches may provide markedly different results because some subjectivity is unavoidable in both, or because of inadequacies in the official figures (which may be used in both top-down and bottom-up analyses), and it would seem likely that neither approach is definitive. The true totals probably lie somewhere between the two. For example, in one study,[34] the cost of lost productivity related to the morbidity of neurotic illness was very different, depending on whether bottom-up or top-down data were used. The cost was 250 million pounds sterling (£) [1985 costs] using the 'number of days' certified absence for which mental disorders were the reason in official statistics, but nearer £2.9 billion when experimental data were used for calculations.[34]

2.3.2 Prevalence and Incidence Rate

The type of rate used for the occurrence of variables, prevalence or incidence, can also affect the conclusions of cost studies. The prevalence rate considers the total *costs* within a defined time period, so that some may originate from *events* that occurred before the study period. The incidence rate is a prospective measure of the total future (time-unlimited) lifetime costs that accrue to new cases in the study period.

Weinstein and Saturno[41] considered the incidence measure to be more suitable for cost-effectiveness and cost-benefit analyses. This is because it can be used to calculate the total savings possible from intervention strategies that occur in a small, defined, time interval. Prevalence data will be confounded by its retrospective component, so that it will incorporate the consequences of changes that have already occurred, and is also confounded by current events. The problems become clear from consideration of the campaigns of the 1990s to improve awareness and diagnosis of depression. These may lead to a larger clinical population which is very different to earlier ones, with more early stage disease. The evolution of disease in these patients will not be accurately reflected in current prevalence data. By contrast, the incidence approach will incorporate the accrual of direct costs over the years for a patient with early onset depression.

Hence, although the incidence approach is more open to inaccuracies from assumptions about the future, it may be a more sensitive tool. Nonetheless, almost all pharmacoeconomic analyses of mental illness, depression or antidepressants have used the prevalence rate of illness.

2.3.3 Discounting

Since the advantages of many of the savings from an intervention will take a long time to be realised, some authors[8,32,35,36,41,44,45] discount costs, weighting them in favour of more immediate savings. There are several arguments in favour of this. Limited empirical evidence supports the subjective notion of time preference, where the individual prefers immediate benefits, but with deferred costs (a notional immediate saving).[46] However, this preference may not be in the interest of future society,[46] and preferences may depend on whether or not the cost is to the individual.[46]

It is generally accepted that discounting of costs should be used when procedures or diseases with different time profiles are being compared, and also for cost-effectiveness analyses, and any other studies that evaluate the effect of intervention or change on future costs.[41] However, a small difference in the discount rate used can make a large difference to the final costing for the same data, when comparing different age groups, and when comparing interventions in which one has a larger deferred cost component than another, and this is not usually satisfactorily dealt with. Standardisation of discount rates used is important to enable comparisons of different studies.[44] The Netherlands has adopted a uniform 5% rate for public projects, while US federal agencies all use a 10% rate. The UK previously recommended a general 5% rate, but by 1992, had decided that health benefits should have a zero rate.[24]

The time profile of benefits is likely to be more variable and larger than for direct costs, increasing the risk of inaccuracy. Interventions with immediate costs and delayed benefits are more sensitive to discounting than those in which costs and benefits are both stepped.

There are arguments in favour of using a different discount rate for direct financial costs and for health benefits,[46] but if a lower discount rate is used for benefits than costs, the logical conclusion is that the greater the delay in starting an intervention, the more cost effective it is.[45]

2.3.4 Sensitivity Analyses

Sensitivity analyses are used to test the robustness of a result over a range of alternative values of parameters for which some uncertainty over accuracy exists. The best- and worst-case scenarios can be discussed and sensitivity analyses should certainly be advocated. However, the selection of both upper and lower limits, and the interpretation of robustness, may be arbitrary or subjective. Such analyses also ignore changes in the interaction of parameters. Some attempt has been made to improve on traditional sensitivity analyses with the so-called 'Monte Carlo simulation' method or nonparametric bootstrapping.[10]

2.3.5 Measures of Outcome

In order to compare 2 treatments, the same outcome measure must be used for both; this is necessary whatever the source of the data. Partly for this reason, it may not be possible to extract an ideal outcome measure from data that are not generated *de novo*, and even with prospective studies, the wrong decision may be made.

A patient who has used an active dosage of antidepressant for the generally recommended time is often recorded as a treatment success.[13,24] But this may be inappropriate. The course of depression is very variable, durations of depressive episodes vary, depression is often cyclical, and relapse can occur even when on therapy.[7,48,49] The choice and dosage of antidepressant therapy is tailored to the individual, and many patients are given subtherapeutic dosages, creating problems in the evaluation of success on the basis of adequate therapy. Moreover, comparisons are hindered by the tendency to quote per-patient or national values, and rarely, both. In any case, this is an indirect measure of health outcome, which essentially equates with compliance.

Direct measures of success, such as percentage of responders according to clinical impression or a rating scale, are less objective than for organic illnesses, and it is difficult to definitively test emotional functioning.

3. Different Pharmacoeconomic Analyses of Antidepressant Use

There are differences not only in the source and collection of data, the study objectives, the analytical approach and the rigorousness of the methodology, but also in the pharmacoeconomic method used. This may depend on the study objectives or on the available data.

3.1 Cost-Effectiveness Analysis

Cost-effectiveness analysis is appropriate when alternative therapies have different effectiveness (not to be confused with efficacy, which is effectiveness as measured under clinical trial conditions), as is the case with antidepressants. Its final statistic is usually the ratio of net costs to net effectiveness (as measured by health outcome). It may be no coincidence that this is similar to the ratio used by Bochner et al.[50] to determine whether a drug should be included in a formulary.

In Jonsson and Bebbington's[2,3] comparison of the direct costs of paroxetine and imipramine in the treatment of depression, the annual cost per successfully treated patient gave an advantage to paroxetine (£785) over imipramine (£1024), and differed from the annual cost per patient treated (around £430 for both paroxetine and imipramine).

Bentkover et al.[4] used the same clinical trial data as Jonsson and Bebbington[2,3] for their cost-effectiveness model, but considered US prices. They determined that treatment failure, measured by noncompliance, as with Jonsson and Bebbington,[2,3] needed to be only 4.1% greater for generic imipramine than branded paroxetine for cost effectiveness to be equal. In fact, the compliance differential was 12% and the 6-month cost per successfully treated patient was $US5713 for paroxetine and $US6424 for imipramine. The savings over 6 months for

1000 patients taking paroxetine rather than imipramine were $US67 188 in hospitalisation costs and $US11 546 in outpatient visit costs, while medication costs increased by $US31 476.

There are problems with the Jonsson and Bebbington data.[2,3] Not only was the choice of outcome measure weak, but it depended on a rather high 20% difference in withdrawal rates between the types of antidepressant.[9] Withdrawal rates vary widely between clinical trials, with a possible range of 0 to 80% for the same drug,[9] depending on factors such as patient selection, previous treatment, methodology and study setting. Use of a meta-analysis would have been more appropriate than Jonsson and Bebbington's pooling of selected data. Meta-analyses undertaken by other authors report a difference in withdrawals related to adverse effects of SSRIs compared with TCAs of between 3.4% and 4.9% in favour of SSRIs.[9,51,52]

Jonsson and Bebbington[2,3] have also been criticised for the practice of extrapolating the results of a 12-week study to 1 year. During longer treatment periods the withdrawal rate will change. Although there is disagreement as to whether it increases[9] or decreases,[10] there is no doubt that cost-effectiveness measures should differ, depending on whether treatment is at an acute or maintenance phase.

Le Pen et al.[53] used a Delphi expert panel and a 4-month decision tree to estimate the expected cost of treatment withdrawal, including suicide, when using fluoxetine or TCAs in the outpatient setting to treat a hypothetical group of patients with either 'dysthymic-neurotic depression' or 'reactive depression'. Withdrawal rates were obtained from 14 clinical trials lasting 4 to 8 weeks. The analysis showed that short term treatment with fluoxetine was cost effective if the value of a human life exceeded FF8600 (1994 values) up to a maximum of FF23 800 (equivalent to $US1500 to $US4300 in 1994); the range is the result of a sensitivity analysis. The cut-off value that determines whether a medical intervention is an appropriate use of resources is usually taken to be in the range of $US50 000[54] to $US100 000[55] per quality-adjusted life year.

However, years of life saved were only approximately computed by Le Pen et al.,[53] who standardised the age of suicide of all patients to 49.4 years for men and 49 years for women. This is important because suicide was the most influential factor affecting results in favour of fluoxetine in this study, and direct costs had only a weak effect. If this reflects reality, the real cost effectiveness of fluoxetine is greater than this study of Le Pen et al.[53] suggests, since it ignored secondary direct costs of suicide. Many other costs were similarly ignored on the assumption that they would have been likely to favour fluoxetine anyway and so would not affect the direction of results. This limits the usefulness of the study.[53]

Brown et al.[55a] based their cost-effectiveness comparison of mirtazapine with amitriptyline and fluoxetine on a meta-analysis, which may have affected the accuracy of their study. They extrapolated the data to 6 months using a Delphi panel and published information, and so their study suffers similar drawbacks to the Jonsson and Bebbington study.[2,3] Their decision tree included time off work because of the depression. They reported that mirtazapine was cost-effective in comparison with amitriptyline in their Austrian setting, with fewer hospitalisations from treatment withdrawals, less time off work, and more patients successfully treated (23.2% compared with 19% for amitriptyline). A study of the French situation, based on published data, an expert panel, and a large multicentre study, examined an 18-month period in order to capture data on relapses and recurrences.[55b] This study found maintenance use of fluvoxamine was less costly than the use of tricyclics in terms of total direct and indirect costs.

Fluvoxamine was associated with a longer depression-free period (79% of the study period compared with 71% for TCAs).

Einarson et al.[56] used the 'number of symptom-free days' in major depressives as their outcome measure of cost effectiveness. SSRIs and venlafaxine were more cost effective in their inpatient model than TCAs and heterocyclic antidepressants, and heterocyclic antidepressants were the most cost effective in outpatients, although none of the advantages were statistically significant. Sclar et al.[57] used healthcare expenditure to measure the cost effectiveness of antidepressant use in a US health maintenance organisation. They found that while the cost of drug used was higher for fluoxetine than TCAs, the direct costs of healthcare expenditure for the treatment of depression were lower for fluoxetine.

3.2 Marginal Cost-Effectiveness Analysis

The most meaningful measure in cost-effectiveness analyses is one that compares the cost-effectiveness ratio of one therapy with that of an alternative, rather than against the zero value of no treatment. Hence the cost-effectiveness ratio for each drug should not be the only result considered for comparison; the average cost-effectiveness ratio (the mean of the cost-effectiveness ratios of all the alternatives), or else the marginal cost-effectiveness value, should also be given.

Marginal cost-effectiveness studies enable an estimate to be made of the price to be paid for a small change in a variable, such as the use of a more effective therapy, or reduced inpatient care. A threshold is reached at which the benefits exceed the marginal costs, and at this point, the substitute therapy is said to dominate. This feature of marginal cost-effectiveness studies is particularly useful in making decisions about resource allocation. For example, Boyer and Feighner[7] compared the direct costs of hospitalisation, drugs and outpatient-clinic attendance of patients treated with SSRIs or TCAs, and found that, during acute (6-month) management, reducing hospitalisation rates for depressed patients from an assumed 11% to a hypothetical 3% still gave each of the chosen SSRIs a cost advantage. The same was true when hospitalisation rates were kept at 11%, but outpatient attendances were reduced to zero. The limitations of this and other studies have already been discussed in section 2.2.

Kind and Sorenson[5] considered the presence or absence of symptoms as the primary outcome measure in their simple model of 1 year of maintenance treatment with a SSRI. They used relapse and compliance estimates from published trial data. Although they acknowledged that the source studies varied in important parameters such as duration, they took simplified measures of median values of unweighted data from these trials. Costs were updated from 1993 to 1994 values from their earlier study of the costs of depression.[30] Estimated costs of SSRI drug therapy ranged from £0.64 to £1.55 for a daily dose (£116.48 to £282.10 for a 6-month period).

Two alternative treatment strategies were modelled in this study,[5] one in which patients were only actively treated for depression when symptoms re-emerged, and a prophylactic one, in which all patients received maintenance SSRI treatment after their initial episode of depression. The average cost per symptom-free patient was estimated to be £271 with the first strategy and £389 to £474 with the second, but with a larger number of symptom-free patients (633 to 846 per 1000 patients with the second strategy, compared with 464 per 1000 patient for the first). Varying the levels of compliance plus response for the second strategy resulted in the following indirect benefits per 1000 patients treated in: 169 to 382 additional symptom-free patients; 18 083 to 40 874 days of lost productivity avoided; £216 996 to £490 488 (1994 values) equivalent income saved (according to previous methodology[30]); and 10 to 24 life-years saved. All measures were subject to the same criticism as their original study,[30] on which they are based. The model was particularly sensitive to changes in the rate of patient admission to psychiatric hospital.

Gross[58] considered the effect of substituting venlafaxine for fluoxetine in hospitalised patients. He calculated direct and indirect costs, but did not consider the effects of a reduced suicide rate with venlafaxine or the cost of treating recurrences and relapse. Gross[58] assumed that venlafaxine was 20% more effective than fluoxetine. The proposed switch of therapy was calculated to result in savings of 11.3%. Even when corrections were made for the high dosage of fluoxetine used (40 mg/day), a switch to venlafaxine still resulted in cost savings.

These types of study have huge implications in the current cost climate. They show that improved treatment may make economic sense, despite initially high financial commitments.

3.3 Cost-Utility Analysis

Cost-utility analysis may be considered as a type of cost-effectiveness study. The difference is that in a cost-effectiveness study, 'life-years' or 'drug failure' may be the index of effectiveness. In a cost-utility analysis, it is the increase in years of life adjusted for their health quality, which are termed quality-adjusted life years (QALYs). One year of good health (QALY 1.0) is equivalent to 10 years of severely impaired health (each of QALY 0.1).

The ultimate aim of all drug treatment (including antidepressants) is to improve and maintain health and well-being, and quality or duration of life, so it might appear that QALYs are an optimal measure that should be preferentially employed in assessing treatment costs. This would make cost-utility analysis the optimal pharmacoeconomic study choice. Like cost-effectiveness studies, they are suited to the allocation of resources within a defined budget, but cost-utility studies are the only type of economic analysis that can combine multiple outcome measures into a single value. The preferred stratagem is the one with the lowest cost per QALY.

QALYs take individual preferences into account. They are generated by assigning common measures of satisfaction, derived from patients or clinicians, and termed 'utilities', to improvements in mortality and morbidity. They can then be used as a simple summary statistic of the change that a treatment produces in expected years of life, reflecting the quality of those years. QALYs are particularly useful when medical intervention has a large impact on morbidity, but not on mortality. They are also useful when considering failed suicide, which may lead to a reduced quality of life, independent of the morbidity of the depressive disease itself.

The QALY as a utility value was used in a study by Kamlet et al.[54] of long term maintenance therapy with trimipramine compared with no maintenance therapy. A Markov model was used to examine lifetime values. The only outcomes of the analysis were 'depressed', 'nondepressed' or 'dead'; there was no direct estimate of utility values and so a range was used, with no particular value highlighted. The model was sensitive to utility values and discount rates. With the utility set at 0.9 and a 3% discount rate, for example, the cost-utility ratio of using maintenance therapy was a favourable $US5427. However, with a 5% discount rate there was a negative benefit from using maintenance therapy (a decrease of 0.31 QALYs compared with not using therapy). This is the consequence of reducing, by means of higher discounting, the impact of an intervention on outcome (section 2.3.3).

3.4 Marginal Cost-Utility Analysis

Since cost utility is a form of cost-effectiveness analysis, it is more appropriate to consider the marginal value. Hatziandreu et al.[6] determined the marginal or incremental cost-utility value of using sertraline as maintenance therapy for patients with recurrent major depression, rather than episodic treatment with dothiepin, a TCA. The treatment regimens compared were very different (which is not a problem for cost-utility analysis) in order to reflect clinical practice. The study restricted itself to only a limited patient group, women aged 35 years at high risk of recurrent major depression. Sensitivity analyses varied the utilities, compliance, drug cost, recurrence and discount rates, and number of years on maintenance therapy.

The main result quoted was an incremental cost per QALY with sertraline of £2172 (in 1994) over dothiepin. This was considered to be economically and clinically supportive of the use of long term maintenance treatment with sertraline in patients at high risk of recurrent depression.[59] The quoted cost depended on the following values in the sensitivity analysis: utilities of 0.72 for sertraline and 0.69 for dothiepin, a 5% discount rate for both costs and outcomes, maintenance therapy lasting 2 years and episodic treatment lasting 3 months. Increasing the QALYs for dothiepin reduced the marginal cost utility of sertraline. By contrast, increasing the QALYs or compliance rate for sertraline or decreasing those for dothiepin was to the advantage of sertraline. However, increasing the duration of dothiepin treatment or sertraline maintenance therapy had very little effect. This reflects the interdependence of other costs. The model was most sensitive to changes in the probabilities and timing of illness recurrences.

One criticism of the model is that the difference in withdrawal rates between the drugs was a little on the high side: 13.5% for sertraline and 23.5% for dothiepin, compared with worldwide experience of 14.8% for sertraline and 20.8% for the TCAs amitriptyline and desipramine.[60] The highest incremental cost-utility ratio of £5260 arose when compliance was assumed to be 100% for both treatments.

Kamlet et al.[61] also undertook a prospective cost-utility study comparing different maintenance treatments for recurrent depression in a customised trial. The treatments they considered were antidepressant (imipramine) use, interpersonal psychotherapy, and a combination of both, with placebo control for drug therapy. Patients who entered the maintenance phase were selected from those who responded to, and were stable on, acute-phase treatments, and so were only representative of a select group of patients in the community.

In this study,[61] 77% of the imipramine group and only slightly fewer of the imipramine plus interpersonal psychotherapy group remained free of recurrence over the 3 years of the study, compared with 28% of those receiving interpersonal psychotherapy alone and 10% of placebo recipients. Attendance at therapy sessions was costed as the sum of professional fees plus 60 to 80% of the average pay of the patient, for the duration of, plus travel to and from, the session, plus parking costs. Costs of drug therapy were the sum of the purchase price plus costs of blood monitoring and physician visits. Cost-utility values were under $US3000 (1994 costs) per QALY for interpersonal psychotherapy, and under $US5000 per QALY for imipramine plus interpersonal psychotherapy. These are well below the cut-off threshold for cost effectiveness.[54,55]

4. Influential Outcomes

Pharmacoeconomic studies do not claim to consider all the costs that may possibly accrue. Sometimes, however, the omissions can and should be rectified, such as when the cost of failed treatment or compliance is not taken into account. Most studies show that these are the most influential parameters in determining whether SSRIs are more cost effective than other antidepressants.[2,3,7,39,53]

4.1 Treatment Failure and Resulting Withdrawals

It is generally accepted that one-third of patients treated with an antidepressant do not respond.[62] Even when relatively few patients experience treatment failure, their contribution to overall costs is high. Anderson and Tomenson,[9] in their re-analysis of Jonsson and Bebbington's[2,3] data, showed that depending on whether the analysis considered only those patients who were successfully treated or the total number of patients treated, different and opposite conclusions could apply.

It is known that about 11% of those who withdraw from, or fail, first-line antidepressant therapy require hospitalisation.[62] Failure of correctly administered TCA therapy has been estimated to result in increased direct healthcare costs of $US1043 per patient in the first year after a depressive episode,[13] with $US227 spent on nursing and $US921 on hospital costs (1994 values). This estimate took into account savings in drug costs associated with treatment withdrawal ($US211). Even when failure merely leads to higher outpatient costs, these can be significant. Bentkover et al.[63] reported that the cost of outpatient visits when first-line drug treatment of depression was successful was $US12, and that failures cost an additional $US35 (1992 values).

More costly treatment failures have been suggested by multiple regression analysis to be associated with older age and prior use of the various items costed, while less costly failures were associated with women. In the model used for the multiple regression analysis,[47] treatment failure was assumed for patients who switched between three or more antidepressants during an episode, those who subsequently began augmentation therapy, or those who were not treated with a sufficient dosage for a sufficient time.[47]

4.1.1 Noncompliance as an Index of Treatment Failure

Noncompliance tends to be an integral part of most cost-analysis models, either explicitly[2,7,53] or through the use of top-down data (section 2.3.1), such as existing published statistics, on actual use and response. But Freemantle et al.[8] excluded compliance and treatment failure from their cost-effectiveness model, which attempted to quantify the marginal cost effectiveness of a switch from current antidepressant prescribing patterns to one in which mainly SSRIs were prescribed. Their conclusions differed markedly from those of other studies,[2,3,7,40,50] and it is notable that Freemantle et al.[8] concentrated their analysis on the market cost of the different drugs. They acknowledged the importance of the advantages of SSRIs in relation to the number of suicides successfully prevented. However, their estimate of the cost per life-year gained for a switch to the SSRIs was £19 000 to £173 000, depending on the values used for parameters, and the model did not support the use of these drugs.

Freemantle et al.[8] claimed that the inclusion of treatment withdrawals in their model would place the SSRIs at an even greater cost disadvantage, because they assumed no difference in compliance between the antidepressant drug groups, on the basis of their own earlier, heavily criticised[64-69] meta-analysis.[51] This contradicted data from other sources which show a statistically significantly better compliance rate for patients using SSRIs.[11,70,71] The model of Freemantle et al.[8] does not reflect the 'real world' situation.

Noncompliance has often been used as an index of treatment failure, but this is inadequate and can lead to unwarranted assumptions. For example, Jonsson and Bebbington[2] wrongly considered that any patient who continued to take their medication had responded, when they estimated the cost of treatment failure in 1992 at £488 per patient.

Another drawback of using noncompliance to indicate failure of treatment is that withdrawals may in fact occur for many different reasons. Errors in calculations also arise when the models do not allow that withdrawals due to treatment failure that occur early on in a course of treatment may be less expensive as treatment 'failures'. This assumption remains to be quantified but is likely because these patients will probably receive a suitable alternative treatment in a timely fashion.[10]

4.2 Noncompliance Related to Adverse Effects

It has been argued that noncompliance caused by adverse effects should be evaluated separately from withdrawals caused by lack of efficacy. However, Le Pen et al.[53] point out that this may not be helpful if lack of efficacy is caused because lower dosages are prescribed in order to reduce adverse effects. Withdrawal rates in placebo groups because of adverse effects also need to be considered. It may be important to compare both the total number of withdrawals and those that may be attributable to specific causes.[9] This helps to correct for the occurrence of less obvious adverse effects, as some withdrawals caused by them may be wrongly attributed to other causes.

Anderson and Tomenson[9] undertook a meta-analysis of 62 randomised controlled trials of 6029 patients with major unipolar depression. They found that the total discontinuation rate was 10% lower with SSRIs than TCAs. The withdrawal rate resulting from adverse effects was 23% lower with SSRIs than TCAs, which compares with 18 to 26% in other studies.[51,52,71]

5. Economic Implications of Adverse Effects

Drugs with fewer adverse effects may be more cost effective simply in terms of compliance.[11,27,72] However, there are a number of costs associated with morbidity and adverse effects that remain to be properly quantified and that could affect the equation. Adverse effects of drugs will reduce quality of life, and antidepressant treatment may cause morbidity that is little recognised, but will add to the hidden costs of treatment.

The direct costs of treatment for adverse effects (especially drug therapy) are not large, but are often omitted; few studies even mention what, if any, treatment is given. Costs may also accrue from hospitalisation following adverse events; this occurred in 217 of 24 624 patients (0.88%) in worldwide clinical trials of fluvoxamine[73] and the figure is likely to be higher for TCAs.

Hidden costs of TCAs may be greatest in the elderly, and include hip fractures.[74-76] Less serious problems with financial implications include tooth decay[77] in TCA users, and body-weight changes, constipation and other gastrointestinal problems with antidepressants generally. Approximately 6% of psychiatric inpatients treated for depression will experience central nervous system (CNS) toxicity because of inadvertent overdosage, at an average cost for TCAs of $US125.[78]

The adverse effects of the SSRIs are comparatively minor and their economic consequences may turn out to be lower than those of other antidepressants. This may offset their relatively high purchase price.

5.1 Cognitive Effects

In 1984, it was reported that over 10% of car drivers in the UK took medicinal drugs that might influence their driving,[79] and in 1993, that psychotropic drug use may have contributed to 10% of the deaths or injuries in UK road traffic accidents.[80] According to a US Medicaid analysis, the risk of road traffic accidents in elderly individuals receiving TCA therapy has been put at 24.4 per 1000 of those on TCAs;[81] this compares unfavourably with the rate of 16.7 per 1000 for patients taking benzodiazepines,[81] which are widely known to be associated with this problem. More specifically, elderly TCA users had a significantly higher (2.2-fold) relative risk for road traffic accidents than nonusers of the same age, after correcting for demographic characteristics and use of medical care, and rejecting alcohol use or driving frequency as possible confounders.[81] A TCA dosage equal to or greater than 125 mg/day (amitriptyline equivalent) resulted in a nearly 6-fold increase in risk.[81]

Cognitive impairments, and hence drug-related road traffic accidents, are less likely with the newer antidepressants.[81-83] Although sertraline and paroxetine affect reaction times in healthy volunteers, fluvoxamine and fluoxetine scarcely do so.[83,84] Nefazodone – especially at low, but clinically effective, dosages – causes less impairment of performance than imipramine.[85,86]

Studies are still needed to validate laboratory performance as a measure of 'real world' driving, [87] although epidemiological assessments of the risk of road traffic accidents provide useful corroboration. Hale[88] attempted to put a figure on the number of deaths that occur each year in the UK as a result of antidepressant-associated road traffic accidents, although such an estimate must remain tentative in the absence of causal data. He assumed a similar risk to that from alcohol (1 road traffic accident death per 263 individuals at risk) and that 200 000 people took antidepressants each year, to arrive at a minimum of 760 fatal road traffic accidents per annum associated with antidepressants. Of these accidents,[88] between 6 and 22 were attributable to SSRIs, and between 738 and 754 to TCAs.

Ray[87] put the cost of road traffic accidents in those aged 65 years or more in the USA in 1986 at $US7 319 255 per death, which allowed for sharing of costs with nonfatal accidents. Hale[88] adopted the same approach, and used a value for a fatality of £420 000, so that his total annual cost for road traffic fatalities in the UK attributable to all antidepressants was £320 million. A single road traffic death in the UK has elsewhere been costed at £811 524.[89] Using Hale's figures, this gives a total cost from the SSRIs each year of £4.8 million to £17.9 million and from the TCAs of £598 million to £612 million.

In a more in-depth study,[90] samples were taken from the bodies of individuals who had died within 12 hours of a road traffic accident. Using established analytical methods the researchers found antidepressants, namely the TCAs amitriptyline and dothiepin, in only 0.2% of cases, and other CNS-active drugs were found in 8.4%; in contrast, alcohol was detected in 35%. Using these figures, the annual cost of road traffic fatalities attributable to all antidepressants, assuming a cost per person of £420 000 to £811 524[88,89] would be of the region of £3.4 to £6.5 million. The difference from the estimate of Hale[88] may partly result from the fact that one study is top-down[88] and the other bottom-up[90] (section 2.3.1), and partly from methodological differences and limitations in each study.

5.2 Drug Interactions

Koenig and Breitner[91] found that 60% of inpatients with major depression who were taking TCAs were receiving other drugs with which the TCAs could interact. This is most likely in elderly patients, who may be taking medication for a variety of illnesses. The cost of this is not possible to determine.

Interactions with other drugs are, on the whole, more likely with the TCAs and the monoamine oxidase inhibitors (MAOIs).[92] However, the serotonergic syndrome is a serious potential interaction of an SSRI with another drug that potentiates serotonin transmission, such as tryptophan, lithium or a MAOI.[93]

5.3 Falls

Falls in the elderly are a known hazard of TCA use because of decreased alertness, dizziness, syncope, orthostatic hypotension, and impaired judgement and balance. Although there is no causal evidence, dothiepin has been particularly implicated (through blockade of histamine H_1 receptors), along with clomipramine, imipramine and trazodone (through α_1-adrenergic receptor blockade); amitriptyline and mianserin may act via both mechanisms.[94]

In a multicentre clinical trial of outpatients aged 60 years or more, the prevalence of reported ataxia was 5% in amitriptyline recipients and 0.6% in sertraline recipients.[94] In another study, just under 5% of imipramine recipients fell and sustained fractures or lacerations requiring sutures;[95] the risk of a fall leading to a hip fracture in the elderly has been put at around 1% overall per person in a lifetime.[96,97] The risk of hip fractures has been estimated to be 60% higher for users of TCAs at normally prescribed dosages, especially amitriptyline, doxepin and imipramine, than for those not taking TCAs,[74,98,99] and there is a dosage-response relationship.[100]

The cost implications can be measured from consideration of the estimated annual cost of hip fractures ($US7.3 billion in 1983[98]) and the annual number of hip fractures (247 000 in 1985) among those aged over 45 years in the US.[101] On the basis of these figures, hip fractures in the US resulting from TCA use cost approximately $US4.5 billion per year (1983 values); this will have increased with recent demographic changes.[96,102] Similar calculations can be made for the UK, where there were 41 274 hip fractures in those aged over 45 years in 1985. Their average length of hospital stay was 30 days, with direct hospital costs of £100 million to £160 million a year.[102,103] From these figures, the estimated cost of hip fractures as a result of TCA use in the UK is £98 million per year (1987 values).

There are secondary effects of hip fractures, which would apply whether or not the fall arose from antidepressant use. Among US patients who had been functionally independent and living at home before sustaining a hip fracture, 15 to 25% remained in long term care institutions for more than a year afterwards, and another 25 to 35% had to depend on other people or mechanical aids for mobility.[101] Mortality in patients who have experienced a hip fracture is 5 to 24% higher than in other persons of similar age and the same sex.[96,104,105]

Moreover, a patient who is immobilised with a hip fracture is at high risk of developing venous thrombosis.[106] This also occurs after hip surgery, when, in the absence of prophylaxis, around 23 to 50% of patients with a hip fracture develop a deep vein thrombosis. 20% of these patients develop a pulmonary embolism, with 59% of these patients[107] dying as a result.

5.4 Ophthalmic Effects

Mydriasis and interference with visual accommodation occur with TCAs and can affect driving. Reduction in lacrimation as a result of TCA use may cause epithelial damage in contact lens wearers,[108] and TCA users should be advised to limit their driving and the use of contact lenses. The economic consequences of this are not easily quantifiable.

5.5 Constipation

It has been suggested that anxiety and depression may result in patients exaggerating problems with defecation. Patients tend to define constipation in terms of the need to strain – which can be affected by psychological distress – rather than using the common clinical definition relating to frequency of bowel movement.[109] Also, constipation is widely regarded as a somatic symptom of depression. However, TCAs are themselves considered to be a cause of constipation.[110]

After psychotropic agents, laxatives are the main drug cost in the pharmacies of many psychiatric hospitals. In the US, they are prescribed for more than 3 million people each year,[111] but, to our knowledge, no study has examined what proportion are depressed or taking antidepressants. Thus, although the cost of treating constipation *per se* is considerable,[112] the cost in relation to antidepressant use is not at present quantifiable.

5.6 Tooth Decay

The anticholinergic effects of the TCAs cause reduced salivation. This leads to dry mouth, and may exacerbate gum disease and dental caries.[113] The economic consequences are not known, but, although quantifiable (especially in the context of institutional care), are probably small.

5.7 Cardiotoxicity

The TCAs can cause cardiac arrhythmias in individuals with pre-existing heart disease, but in practice, prescribing exclusions mean that this should not be a problem, except when an acute overdose of a TCA is ingested.[114] The cost implications of the cardiac effects of antidepressants are likely to be difficult to calculate, speculative and small in comparison with other areas, such as compliance.

5.8 Overdose

Both completed and failed suicide attempts are an important cause of direct and indirect costs. As the likelihood of serious effects from overdose, including death, are greater for some antidepressants than others, consideration of overdose can influence the outcome of a cost analysis. However, the costs are hard to quantify, and they are frequently ignored. This is particularly true when overdose results in death and the main cost is lost productivity potential. Indirect costs of suicide were considered in Part 1 of this review (page 167).[1]

Table II. Antidepressant drugs available in the UK and their rates of fatal toxicity (deaths per million prescriptions) between 1987 and 1992. Data for the fatal toxicity of drugs introduced after 1992 are not included. Year of introduction and availability of generic versions pertain to the UK

Drug	Year introduced	Generics available?	Fatal toxicity
Tricyclic antidepressants			
Imipramine	1959	Yes	157.18
Amitriptyline	1961	Yes	75.76
Desipramine	1963	No	51.77
Nortriptyline	1963	No	47.86
Protriptyline	1966	No	38.94
Trimipramine	1966	No	31.45
Iprindole	1968	No	23.99
Dothiepin	1969	Yes	13.93
Doxepin	1969	No	7.26
Clomipramine	1970	Yes	2.42
Butriptyline	1975	No	0.00
Lofepramine	1983	No	0.00
Amoxapine	1989	No	0.00
Monoamine oxidase inhibitors			
Iproniazid	1958	No	27.87
Phenelzine	1959	No	7.86
Isocarboxacid	1960	No	0.00
Tranylcypromine	1960	No	0.00
Moclobemide	1993	No	
Atypical antidepressants			
Viloxazine	1974	No	63.17
Maprotiline	1974	No	16.22
Mianserin	1976	Yes	7.83
Trazodone	1980	No	4.11
Selective serotonin reuptake inhibitors and serotonin/noradrenaline reuptake inhibitors			
Fluvoxamine	1987	No	6.23
Fluoxetine	1989	No	2.60
Sertraline	1990	No	4.78
Paroxetine	1991	No	0.66
Nefazodone	1995	No	
Venlafaxine	1996	No	

5.8.1 Differences in Completed Suicide

In England and Wales, the most common method of suicide is self-poisoning, which accounted for 39% of known suicides in 1994 (35% of male suicides and 53% of female suicides). Antidepressants account for 9% of poisoning deaths in England and Wales.[115]

Overall, about 1% of depressed patients who are prescribed antidepressants will attempt or complete suicide,[116] and about one-third of these will use the prescribed drug in the attempt.[117] In a doctors' questionnaire analysis of patients in general practice, 246 of 42 082 amitriptyline recipients (0.6%) had attempted suicide with their antidepressant.[117] Some antidepressants, such as fluoxetine, are less likely than this to be used in overdose;[118] the reasons are complex and relate both to the mechanism of action and to indirect factors such as lower perceived toxicity for the SSRIs than the TCAs.

The mortality figure generally accepted after overdose with any antidepressant, excluding the SSRIs, is 2 to 3%.[119,120] But toxicity is lower for the SSRIs than the TCAs in general. The consequence is that there is a range of risk of fatal toxicity from antidepressant use (table II). This is supported by a 5-year study of a UK general practice database.[121] Although the suicide rate among people taking antidepressants was highest for those on fluoxetine, this appeared to be due solely to selection biases such as increased baseline suicidality in these patients. Moreover, once deaths from antidepressant overdoses alone were considered, dothiepin was responsible for almost twice the number of suicides per person-years at risk as fluoxetine, and amitriptyline was only slightly less lethal than dothiepin. TCAs are associated with 36 deaths per million prescriptions in the UK.[122]

The majority of individuals may not intend to die,[123] so that if they are prescribed the less toxic antidepressants such as fluoxetine and make a failed attempt using this, they may never try again. However, some individuals may substitute a more lethal method of suicide[124] and cannot be considered as saved lives.

5.8.2 Differences in Direct Costs of Suicide Attempts

Acute hospital admissions related to attempted suicide lead to 'hidden' costs of antidepressant use. In the UK, about 3890 admissions occur each year for antidepressant poisoning, a rate of 79 per million of the male population and 109 per million of the female population.[30] Overall, acute hospital admissions associated with depression (including overdose) have been suggested to take up almost 100 000 bed days each year in the UK, at a cost of almost £12 million, based on hospital bed day charges.[30]

Consideration of hospital admissions for overdose from the antidepressants and prescribing figures show that several patients out of every million prescribed an antidepressant will be hospitalised because of an overdose. In one study, 75% of patients who had taken an overdose and were known to their general practitioner were referred to hospital.[125] But in another study, only 24.3% of suicide attempts led to contact with professional health services of any kind (17.7% of contacts were in hospitals).[126] Others have reported that only 1 in 10 suicide attempts lead to contact with healthcare professionals.[127] Even when medical intervention is invoked, because of their great toxicity, 70 to 80% of those patients who die from TCA overdose do so before reaching hospital.[128] Thus, in a proportion of suicide attempts, the patients never make contact with medical services of any kind,[129] incurring autopsy-related costs, but not treatment costs. The safety record of the SSRIs in overdose[122,130] suggests that the percentage who reach hospital is much higher for the SSRIs.

Clearly, the difference in direct costs between a fatal and nonfatal overdose depends largely on when the patient dies following the overdose. The main costs of treatment for an overdose are related to the journey to and from hospital, emergency department care (including resuscitation and gastric decontamination), hospital stay in the ward and intensive care unit, and psychiatric assessment and counselling. The hospital costs of overdoses that do not result in early death are obviously greater.

A proportion of patients who take a TCA overdose will have a lengthy stay in an intensive care unit and in hospital generally; those who overdose on an SSRI usually do not. Although one study reported (in 1990) that 10 of 37 patients who took overdoses of fluoxetine alone were admitted to an intensive therapy unit, with a mean time to discharge of 24.4 hours,[119] experience of overdose with this drug was limited at the time. Unlike the SSRIs, over 50% of TCA overdoses are associated with significant cardiac complications.[131] As a result, recommended management for any intensity of TCA overdose has, in the past, involved admission to a cardiac monitored bed for at least 72 hours. In the 1980s, attempts were made to modify the management of low-risk patients, and so reduce the burden on hospitals. For example, between 1985 and 1988, only 10 of 33 TCA overdose admissions to one US hospital were admitted to a cardiac unit for monitoring.[120] In the US, before the SSRIs became available, antidepressants often accounted for more than 24 to 50% of all admissions to intensive therapy units for any type of drug overdose.[132,133] The proportion due to antidepressants could well reduce with widespread adoption of more selective management of TCA overdose and increasing use of the SSRIs.

6. Discussion

Most studies of the cost effectiveness of antidepressants only give an indication of trends and directions. As such, they may not go far enough. The balance must be drawn between restricting a study to only the most clear data, and providing sufficiently accurate end figures that adequately put across a message and that can have a bearing on future policies. Moreover, most studies have tended to ignore the costs of adverse effects, although it is precisely these that most influence the prescriber to switch between antidepressant drugs[134] and have a major influence on the overall cost of treatment.[2,3,7] However, care must also be taken that in the search for precision, detailed calculations on both major and minor parameters do not simply increase the sources of inaccuracy, making the work appear authoritative, while in reality it suffers from 'pseudo-precision'.

Clearly, a lack of generalisability, together with important omissions from studies and the absence of a standardised methodology – despite attempts by Drummond and Davies[135] in particular – means that there are no clear answers; each cost analysis of depression and its treatment has differed from the last. The situation might be improved if a clearer indication of margins of error was given in studies. In fact, sensitivity analyses are often not made explicit, with consideration of alternatives either omitted or left to a brief mention in the discussion.

Moreover, while current costs can be determined from existing statistics, the effects of putative changes can only be hypothetical and subject to various assumptions. Their accuracy is only slightly improved by small-scale experimental studies of the substitute. They are difficult to identify, measure and evaluate. A major objective in assessing healthcare economics should be to have robust methodology that provides a clear indication of which cost-analysis conclusions hold good across time and place, and that enables studies to be compared.

The British Association for Psychopharmacology states in its Guidelines that the 'cost of a drug should be a secondary issue since the major costs to the country in treating depression are hospital inpatient and outpatient care and in general practice follow-up'.[18] One of the purposes of pharmacoeconomics should be to establish this and to enable doctors to justify the initial expense when prescribing a drug. Although it would be logical to prescribe the cheapest treatment, the prescriber should be made more aware of the many arguments that are put forward to show, for example, that the benefits of the SSRIs outweigh their costs. However, these arguments may only be accepted when pharmacoeconomic studies develop a standardised methodology and greater local relevance.

For example, there is the problem that when direct cost comparisons of the new SSRIs with the older TCAs are made, it is natural, where possible, to use the much cheaper generic price. This biases costs against the new drugs, for which generic forms are not yet marketed. Boyer and Feighner[7] considered both branded and generic prices of the TCAs against the (branded) prices of the SSRIs. They found that, because of the advantages of the SSRIs in clinical use, they were in fact less expensive than generic TCAs in hypothetical acute and acute-plus-maintenance therapy courses.

Thus, market price should not be the overriding consideration in prescribing antidepressants that it currently appears to be. The exception may be situations in which patients have to pay at least some of the cost of treatment themselves. This is increasingly true of insurance-based healthcare,[136] as in the US. A higher purchase price can affect compliance by paying patients, regardless of the severity of their illness and the benefits of the treatment.[136]

7. Conclusion

The compilation of the two parts of this review leads us to conclude that there are many shortcomings and pitfalls in healthcare costing in general, but that the cost-effectiveness analysis of the treatment of depression is, because of the nature of the illness and of the interventions, one of the most difficult areas of all. Simple generalisations from changes in a single parameter, while illustrative, are often unhelpful.

However, some conclusions may be drawn. The work of authors such as Jonsson and Bebbington,[2,3] Brown et al.,[55a] Nuijten et al.[55b] and Boyer and Feighner[7] suggests that the newer antidepressants may provide overall savings to healthcare budgets. Even at this stage, it is apparent that differences in compliance and safety in overdose are important factors that deserve thorough investigation so that appropriate economic and clinical decisions can be made at governmental, local and individual levels. These studies, combined with the magnitude of direct and indirect costs of depression, and their ratio (table I), which may be dynamic,[32] also suggest that a relatively small extra outlay in terms of drug purchase costs could lead to a significant reduction in the total costs of depressive illness to society. Estimates of the savings will tend to remain conservative, as many indirect costs cannot be definitively calculated.

It is clear that a considerable amount of work is required in order to identify, beyond all reasonable doubt, the areas in which changes in drug prescribing in everyday practice might lead to major differences in the distribution of resources in healthcare systems. Current studies are moving in the right direction.

References

1. Henry JA, Rivas CA. Constraints on antidepressant prescribing and principles of cost-effective antidepressant use. Part 1: depression and its treatment. Pharmacoeconomics 1997; 11 (5): 419-43
2. Jonsson B, Bebbington P. Economic studies of the treatment of depressive illness. In: Jonsson B, Rosenbaum J, editors. Health Economics of Depression. New York: John Wiley, 1993: 35-48
3. Jonsson B, Bebbington P. What price depression? The cost of depression and the cost-effectiveness of pharmacological treatment. Br J Psychiatry 1994; 164: 665-73
4. Bentkover J, Capierre Y. Cost-effective antidepressant therapy. Hum Psychopharmacol 1994; 9: S22
5. Kind P, Sorensen J. Modelling the cost-effectiveness of the prophylactic use of SSRIs in the treatment of depression. Int Clin Psychopharmacol 1995; 10: 41-8
6. Hatziandreu EJ, Brown RE, Revicki DA, et al. Cost utility of maintenance treatment of recurrent depression with sertraline versus episodic treatment with dothiepin. Pharmacoeconomics 1994; 5 (3): 249-64
7. Boyer WF, Feighner JP. The financial implications of starting treatment with a selective serotonin reuptake inhibitor or tricyclic antidepressant in drug-naive depressed patients. In: Jonsson B, Rosenbaum J, editors. Health Economics of Depression - perspectives in psychiatry. Vol. 4. Chichester: John Wiley, 1993: 65-76
8. Freemantle N, House A, Song F, et al. Prescribing selective serotonin reuptake inhibitors as strategy for prevention of suicide. BMJ 1994; 309: 249-53
9. Anderson IM, Tomenson BM. Treatment discontinuation with selective serotonin reuptake inhibitors compared with tricyclic antidepressants: a meta-analysis. BMJ 1995; 310: 1433-8
10. O'Brien JT. Cost-effectiveness of antidepressants. Br J Psychiatry 1994; 164: 665-73
11. Katon W, von Korff M, Lin E, et al. Adequacy and duration of antidepressant treatment in primary care. Med Care 1992; 30: 67-76
12. Simon G, Wagner E, Vonkorff M. Cost-effectiveness comparisons using 'real world' randomized trials: the case of new antidepressant drugs. J Clin Epidemiol 1995; 48: 363-73
13. McCombs JS, Nichol MB, Stimmel GL, et al. The cost of antidepressant drug therapy failure: a study of antidepressant use patterns in a Medicaid population. J Clin Psychiatry 1990; 51 (6): 60-72
14. Begg D. Do patients cash prescriptions? An audit in one practice. J R Coll Gen Pract 1984; 34: 272-4
15. Johnson DAW. Depression: treatment compliance in general practice. Acta Psychiatr Scand 1981; 63: 447-53
16. Johnson DAW. Antidepressant treatment observed: some problems of compliance by doctors and patients. In: Sims, Ottofson, editors. Antidepressants: progress in problem areas. London: Franklin Scientific Projects, 1984
17. Chrischilles EA. The contribution of epidemiology to pharmacoeconomic research. Drug Inf J 1992; 26: 219-29
18. Montgomery SA, Bebbington P, Cowen P, et al. Guidelines for treating depressive illness with antidepressants. J Psychopharmacol 1993; 7 (1): 19-23
19. Katona C. Rationalizing antidepressants for elderly people. Int Clin Psychopharmacol 1995; 10: 37-40
20. Paykel ES, Freeling P, Hollyman JA. Are tricyclic antidepressants useful for mild depression? A placebo controlled trial. Pharmacopsychiatry 1988; 21: 15-8
21. Gotschke PC. Methodology and overt and hidden bias in reports of 196 double-blind trials of nonsteroidal antiinflammatory drugs in rheumatoid arthritis. Control Clin Tials 1989; 10: 31-56
22. Strom BL. Pharmacoepidemiology. New York: Churchill Livingstone, 1989

23. Lewis NJW, Patwell JT, Briesacher BA. The role of insurance claims database in drug therapy outcome research. Pharmaco-economics 1993; 4 (5): 323-30
24. Drummond M, Torrance G, Mason J. Cost-effectiveness league tables: more harm than good? Soc Sci Med 1993; 37: 33-40
25. Drummond MF, Bloom BS, Carrin G, et al. Issues in the cross-national assessment of health technology. Int J Technol Assess Health Care 1992; 8: 671-82
26. Frank RG, Kamlet MS. Economic aspects of patterns of mental health care: cost variation by setting. Gen Hosp Psychiatry 1990; 12: 11-8
27. Johnson DAW. Non-compliance with antidepressant therapy: an underestimated problem. Intern Med 1986; 11 Suppl.: 14-7
28. Johnson DAW. Treatment of depression in general practice. BMJ 1973; ii: 18-20
29. Montgomery SA. Prophylactic treatment of depression [editorial]. Br J Hosp Med 1994; 52 (1): 5-7
30. Kind P, Sorensen J. The costs of depression. Int Clin Psycho-pharmacol 1993; 7 (3-4): 191-5
31. West R. Depression. London: Office of Health Economics, 1992
32. Rice DP, Kelman S, Miller LS. Estimates of economic costs of alcohol and drug abuse and mental illness, 1985 and 1988. Public Health Rep 1991; 106 (3): 280-92
33. Weisbrod BA. Economics of mental illness: costs, benefits and incentives. In: Jonsson B, Rosenbaum J, editors. Health economics of depression – perspectives in psychiatry. Vol. 4. Chichester: John Wiley, 1993: 15-34
34. Croft-Jeffreys C, Wilkinson G. Estimated costs of neurotic disorder in UK general practice 1985. Psychol Med 1989; 19: 549-58
35. Hertzman P. The economic costs of mental illness in Sweden 1975. Acta Psychiatr Scand 1983; 68: 359-67
36. Stoudemire A, Frank R, Hedemark N, et al. The economic burden of depression. Gen Hosp Psychiatry 1986; 8: 387-94
37. Abraham IL, Bryant Neese J, Westerman PS. Depression: nursing implications of a clinical and social problem. Nurs Clin North Am 1991; 26 (3): 527-36
38. Feighner JP. A comparative trial of fluoxetine and amitriptyline in patients with major depressive disorders. J Clin Psychiatry 1985; 46: 369-72
39. Greenberg PE, Stiglin LE, Finkelstein SN, et al. The economic burden of depression in 1990. J Clin Psychiatry 1993; 54 (11): 405-18
40. Mendlewicz J. The social burden of depressive disorders. Neuropsychobiology 1989: 22: 178-80
41. Weinstein MC, Saturno PJ. Economic impact of youth suicide and suicide attempts. Rockville: Department of Health and Human Services, US DHSS Publication, 1989; ADM 89-1264: 4/82-4/89
42. Montgomery SA, Doogan DP, Burnside R. The influence of different relapse criteria on the assessment of long term efficacy of sertraline. Int Clin Psychopharmacol 1991; 6 (2 Suppl.): 37-46
43. Paykel ES, Priest RG. Recognition and management of depression in general practice: consensus statement. BMJ 1992; 305: 1198-202
44. Russell L. Is prevention better than cure? Washington (DC): Brookings Institution, 1986
45. Keeler E, Cretin S. Discounting of life-saving and other non-monetary effects. Manage Sci 1983; 29: 300-6
46. Katz DA, Welch HG. Discounting in cost-effectiveness analysis of healthcare programmes. Pharmacoeconomics 1993; 3 (4): 276-85
47. McCombs JS, Nichol MB. The cost of treatment failure. In: Jonsson B, Rosenbaum J, editors. Health economics of depression – perspectives in Psychiatry. Vol. 4. Chichester: John Wiley, 1993: 49-64
48. Mindham RH, Howland C, Shepherd M. Continuation therapy with tricyclic antidepressants in depressive illness. Lancet 1987; II: 854-5
49. Prien R, Kupfer D. Continuation drug therapy for major depressive episodes: how long should it be maintained? Am Psychiatry 1986; 143: 18-23
50. Bochner F, Martin DE, Burgess NG, et al. Drug rationing in a teaching hospital: a method to assign priorities. BMJ 1994; 308: 901-5
51. Song F, Freemantle N, Sheldon TA, et al. Selective serotonin reuptake inhibitors: meta-analysis of efficacy and acceptability. BMJ 1993; 306: 683-7
52. Montgomery SA, Kasper S. Comparison of compliance between serotonin reuptake inhibitors and tricyclic antidepressants: a meta-analysis. Int Clin Psychopharmacol 1995; 9 Suppl. 4: 33-40
53. Le Pen C, Levy R, Ravily V, et al. The cost of treatment dropout in depression. J Affect Disord 1994; 31: 1-18
54. Kamlet MS, Wade M, Kupfer D, et al. Cost-utility analysis of maintenance treatment for recurrent depression: a theoretical framework and numerical illustration. In: Frank R, Manning W, editors. Essays in honor of Carl Taube. Baltimore: John Hopkins University Press, 1992: 267-91
55. Drummond M, O'Brien B. Clinical importance, statistical significance and the assessment of economic and quality-of-life outcomes. Health Econ 1993; 2: 205-12
55a. Brown MC, Nimmerrichter AA, Guest JF. Cost-effectiveness of mirtazapine compared to amitriptyline and fluoxetine in the treatment of moderate and severe depression in Austria. Eur Psychiatry 1999; 14: 230-44
55b. Nuijten M, Hadjadjeba L, Evans C, et al. Cost effectiveness of fluvoxamine in the treatment of recurrent depression in France. Pharmacoeconomics 1998; 14 (4): 433-45
56. Einarson TR, Arikian S, Sweeney S, et al. A model to evaluate the cost-effectiveness of oral therapies in the management of patients with major depressive disorders. Clin Ther 1995; 17: 136-53
57. Sclar DA, Robinson LM, Skaer TL, et al. Antidepressant pharmacotherapy: economic outcomes in a health maintenance organization. Clin Ther 1994; 16: 715-30
58. Gross PF. Potential economic effects of a new antidepressant (venlafaxine) in treating major depressive disorder in France. Sydney: Institute of Health Economics and Technology Assessment, 1994. Health economics monograph no. 62

59. Laupacis A, Feeny D, Decsky AS, et al. How attractive does a new technology have to become to warrant adoption and utilization? Tentative guidelines for using clinical and economic evaluations. Can Med Assoc J 1992; 146: 473-81
60. Doogan DP, Caillard V. Sertraline in the prevention of depression. Br J Psychiatry 1992; 160: 217-22
61. Kamlet MS, Paul N, Greenhouse J, et al. Cost utility analysis of maintenance treatment for recurrent depression. Control Clin Trials 1995; 16: 17-40
62. Gerner R, Estabrook W, Steuer J, et al. Treatment of geriatric depression with trazodone, imipramine and placebo: a double-blind study. J Clin Psychiatry 1980; 41: 216-20
63. Bentkover JD, Baker AM, Feighner JP, et al. 18th CINP Conference, Nice; 1992 Jun 28 - Jul 2
64. Hale AS. Effective and acceptable treatment for depression [letter]. BMJ 1993; 306: 1124
65. Cialdella P. Effective and acceptable treatment for depression [letter]. BMJ 1993; 306: 1125
66. Foulds RA. Effective and acceptable treatment for depression [letter]. BMJ 1993; 306: 1125
67. Nakielny J. Effective and acceptable treatment for depression [letter]. BMJ 1993; 306: 1125
68. Robertson MM, Katone CLE. Effective and acceptable treatment for depression [letter]. BMJ 1993; 306: 1126
69. Madeley P, Wattis JP. Effective and acceptable treatment for depression [letter]. BMJ 1993; 306: 1126
70. Katon W, von Korff M, Line E, et al. A randomized trial of psychiatric consultation with distressed high utilizers. Gen Hosp Psychiatry 1992; 14 (2): 86-98
71. Montgomery SA, Henry JA, McDonald G, et al. Selective serotonin reuptake inhibitors: meta-analysis of discontinuation rates. Int Clin Psychopharmacol 1994; 9: 47-54
72. Thompson C, Thompson CM. The prescription of antidepressants in general practice: I. A critical review. Hum Psychopharmacol 1989; 4: 91-102
73. Wagner W, Plekkenpol B, Gray TE, et al. Review of fluvoxamine safety database. Drugs 1992; 43 (2): 48-54
74. Glassman AH, Bigger JT. Cardiovascular effects of therapeutic doses of tricyclic antidepressants: a review. Arch Gen Psychiatry 1981; 38: 815-20
75. Tesar GE, Rosenbaum JF, Biederman J, et al. Orthostatic hypotension and antidepressant pharmacotherapy. Psychopharmacol Bull 1987; 23: 182-6
76. Ray RA, Griffin R, Schaffner W, et al. Psychotropic drug use and the risk of hip fracture. N Engl J Med 1987; 316: 363-9
77. Stevens JB, Wilkinson EG. Drugs, dry mouth and dental disease. Psychosomatics 1971; 12: 310-12
78. Preskorn SH, Dorey RC, Jerkovich GS. Therapeutic drug monitoring of tricyclic antidepressants. Clin Chem 1988; 34 (5): 822-8
79. The House of Commons Transport Committee. Report on road safety: drugs and driving. Vol. 1, para 39. London: HMSO, 1984
80. De Gier JJ. Driving licences and known use of licit or illicit drugs (IHP 93-39). Maastricht: University of Limberg, 1993
81. Ray WA, Fought RL, Decker MD. Psychoactive drugs and the risk of injurious motor vehicle crashes in elderly drivers. Am J Epidemiol 1992; 136: 873-83
82. Hindmarch I. The effects of psychoactive drugs on car handling and related psychomotor ability: a review. In: O'Hanlon JF, de Gier JJ, editors. Drugs and driving. London: Taylor and Francis, 1986: 71-9
83. Hindmarch I. A review of the psychomotor effects of paroxetine. Int Clin Psychopharmacol 1992; 6 Suppl. 4: 65-7
84. Hindmarch I, Kerr J. Behavioural toxicity of antidepressants with particular reference to moclobemide. Psychopharmacology 1992; 106 Suppl.: 49S-55S
85. Fontaine R. Novel serotonergic mechanisms and clinical experience with nefazodone. Clin Neuropharmacol 1993; 16: S45-50
86. Preskorn SH. Comparison of the tolerability of bupropion, fluoxetine, imipramine, nefazodone, paroxetine, sertraline and venlafaxine. J Clin Psychiatry 1995: 56: 12-21
87. Ray WA. Psychotropic drugs and injuries among the elderly: a review. J Clin Psychopharmacol 1992; 12: 386-96
88. Hale AS. The importance of road traffic accidents in evaluating the cost of SSRIs. Int J Psychopharmacol 1994; 9 (3): 195-201
89. Currie DJ, Fairweather DB, Hindmarch I. Social aspects of treating depression. In: Jonsson B, Rosenbaum J, editors. Health economics of depression – perspectives in psychiatry, Vol. 4: John Wiley: Chichester, 1993: 129-40
90. Everest JT, Tunbridge RJ, Widdop B. The incidence of drugs in road accident fatalities. Transport and Road Research Laboratory Research Report 202. London: Department of Transport, 1989
91. Koenig HG, Breitner JC. Use of antidepressants in medically ill older patients. Psychosomatics 1990; 31 (1): 22-32
92. Warrington SJ. Clinical implications of the pharmacology of sertraline. Int Clin Psychopharmacol 1991; 6 Suppl. 2: 11- 21
93. Sternbach H. The serotonin syndrome. Am J Psychiatry 1991; 184: 705-13
94. Cohn CK, Shrivastava R, Mendels J, et al. Double-blind, multicenter comparison of sertraline and amitriptyline in elderly depressed patients. J Clin Psychiatry 1990; 51 (12 Suppl. B): 28-33
95. Glassman AH, Giardina EGV, Perel JM, et al. Clinical characteristics of imipramine-induced orthostatic hypotension. Lancet 1979; I: 468-72
96. Cummings SR. Epidemiology of hip fractures. In: Christainsen, et al., editors. Osteoporosis. Copenhagen: Osteopress, 1987: 40-4
97. Baker SP, Harvey AH. Fall injuries in the elderly. In: Radebaugh TS, editor. Clinics in geriatric medicine. Vol. 1, no. 3. Philadelphia: WB Saunders, 1985
98. Davie JW, Blumenthal MD, Robinson-Hawkins S. A model of risk of falling for psychogeriatric patients. Arch Gen Psychiatry 1981; 38: 463-7
99. Holbrook TL, Grazier K, Kelsey JL, et al. The frequency of occurrence, impact and cost of musculoskeletal conditions in the United States. Chicago: American Academy of Orthopedic Surgeons, 1985

100. Ray WA, Griffin MR, Malcolm E. Cyclic antidepressants and the risk of hip fracture. Arch Intern Med 1991; 151 (4): 754-6
101. Cummings SR, Kelsey JL, Nevitt MC, et al. Epidemiology of osteoporosis and osteoporotic fractures. Epidemiol Rev 1985; 7: 178-208
102. The Royal College of Physicians of London. Fractured neck of femur – prevention and management. London: Royal College of Physicians, 1989
103. Dreghorn CR, Roughneen P, Graham J, et al. The real cost of joint replacement. BMJ 1986; 292: 1636-7
104. Bergqvist D, Jendteg S, Lindgren B, et al. The economics of general thromboembolic prophylaxis. World J Surg 1988; 12: 349-55
105. Ray WA, Griffin MR, Baugh DK. Mortality following hip fracture before and after implementation of the prospective payment system. Arch Intern Med 1990; 150: 2109-14
106. Fenech A, Winter JH, Bennet B, et al. Preoperative frequency of deep venous thrombosis in patients with fractured neck of the femur. Lancet 1981; I: 1212
107. Mol WEM, Egberts TCG. Prophylaxis for venous thromboembolism in hip fracture surgery: total cost and cost effectiveness in the Netherlands. Pharmacoeconomics 1994: 5 (1): 48-55
108. Litovitz GL. Amitriptyline and contact lenses [letter]. J Clin Psychiatry 1984; 45 (4): 188
109. Wald A. Constipation in elderly patients: pathogenesis and management. Drugs Aging 1993; 3 (3): 220-31
110. Robertson MM, Abou-Saleh MT, Harrison DA, et al. A double-blind controlled comparison of fluoxetine and lofepramine in major depressive illness. J Psychopharmacol 1994; 8: 98-103
111. Johanson JF, Sonnenberg A, Koch TR. Clinical epidemiology of chronic constipation. J Clin Gastroenterol 1989; 11: 525-36
112. Gibson P, Liversedge S, Moriarty K. The management of constipation. Gastroenterology in Practice 1993; June/July: 18-22
113. Stevens JB, Wilkinson EG. Drugs, dry mouth and dental disease. Psychosomatics 1971; 12: 310-2
114. Goldney RD, Trowse MM, Chia MM. Direct cost saving of SSRI overdose. Med J Aust 1995; 162: 668-9
115. Office of Population Censuses and Surveys. Mortality statistics – accidents and violence (England and Wales), Series DH4. London: HMSO, 1990, 1991, 1992
116. Bulik CM, Carpenter LL, Kupfer DJ, et al. Features associated with suicide attempts in recurrent major depression. J Affect Disord 1990; 18 (1): 29-37
117. Inman WHW. Blood disorders and suicide in patients taking mianserin or amitriptyline. Lancet 1988; II: 90-2
118. Kapur S, Mieczkowski T, Mann JJ. Antidepressant medications and the relative risk of suicide attempts and suicide. JAMA 1992; 268 (24): 34-41
119. Borys DJ, Setzer SC, Ling LT, et al. The effects of fluoxetine in the overdose patient. Clin Toxicol 1990; 28: 331-40
120. Banahan BF, Shelkun PH. Tricyclic antidepressant overdose: conservative management in a community hospital with cost saving implications. J Emerg Med 1990; 8: 451-4
121. Jick SS, Dean AD, Jick H. Antidepressants and suicide. BMJ 1995; 310: 215-8
122. Henry JA, Alexander CA, Sener EK. Relative mortality from overdose of antidepressants. BMJ 1995; 310: 221-4
123. Bancroft J, Skrimshire A, Casson J, et al. People who deliberately poison or injure themselves: their problems and their contacts with helping agencies. Psychol Med 1977; 7: 289-303
124. Lester D. The association between platelet imipramine binding sites and suicide [letter]. Pharmacopsychiatry 1991; 24: 232
125. Kennedy P, Kreitman N. An epidemiological survey of parasuicide ('attempted suicide') in general practice. Br J Psychiatry 1973; 123: 23-34
126. Diekstra RFW, Moritz B. Suicidal behaviour among adolescents. In: Diekstra RFW, Hawton K, editors. Suicide in adolescence. Boston: Kluwer, 1987
127. Diekstra RF. Suicide and attempted suicide: an international perspective. Acta Psychiatr Scand Suppl 1989; 354: 1-24
128. Callaham M, Kassel D. Epidemiology of fatal tricyclic antidepressant ingestion: implications for management. Ann Emerg Med 1985; 14: 1-9
129. Montgomery SA, Lambert MT, Lynch SP. The risk of suicide with antidepressants. Int Clin Psychopharmacol 1988; 3 (2 Suppl.): 15-24
130. Molcho A, Stanley M. Antidepressants and suicide risk: issues of chemical and behavioral toxicity. J Clin Psychopharmacol 1992; 12: 13S-7S
131. Frommer DA, Kulig KW, Marx JA, et al. Tricyclic antidepressant overdose: a review. JAMA 1987; 257 (4): 521-6
132. Dec GW, Stern TA. Tricyclic antidepressants in the intensive care unit. J Intensive Care Med 1990; 5: 69-81
133. Kathol RG, Henn FA. Tricyclics – the most common agent used in potentially lethal overdoses. J Nerv Ment Dis 1983; 171 (4): 250-2
134. Rosenbaum JF. Clinical choices, cost-effectiveness and antidepressant treatment. In: Jonsson B, Rosenbaum J, editors. Health Economics of Depression. New York: John Wiley, 1993: 141-8
135. Drummond MF, Davies L. Economic analysis alongside clinical trials. Int J Technol Assess Health Care 1991; 7: 561-73
136. Drummond MF, Jefferson TO. Guidelines for authors and peer reviewers of economic submissions to the BMJ. BMJ 1996; 313: 275-82

Correspondence: Prof. *John A. Henry*, Accident and Emergency, St Mary's Hospital, London W2, England.